Pandemic Influenza

2nd Edition

Edited by

Jonathan Van-Tam

MBE BMedSci(Hons) BMBS DM FFPH FRSPH
Professor of Health Protection, University of Nottingham, UK
Honorary Consultant Epidemiologist, Health Protection Agency, UK

Chloe Sellwood

BSc(Hons), PhD, FRSPH, DipHEP
Pandemic and Seasonal Influenza Resilience Manager, NHS London, UK

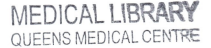
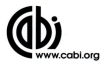
www.cabi.org

CABI is a trading name of CAB International

CABI	CABI
Nosworthy Way	38 Chauncey Street
Wallingford	Suite 1002
Oxfordshire OX10 8DE	Boston, MA 02111
UK	USA
Tel: +44 (0)1491 832111	Tel: +1 800 552 3083 (toll free)
Fax: +44 (0)1491 833508	Tel: +1 (0)617 395 4051
E-mail: info@cabi.org	E-mail: cabi-nao@cabi.org
Website: www.cabi.org	

A catalogue record for this book is available from the British Library, London, UK.

Library of Congress Cataloging-in-Publication Data

1008807139

Pandemic influenza / edited by Jonathan Van-Tam and Chloe Sellwood. -- 2nd ed.
    p. ; cm. -- (Modular texts)
  Rev. ed. of: Introduction to pandemic influenza. c2010.
  Includes bibliographical references and index.
  ISBN 978-1-84593-856-7 (hardback) -- ISBN 978-1-84593-857-4 (pbk.)
  I. Van-Tam, Jonathan. II. Sellwood, Chloe. III. C.A.B. International. IV. Introduction to pandemic influenza. V. Series: Modular texts.
  [DNLM: 1. Influenza, Human--epidemiology. 2. Communicable Disease Control. 3. Influenza, Human--prevention & control. 4. Pandemics--prevention & control. WC 515]

  614.5'18--dc23

                      2012026677

ISBN: 978 1 84593 857 4 (paperback)
ISBN: 978 1 84593 856 7 (hardback)

Commissioning editor: Rachel Cutts
Editorial assistant: Chris Shire
Production editor: Tracy Head

Typeset by SPi, Pondicherry, India.
Printed and bound by Gutenberg Press Ltd, Tarxien, Malta.

Contents

Contributors

Thomas Abraham, *Associate Professor of Practice and Director Public Health Communication Project, Journalism and Media Studies Centre, The University of Hong Kong, Hong Kong*

Dr Patricia R. Blank, PhD, *Senior Research Scientist, Institute of Social and Preventive Medicine, Medical Economics, University of Zurich, Hirschengraben 84, 8001 Zurich, Switzerland and Institute of Pharmaceutical Medicine/European Center of Pharmaceutical Medicine, University of Basel, Klingelbergstrasse 61, 4056 Basel, Switzerland*

Dr Caroline S. Brown, *Programme Manager, Influenza & other Respiratory Pathogens, Division of Communicable Diseases, Health Security, & Environment, WHO Regional Office for Europe, Copenhagen, Denmark*

Peter Carrasco, MPA, *Former Policy Adviser – Vaccines and Immunization, World Health Organization, Geneva, Switzerland; retired 2010, USA*

Dra Jeannette Dabanch, *Universidad de los Andes Hospital Militar, Santiago, Chile*

Prof Lindsey Davies, CBE FFPH FRCP, *President, Faculty of Public Health, 4 St Andrews Place, London NW1 4LB, UK*

Ms Joanne Enstone, BSc MPhil MPH RGN, *Influenza Studies Research Nurse, University of Nottingham, Room A40d, Clinical Sciences Building, City Hospital, Nottingham NG5 1PB, UK*

Elaine M. Gadd, MA FRCPsych FFFLM, *Honorary Professor, School of Law, Queen Mary University of London, Mile End Road, London E1 4NS, UK*

Stephen D. Gardner, *Former Chair of the Influenza Working Group of the European Vaccine Manufacturers (EVM). Retired 2011*

Dr Peter G. Grove, *Senior Principal Analyst, Health Protection Analytical Team, Department of Health, 3rd Floor, Wellington House, 133–155 Waterloo Road, London SE1 8UG, UK*

Dr Lars R. Haaheim, DPhil, *Retired in 2008 from the position of Professor and Head of the Influenza Centre, The Gade Institute, University of Bergen, Bergen, Norway*

Dr David Hagen, BSc MD FFPH FRSPH, *Consultant in Communicable Disease Control, Health Protection Agency (South-East), County Hall North, Chart Way, Horsham RH12 1XA, UK*

Dr Michala Hegermann-Lindencrone, *Technical Officer, Influenza & other Respiratory Pathogens, Division of Communicable Diseases, Health Security, & Environment, WHO Regional Office for Europe, Copenhagen, Denmark*

Dr Bernadette Hendrickx, MD, *Chair of the Regulatory Working Group of the European Vaccine Manufacturers (EVM), Sanofi Pasteur, 2 Avenue Pont Pasteur, 69367 Lyon Cedex 07, France*

Dr Seema Jain, MD, *Medical Epidemiologist, Epidemiology and Prevention Branch, Influenza Division, National Center for Immunization and Respiratory Diseases, Centers for Disease Control and Prevention, 1600 Clifton Road, MS A-32, Atlanta, GA 30329, USA*

Dr Lance C. Jennings, QSO PhD FRCPath FFSc(RCPA), *Clinical Virologist, Department of Microbiology, Virology & Serology Section, Canterbury Health Laboratories, Cnr Hagley Ave & Tuam Street, Christchurch*

8011, *New Zealand and Clinical Associate Professor, Pathology Department, University of Otago, Christchurch, New Zealand*

Dr Daniel B. Jernigan, MD MPH, *Deputy Director, Influenza Division, National Center for Immunization and Respiratory Diseases, Centers for Disease Control and Prevention, 1600 Clifton Road, MS A-20, Atlanta, GA 30333, USA*

Dr Ben Killingley, BSc MBChB MRCP, *Infectious Diseases Physician, University of Nottingham, Room A40d, Clinical Sciences Building, City Hospital, Nottingham NG5 1PB, UK*

Dr Vernon Lee, MBBS PhD MPH MBA, *Adjunct Associate Professor, Saw Swee Hock School of Public Health, National University of Singapore, Singapore MD3, 16 Medical Drive, Singapore 117597*

Prof Geert Leroux-Roels, MD PhD, *Director, Centre for Vaccinology, Ghent University and Hospital, Ghent, Belgium*

Dr Wei Shen Lim, DM FRCP, *Consultant in Respiratory Medicine, Nottingham University Hospitals NHS Trust, City Hospital Campus, Nottingham NG5 1PB, UK*

Vicente Lopez Chavarrias, DVM MSc, *Scientific Officer – Influenza and Other Respiratory Viruses Programme, European Centre for Disease Prevention and Control (ECDC), Tomtebodavägen 11A, Solna 171 83 Stockholm, Sweden*

Dr Jim McMenamin, MBChB MRCP MPH MFPMI FFPH, *Consultant Epidemologist, Health Protection Scotland, NHS National Services Scotland, 4th Floor, Meridian Court, 5 Cadogan Street, Glasgow G2 6QE, UK*

Prof Ziad A. Memish, MD FRCP(Can) FRCP(Edin) FRCP(Lond) FACP, *Deputy Minister for Public Health, Ministry of Health, PO Box 54146, Riyadh 11514 and Professor, College of Medicine, Alfaisal University, Riyadh, Kingdom of Saudi Arabia*

Dr Kåre Mølbak, MD DMSC, *Director, Department of Infectious Disease Epidemiology, Statens Serum Institut, 5 Artillerivej, DK-2300 Copenhagen S, Denmark*

Prof Arnold S. Monto, MD, *Thomas Francis Jr. Professor of Epidemiology, School of Public Health, University of Michigan, 1415 Washington Heights, Ann Arbor, MI 48109, USA*

Prof Abdulsalami Nasidi, MD PhD, *Director, Nigeria Centre for Disease Control (NCDC), Federal Ministry of Health, 50 Haile Selasie Street, Asokoro, Abuja, Nigeria*

Prof Angus Nicoll, CBE, *Senior Expert – Head of Influenza and Other Respiratory Viruses Programme, European Centre for Disease Prevention and Control (ECDC), Tomtebodavägen 11A, Solna 171 83 Stockholm, Sweden*

Prof Albert D.M.E. Osterhaus, DVM PhD, *Head, Department of Virology, Erasmus Medical Centre, PO Box 2040, 3000 CA Rotterdam, the Netherlands and Artemis Research Institute for Wildlife Health in Europe, Utrecht, the Netherlands*

Prof John S. Oxford, DSc FRCPE, *Blizard Institute of Cell and Molecular Science, Bart's and The London School of Medicine and Dentistry, Queen Mary College and Retroscreen Virology Ltd, 4 Newark Street, London E1 2AT, UK*

Dr Chris Packham, MMedSci DM FRCP FFPH MRCGP, *General Practitioner and Consultant Public Health Physician, Director of Public Health, Nottingham, UK and Associate Medical Director, Highbury Hospital, Highbury Vale, Nottingham NG6 9DR, UK*

Vincent Junxiong Pang, MSc, *Research Associate, Centre for Infectious Disease Epidemiology, Saw Swee Hock School of Public Health, National University of Singapore, Singapore MD3, 16 Medical Drive, Singapore 117597*

Dr Irina Papieva, MD MPH, *Health Systems Programme Coordinator, WHO Country Office in Armenia, 9 Alek Manoukyan Street, AUA Business Centre, Yerevan 0070, Armenia*

Dr Richard G. Pebody, BSc DTMH MSc MRCP FFPH PhD, *Consultant Epidemiologist, Respiratory Diseases Department, Health Protection Agency (Colindale), 61 Colindale Avenue, London NW9 5EQ, UK*

Daniel Pople, *Senior Communications and Media Manager, Communications and Public Affairs, NHS London, Southside, 105 Victoria Street, London SW1E 6QT, UK*

Prof Martyn Regan, MSc PhD FFPH MRCGP DRCOG, *Regional Director, Health Protection Agency (East Midlands), City Hospital, Nottingham NG5 1PB, UK*

Dr Leslie A. Reperant, DVM PhD, *Scientific Researcher, Department of Virology, Erasmus Medical Centre, PO Box 2040, 3000 CA Rotterdam, the Netherlands*

Dr Chloe Sellwood, PhD FRSPH, *Pandemic and Seasonal Influenza Resilience Manager, Emergency Preparedness, NHS London, Southside, 105 Victoria Street, London SW1E 6QT, UK*

Dr John Simpson, MB BS FFPH, *Deputy Director, Emergency Response and Head of Emergency Response Department, Health Protection Agency, Porton Down, Salisbury SP4 0JG, UK*

Dr James R. Smith, *International Medical Leader: Tamiflu, F. Hoffmann-La Roche Ltd, Pharmaceuticals Division, PBMT Bldg 74/3O Z1.06, CH-4070, Basel, Switzerland*

Dr Richard South, MBChB, *Medical Director, Pandemic Centre of Excellence, GlaxoSmithKline, 980 Great West Road, Brentford TW8 9GS, UK*

Dr Gwen M. Stephens, MD MSc FRCPC, *Senior Consultant, Public Health Directorate, Saudi Arabia Ministry of Health, PO Box 54146, Riyadh 11514, Kingdom of Saudi Arabia 11176*

Dr Norio Sugaya, MD, *Director, Department of Pediatrics, Keiyu Hospital, 3-7-3 Minatomirai, Nishi-ku, Yokohama, 220-0012 Kanagawa, Japan*

Prof Thomas D. Szucs, MD MPH LLM MBA, *Director, Institute of Pharmaceutical Medicine/European Center of Pharmaceutical Medicine, University of Basel, Klingelbergstrasse 61, 4056 Basel, Switzerland*

Prof Jonathan Van-Tam, MBE DM FFPH FRSPH, *Professor of Health Protection, University of Nottingham, Room A40d, Clinical Sciences Building, City Hospital, Nottingham NG5 1PB, UK and Honorary Consultant Epidemiologist, Health Protection Agency (East Midlands), UK*

Diana Vilar-Compte, MD MSc, *Hospital Epidemiologist, Departamento de Infectología, Insituto Nacional de Cancerología, Av. San Fernando 22, Col. Sección XVI, México DF, 14080 México*

Patricia Volkow, MD, *Underdirector of Ancillary, Diagnostic and Treatment Division, Insituto Nacional de Cancerología, Av. San Fernando 22, Col. Sección XVI, México DF, 14080 México*

Andy Wapling, OStJ MSc FICPEM FRSPH, *Head of Emergency Preparedness, NHS London, Southside, 105 Victoria Street, London SW1E 6QT, UK*

Prof John M. Watson, *Head Respiratory Diseases Department, Health Protection Agency (Colindale), 61 Colindale Avenue, London NW9 5EQ, UK*

Dr Isaac B. Weisfuse, *Deputy Commissioner, Office of Emergency Preparedness and Response, New York City Department of Health and Mental Hygiene, Office of Emergency Preparedness and Response, Gotham Center, 42-09 28th Street, Queens, NY 11101, USA*

Editor Biographies

Jonathan Van-Tam, MBE BMedSci(Hons) BMBS DM FFPH FRSPH, is Professor of Health Protection at the University of Nottingham. He graduated in medicine in 1987 and after several years of clinical work, completed an academic training in epidemiology and public health, with a special interest in influenza that now spans over 20 years. He brings a wealth of experience to this book, including formative early training in influenza under the mentorship of Prof Karl G. Nicholson and private sector experience with two major pharmaceutical companies (both manufacturers of neuraminidase inhibitors) and a large European influenza vaccines company. He returned to the public sector in 2004 and was Head of the Health Protection Agency Pandemic Influenza Office during the most frenetic period of UK preparedness activity from 2004 to 2007. He has served as both Temporary Adviser and Short Term Consultant to the World Health Organization (WHO) regarding pandemic preparedness on numerous occasions, and has also undertaken related scientific work for the European Centre for Disease Prevention and Control (ECDC). He is a serving member of the UK national Scientific Pandemic Influenza Committee (SPI), its Clinical Countermeasures Sub-Group and during the 2009 pandemic served on the UK Scientific Advisory Group for Emergencies (SAGE). Since 2010, his unit at the University of Nottingham has been an official WHO Collaborating Centre for pandemic influenza and research.

Chloe Sellwood, BSc(Hons) PhD FRSPH DipHEP, works for the UK National Health Service (NHS) Strategic Health Authority (SHA) in London (NHS London) where she is the Pandemic and Seasonal Influenza Resilience Manager. She graduated in biochemistry in 1998 and completed a PhD in plant biochemistry in 2001. Her experience in pandemic preparedness ranges from the international to local level, and encompasses scientific, strategic and operational aspects. She spent over 7 years at the Health Protection Agency, including 3 years as the Senior Scientist and Coordinator of the Pandemic Influenza Office from 2005 to 2008. She has worked with the World Health Organization (WHO) and European Centre for Disease Prevention and Control (ECDC) on international consultations, as well as on secondment to the Department of Health (England) Pandemic Influenza Preparedness Programme. She has held her present role since 2008, and is responsible for the strategic overview of influenza pandemic preparedness and for seasonal influenza response within the NHS in London. During the 2009 pandemic, she provided strategic, operational and scientific support and advice to the NHS in London, as well as to inter-agency partners. Whilst at NHS London she has obtained a Diploma in health emergency preparedness and broadened her experience to encompass wider aspects of health emergency preparedness, resilience and response.

Foreword

It's tough to make predictions, especially about the future.

Lawrence (Yogi) Berra

When the first edition of this book was planned in late 2007 who could predict that by the time it came to print, in the autumn of 2009, the first pandemic of the 21st century would be well under way?

At the time, the perceived major threat was the A(H5N1) avian influenza virus, but in reality it was an A(H1N1) swine virus (now designated A(H1N1)pdm09) that emerged in 2009. This is not to say that the threat from A(H5N1) has diminished – the threat is ever present and has probably neither increased nor decreased since 2007. In 2007, the most likely geographical origin of the next pandemic was thought to be South-east Asia when in fact it was Central America, probably Mexico; the virus may have undergone evolutionary changes some time in mid to late 2008, leading to its emergence in March 2009.

Although I made some early remarks in my previous Foreword about the emerging epidemiology of A(H1N1)pdm09, we could not have foreseen the difficulties associated with even so mild a pandemic. For example, the high pressure on intensive care beds worldwide, difficulties with communication, public ambivalence towards pandemic vaccination, the prominence of the illness in pregnant women, the emergence of morbid obesity as a new risk factor, and the large variation in case numbers across different regions of the same country.

Much has been made in the media of a supposed overreaction by the World Health Organization (WHO) and individual governments. However, it is worth reflecting that publications such as that by Mark Miller and colleagues point out the particularly young age distribution of deaths in 2009, meaning that in the USA alone between 334,000 and 1,973,000 potential years of life were lost during the pandemic, even if the absolute number of deaths was relatively small. Likewise the 'Fineberg Report' has roundly concluded that with regard to WHO's role in the crisis there was 'no evidence of malfeasance'.

What is certain about the 2009 pandemic is that it was the first since the start of widespread pandemic preparedness activity in 2004, a test of whether such planning was worthwhile and a good, if unwanted, rehearsal for a more severe pandemic that could occur in the future. Many national and international evaluations concluded that pandemic preparedness significantly improved our response in 2009. It is equally clear that a virus causing more severe disease (as a human transmissible A(H5N1) might be) would have 'stressed the system' far more heavily. However, valuable lessons have been learned from A(H1N1)-pdm09.

To paraphrase Field Marshall Helmut von Moltke, 'no plan survives contact with the enemy'. Planning should be seen as a system of options to be tested against an unfolding reality. The response to an influenza pandemic must first be *precautionary* until the rate of spread, severity of the illness and groups most at risk can be established, thereafter it should be *flexible* and *proportionate*.

Jonathan Van-Tam and Chloe Sellwood quickly recognized the need for an expanded second edition of this highly successful text, to bring into focus many of the key lessons from the 2009 pandemic. They have assembled a remarkable cast of authoritative experts from around the world to contribute individual chapters. Of great interest, these are placed alongside case studies from different countries and regions across the globe to add real-world perspectives.

We are now in an immediate post-pandemic phase when many individuals, organizations and governments might feel a false sense of security that the pandemic has 'come and gone'. Sadly, however, it remains a fact that the timing of the next pandemic is entirely unpredictable, as is its place of origin and its severity. In early 2012, the UK Cabinet Office continued to rank pandemic influenza in the highest impact category and the most likely category of all natural disasters in the next 5 years.

Influenza continues to surprise. As we go to press, experts are once again tracking an outbreak of a novel influenza A(H3N2) infection in pigs in the North American Midwest. The virus contains the matrix (*M*) gene from A(H1N1)pdm09 and has so far given rise to over 300 human cases mainly resulting from direct exposure to pigs, although limited human–human transmission has been documented.

Against this backdrop, the new second edition of *Pandemic Influenza* offers an important update on the lessons identified from the 2009 pandemic and once again blends science and public health policy into an accessible, appealing and highly practical handbook, especially for those new to the field or requiring a broad overview of this multi-faceted subject.

This second edition of an important book is very timely, and the book is without parallel as a practical manual of relevance to policy makers, public health officials, healthcare professionals, epidemiologists, health correspondents and interested members of the public.

The editors, Van-Tam and Sellwood, are to be congratulated for creating such an excellent resource, as are the publishers and the distinguished authors of each of the chapters.

Sir Gordon Duff, FRCP, FMedSci, FRSE
Florey Professor of Molecular Medicine, University of Sheffield, UK;
Chairman, UK Scientific Pandemic Influenza Advisory Committee (SPI);
Co-Chairman, UK Scientific Advisory Group for Emergencies (SAGE) during the 2009/10 pandemic.

Further Reading

Centers for Disease Control and Prevention (CDC) (2012) Notes from the Field: Outbreak of Influenza A(H3N2) Virus Among Persons and Swine at a County Fair – Indiana, July 2012. *Morbidity and Mortality Weekly Report* 61, 561. Available at: http://www.cdc.gov/mmwr/preview/mmwrhtml/mm6129a5.htm (accessed 12 September 2012).

Hine, D. (2010) The 2009 Influenza Pandemic – An independent review of the UK response to the 2009 influenza pandemic. Available at: http://www.cabinetoffice.gov.uk/resource-library/independent-review-response-2009-swine-flu-pandemic (accessed 14 June 2012).

Miller, M., Olson, D., Osterholm, M., Simonsen, L. and Viboud, C. (2010) Preliminary Estimates of Mortality and Years of Life Lost Associated with the 2009 A/H1N1 Pandemic in the US and Comparison with Past Influenza Seasons. *Public Library of Science Currents: Influenza* RRN1153. Available at: http://currents.plos.org/influenza/article/preliminary-estimates-of-mortality-and-35hpbywfdwl4n-8/ (accessed 14 April 2012).

UK Cabinet Office (2012) National Risk Register for Civil Emergencies – January 2012 Edition. Available at: http://www.cabinetoffice.gov.uk/resource-library/national-risk-register (accessed 14 April 2012).

World Health Organization (2011) Implementation of the International Health Regulations (2005) Report of the Review Committee on the Functioning of the International Health Regulations (2005) in relation to Pandemic (H1N1) 2009. Available at: http://www.who.int/ihr/review_committee/en/index.html (accessed 14 April 2012).

Acknowledgements

When we set about producing the first edition of this book in late 2007, we had no idea that by the time we had finished the first influenza pandemic of the 21st century would be well under way. Indeed, having worked intensively together in the area of pandemic preparedness for a number of years, we had no idea that such an event would happen 'on our watch'; but it did.

Although the 2009 pandemic has been described as the mildest in recent human history, it nevertheless gave rise to many challenges, such as the unprecedented pressure on intensive care facilities and difficulties with vaccine logistics and communication. It also taught us, once again, to expect the unexpected.

Despite the extensive global preparedness efforts undertaken since 2004 (which definitely paid off), we felt so many new lessons had been identified in 2009 that we should waste no time in getting started on a second edition of this book that incorporates many of these into what is already known. As such, the new version of the book is more expansive than the first; but we hope it retains a freshness and style that will appeal to a wide range of readers, especially those who are self-confessed 'non-experts' but who have been tasked with 'picking up the baton' of pandemic preparedness in what is now a new 'post-pandemic' era.

Again we have relied heavily on a wonderful 'international college' of experts, many of whom are also our friends and all of whom were in some way right there, on the front line, alongside us in 2009. Thank you for your help; without it, assembling this volume would have been a truly daunting task.

The opinions expressed by the editors and authors contributing to this book do not necessarily reflect the opinions of the institutions or organizations with which they are affiliated or by whom they are employed.

JVT and **CS**
April 2012

Glossary

Adjuvant. A compound or agent deliberately added to a vaccine in order to increase the antibody response while having few, if any, direct effects of its own. Especially useful in situations where a 'plain' vaccine produces only a modest antibody response; or for public health reasons the available antigen needs to be eked out to produce more doses (known as an 'antigen sparing' strategy).

Adverse effects/adverse events. Unwanted side-effects caused by a medicine (or vaccine).

A(H1N1)pdm09. Official term used by the World Health Organization to denote the virus, A/California/7/2009(H1N1), which caused the 2009 pandemic.

Antigenic drift. Changes to viral antigens which occur through a process of random genetic mutation. Such changes are relatively frequent in RNA viruses such as influenza. Antigenic drift drives the production of new annual seasonal influenza vaccines, because pre-existing antibodies become poorly matched against the new drifted virus strains.

Antigenic shift. Reassortment of two or more influenza virus subtypes that causes a phenotypic change and the formation of a new subtype having a mixture of the surface antigens of the original viruses (e.g. $A(H1N1) + A(H3N2) = A(H1N2)$).

Antigenic recycling. A pattern of sequential re-emergence of a limited number of novel influenza subtypes in humans, e.g. H1 in 1918, H2 in 1957, H3 in 1968, H1 (again) in 2009. This phenomenon suggests that antigens are 'recycled' and might indicate that relatively few influenza A subtypes have the propensity to cause widespread disease in humans; however this cannot be known for certain.

Antiviral resistance. Development of reduced drug effectiveness (e.g. antivirals) in curing a disease (e.g. influenza), often due to reduced ability to neutralize the pathogen. This phenomenon may be caused by antigenic drift, natural selection or drug pressure (where widespread use of the drug causes frequent exposure of the organism to the drug and accelerates the emergence of resistant variants).

Asymptomatic infections. Infections that do not cause any symptoms, however some asymptomatic patients may still be infectious.

Booster (dose). Re-exposure to an immunizing antigen (usually by means of an additional dose of vaccine) after a period of time, that raises immunity (antibodies) against that antigen back up to protective levels, sometimes enhancing these above the levels produced by the primary immunization.

Business continuity planning (BCP). The development and testing of a plan for organizational continuity of critical functions during an incident or period of extended disruption, including the post-incident recovery phase and return to normality within a pre-defined time.

Case–control study. An epidemiological study or method of analysis based on defining 'cases' – people with a disease – and 'controls' – similar people who do not have the disease – and examining, retrospectively, the exposure of both groups to a range of influencing factors (e.g. vaccination). Increasingly used as a method for the rapid determination of influenza vaccine effectiveness.

Case fatality rate (CFR). The proportion of people who become ill with symptoms that subsequently die as a consequence of their infection. For pandemic influenza this is frequently expressed as a percentage, e.g. CFR in $1918 = 2.5\%$.

Cell-mediated immunity (CMI). Immunity which is not dependent on the raising of antibodies.

Clade. A group of influenza virus strains from a single common ancestor (analogous to a human family, tribe or clan); for example, there are at least 20 clades within the influenza A(H5N1) subtype. Important in relation to pre-pandemic vaccination and cross-protective immunity.

Clinical attack rate (CAR). The infection rate in a population as measured by the development of symptoms; this tends to be measured in a cumulative way to track the progress of a pandemic or epidemic, and is often expressed as a percentage.

Cohorted care. A configuration of healthcare delivery used in situations where infection control is of paramount importance. Patients with the same illness are separated from patients who do not have the illness. Staff are also divided into two teams: those caring for 'ill' patients and those caring for 'not ill' patients.

Co-morbidity. A pre-existing chronic illness or condition, usually used to define medical conditions that are known to place the individual at greater risk from complications, hospitalizations and death.

Critical national infrastructure (CNI). Blanket and rather imprecise term used in emergency preparedness to denote national functions and industries (assets) such as (but not limited to) healthcare, law and order, water supplies, transportation, food, fuel and power distribution, etc. that are considered essential to maintain throughout a disruptive period such as a pandemic (especially if severe) to maintain human society and the economy.

Cross-protective immunity. A situation where immunity to one antigen (stimulated by vaccination or wild infection) provides partial or complete protection against a range of similar antigens, e.g. when a vaccine containing A(H5N1) clade 2 antigens is capable of providing partial or complete protection against clade 1 and clade 3 viruses of the same A(H5N1) subtype.

Cytokine storm. Pro-inflammatory proteins known as cytokines and chemokines, which activate T-cells and macrophages, can be released in response to severe infection. If released in large enough quantity (a cytokine 'storm'), these have the effect of producing an intense immune response which is in itself potentially life threatening. Cytokine storm is implicated in the severe manifestation of some human A(H5N1) infections and may have played a role in severe A(H1N1) infections in young adults during the 1918 pandemic, when paradoxically a young and vigorous immune system may have been disadvantageous.

Defence in depth. Combinations of countermeasures that, when taken together, will most likely be more effective than single measures, and offer assurance that if some measures fail altogether, others will 'hold'. Also known as 'layered interventions' or 'layered containment' (though it is unlikely that pandemic influenza can ever be truly 'contained').

Double-blind placebo controlled trial. A way of carrying out an experiment that is designed to remove subjective bias on the part of the researcher and subject, where allocation to treatment or placebo is on the basis of chance alone, and neither knows who belongs to the control or experimental groups. The use of a placebo or 'dummy' in the control or comparison group ensures that the behavioural effect of being treated is the same in both groups.

Effectiveness. The capability of a treatment or countermeasure to produce the desired effect under 'real life' conditions, e.g. use of face masks by people in their own homes.

Efficacy. The capability of a treatment or countermeasure to produce the desired effect under 'ideal' or perfectly controlled conditions, e.g. use of face masks by supervised, motivated volunteers in a quarantine unit study.

Emergency preparedness. A process of identifying, assessing and addressing risks through preparing for a range of emergency scenarios before they occur. This should include exercising the response and incorporating lessons identified to continually improve arrangements.

Endemic. When a disease is endemic, the illness or infection is persistently present in a certain fraction of a population group. For influenza the term endemic is not especially applicable, as the virus usually afflicts a population group in a wave of acute infections and thereafter returns to baseline in a classical epidemic pattern.

Enzootic. Equivalent of endemic, but a term applied to animals, e.g. avian influenza is enzootic for some bird species in many areas in South-east Asia.

Epidemic. A sudden surge of new cases rising sharply above baseline, before returning again. For a given geographical location, an influenza epidemic period typically lasts for about 8 to 10 weeks, the incidence rate taking a bell-shaped form.

Epidemiology. A formal branch of science and medicine devoted to the study of the patterns of disease, health events and their determinants in human and animal populations.

Epizootic. Equivalent of epidemic, but a term applied to disease in animals.

Excess mortality. A term applied to the number of extra deaths caused by a period of influenza activity, i.e. deaths due to influenza that would not have occurred anyway due to background factors such as winter temperature, etc. Note that excess mortality does not on its own give any clues about the age group of persons who died; pandemics without massive excess mortality may still result in substantial years of life lost if the average age of casualties is young.

Exercise. A process of testing and refining plans and preparedness through simulating the event and testing how organizations and individuals would respond.

Fomite. Inanimate object or substance capable of transmitting an infectious organism from one person to another. In the case of influenza, examples might include: door handles, handrails, shared cups, computer keypads, telephone handsets, etc.

Haemagglutinin. A glycosylated surface protein on the influenza virus that initiates infection by binding to receptors on the host cell.

Infection control measures. A collection of measures intended to reduce the risk of disease transmission from an infected person to uninfected persons (e.g. hand and respiratory hygiene, masks and respirators, disinfection). A term traditionally used in health and social care settings but in an influenza pandemic has potentially far wider applicability.

Influenza-like illness (ILI). Term used to describe a syndrome commonly associated with influenza infection. It is well recognized that the syndrome is fairly non-specific and without laboratory confirmation may inadvertently capture many other acute respiratory virus infections; however ILI becomes much more predictive of true influenza at times of known virus activity, e.g. during epidemic and pandemic periods. Some countries, e.g. the USA, have formal definitions for ILI.

Interpandemic influenza. See Seasonal influenza.

Interoperability. An imprecise term applied to how countries and organizations might plan to act before and during a pandemic in a way that is compatible with each other, or at least does not produce conflicting ideas and responses.

Layered containment. See Defence in depth.

Live-attenuated influenza vaccine (LAIV). A type of influenza vaccine made with virus that has not undergone a process of inactivation (i.e. has not been killed); instead the virus has been cultured to introduce mutations that weaken the virus, preserving its basic ability to induce an antibody response but without making the recipient ill.

M2 channel blockers (adamantanes). Antiviral drugs specific to influenza, which work by preventing the influenza virus from inserting its RNA into the host cell nucleus, e.g. amantadine or rimantadine.

Magistral. Referring to a drug or medicine: formulated extemporaneously or for a special purpose. Taken to mean a non-standard method of presentation or reconstitution of the drug, e.g. Tamiflu® magistral formulation – the dry active granules can be reconstituted with water for mass deployment in an emergency.

Mathematical modelling. Techniques using broad knowledge of the system under investigation to construct simplified, idealized versions (models) that can then be analysed in detail using complex mathematical techniques, to predict what might happen given certain assumptions. Extensively used in pandemic preparedness to scope the possible extent of spread of disease and the effects of interventions.

Mock-up pandemic influenza vaccine. A vaccine that contains any influenza virus subtype to which humans have not yet been widely exposed, with vaccine composition and manufacturing methods identical to those that will eventually be used for future pandemic influenza vaccine. This product is then licensed in advance. When a pandemic virus is identified, a suitable antigen (the vaccine seed virus) is decided upon and vaccine production begins without the need for a further lengthy licensing process. This speeds up the availability of pandemic-specific vaccine.

Monovalent vaccine. A type of influenza vaccine containing only one strain of influenza virus (e.g. a pandemic strain) as opposed to trivalent seasonal influenza vaccines that contain three strains.

Morbidity. Poor health, illness or disability falling short of death (mortality). In relation to influenza, the term is frequently used fairly loosely to describe significant illness, complications and hospitalizations.

Neuraminidase. A glycosylated surface protein on the influenza virus that allows newly made virions to detach from the infected host cell and spread to infect other cells.

Neuraminidase inhibitors. Antiviral drugs specific to influenza that bind to the influenza neuraminidase, thereby blocking the release of newly formed virus particles from infected host cells.

Non-pharmaceutical interventions. Measures of influenza control that do not include pharmaceutical products such as vaccines and drugs. Also referred to as public health measures, public health countermeasures or public health interventions.

Nosocomial infection. Infections that are acquired by patients or staff via a healthcare setting. Includes patient-to-staff transmission, staff-to-patient transmission and patient-to-patient. Nosocomial transmission of influenza by these three means is well recognized.

Pandemic. When a novel influenza A subtype spreads worldwide it is termed a pandemic. A clinical attack rate of 30–50% would be expected.

Peak illness rate. The maximum proportion (usually expressed as a percentage) of the population who will be ill at the same time.

Personal protective measures. Infection control measures that individual people can undertake, e.g. hand washing and respiratory hygiene.

Pre-pandemic vaccine. Vaccine produced in advance of a pandemic, containing antigens against a novel virus considered likely to cause a pandemic. The vaccine is procured in advance and might also be given in advance based on the likelihood that it may confer some protection against the actual pandemic virus; note that an A(H5N1) pre-pandemic vaccine would not offer any protection against a pandemic vaccine caused by a different subtype, such as A(H1N1).

Priming. Exposure of naïve immune cells to a specific antigen (e.g. the influenza A(H5N1) virus) that enables them to differentiate into immune response cells (e.g. antibodies) or memory cells allowing a more rapid response upon re-exposure.

Prophylaxis. An intervention designed to prevent, rather than cure or treat a disease. This can either be 'post' exposure prophylaxis following exposure to the pathogen (termed PEP) or 'pre' exposure (i.e. in advance of exposure). The term is most commonly applied to the use of neuraminidase inhibitors for PEP to prevent or reduce the occurrence of secondary cases in a defined setting such as a household, health facility or school. Note that antiviral PEP does not provide long-lasting immunity and once discontinued, individuals remain susceptible to infection (unless vaccinated in the interim).

Protective sequestration. A term used to describe when healthy people attempt to isolate themselves to reduce the risk of exposure to an infection. Rarely practical in relation to pandemic influenza, and leaves the individual susceptible unless vaccinated in the intervening period.

Public health measures (or countermeasures). Group actions taken that are intended to reduce human-to-human transmission of influenza and thereby mitigate the adverse effects of an epidemic or pandemic.

Quarantine. Applied to people exposed who may or may not be infected but are *not* ill. Separation or restriction of movement is then practised or applied, so that if any of these people subsequently become ill they will not pose a risk of infection to others.

Randomized controlled trial. A type of experiment, used to test the efficacy of an intervention or medicine, which randomly allocates different interventions or medicines to the subjects in the trial, thereby reducing the chances of a biased result.

Real-time modelling. Real-time modelling, or 'nowcasting', is short-range forecasting based on current events to understand an evolving situation.

Reassortment. The mixing of genetic material between influenza viruses. This may occur in nature when an animal or human is simultaneously infected with two genetically different influenza viruses. Deliberate reassortment is also undertaken in laboratories, especially in relation to the development of 'high yield reassortant' viruses optimized for influenza vaccine manufacture.

Reproductive number or R_0. Epidemiological term which describes the average number of people that one person with infection subsequently infects before they themselves recover (or die). If $R_0 > 1$, the number of infected people increases over time and transmission is sustained; if $R_0 < 1$ transmission is not sustained. The underlying R_0 of a pandemic virus affects the effectiveness of interventions and countermeasures.

Respiratory and hand hygiene. Use of tissues to cover mouth and nostrils when coughing and sneezing and their correct disposal, followed by hand washing.

Respirators. Face pieces that often have the external appearance of a simple 'mask' but are in fact specialist filtering devices that prevent the ingress of very small particles, e.g. infectious organisms transmitted via aerosols (droplet nuclei typically ≤5μm diameter). Some respirators are visually and physically substantial pieces of equipment for the wearer and require careful fit-testing in advance.

Seasonal influenza. A term used to refer to influenza that occurs during interpandemic periods, i.e. 'everyday flu'. Used interchangeably with the technically more correct term 'interpandemic influenza'. However the demarcation line between pandemic and seasonal influenza is somewhat artificial and in tropical zones influenza does not have such a distinct seasonal (winter–summer) pattern.

Secondary effects. The costs, risks and consequences of applying public health measures and other interventions.

Secondary attack rate (SAR). Term used to describe the intensity of spread of infection or risk among the susceptible contacts, after exposure to an infective case of influenza. Mathematically expressed as: new illnesses within the range of the incubation period among those exposed, divided by subjects exposed to the primary case(s). Strictly, the denominator and the numerator are restricted to the susceptible contacts; but in practice data on susceptibility are often not known at the time of measurement (e.g. in a household outbreak setting).

Self-isolation. Applies to people experiencing symptoms restricting their movements (in most cases, staying at home) and reducing their level of contact with other people until symptom free in order to reduce the likelihood of onward transmission. This is usually a voluntary action.

Serological attack rate. The influenza infection rate in a population as measured by the development of bloodstream antibodies to the virus. Not all people who demonstrate evidence of infection via antibodies have experienced a symptomatic illness.

Social distancing. An imprecise term often applied to the collection of measures intended to decrease the frequency of close contact among people and so possibly reduce influenza transmission. Most experts consider it better to describe the range of specific interventions within this blanket term.

Strain. Term used to describe sub-classifications of influenza B or influenza A subtypes. New strains of influenza viruses appear and replace older strains over time, through the process of antigenic drift (see above). When a new strain of a human influenza virus emerges, antibody protection that may have developed after infection or vaccination with an older strain may not persist, and the vaccine composition may need changing. Typically new strains of influenza A and B are described annually whereas new subtypes of influenza A appear extremely rarely.

Subtype. Term used to describe sub-classifications of influenza A viruses according to the configuration of the two major surface antigens: haemagglutinin (HA) and neuraminidase (NA).

Surgical masks. Masks worn when undertaking surgical procedures, mostly intended to prevent droplet transmission of respiratory pathogens *from* the wearer (not able to protect fully against aerosol (droplet nuclei) transmission). Also often termed 'face masks'. In practice, often used 'in reverse' with the primary intention of protecting the wearer.

Surveillance. The ongoing systematic collection and analysis of data, and the provision of information which leads to action being taken to prevent and control a disease, usually one of an infectious nature.

Syndrome. A group of symptoms that consistently occur together or a condition characterized by a set of associated symptoms. In relation to influenza (syndromic surveillance), when recognition and counting of the illness is based upon recognition of symptoms without laboratory confirmation.

Zoonosis. When a disease is passed from an animal to a human, it is called a zoonosis.

Epidemiology and Clinical Features of Interpandemic Influenza

JONATHAN VAN-TAM[1] AND CHLOE SELLWOOD[2]

[1]University of Nottingham and Health Protection Agency (East Midlands), Nottingham, UK; [2]NHS London, London, UK

- What is the public health importance of interpandemic influenza?
- What is the relationship between pandemic and interpandemic influenza?
- What are the characteristic epidemiological features of interpandemic influenza?
- Who carries the main burden of interpandemic influenza?

1.1 Pandemic and Seasonal Influenza are Related Diseases

Developing a thorough understanding of pandemic influenza hinges upon first having a sound grasp of influenza as an 'everyday' illness. Influenza pandemics are relatively rare events, when compared with seasonal influenza, which inflicts human illness on a frequent basis. In this context, use of the term 'seasonal influenza' requires qualification. It is well recognized that influenza in temperate zones of the world occurs mainly in winter, justifying the reference to a seasonal illness. However, the seasonal distribution of influenza is far less consistent in the tropics and equatorial zones. Technically, the term 'interpandemic' influenza would be more accurate, but in everyday parlance 'seasonal influenza' is an established expression. Furthermore, many inappropriate comparisons are drawn between pandemic influenza and avian influenza, especially when in reality a pandemic is more likely to resemble seasonal influenza than avian influenza as evidenced by the recent 2009 pandemic.

Indeed, pandemic and seasonal influenza are not separate entities; they represent a continuum of disease, from the emergence of a novel virus in humans (a pandemic) to the continued circulation of closely related viruses (of the same subtype) in subsequent years (seasonal influenza), sometimes several decades. For example, the A(H1N1) viruses which circulated from 1920 to 1956 were, in virological terms, descendants of the A(H1N1) virus which emerged in 1918 and caused the 'Spanish influenza' pandemic (Chapter 5); however the epidemiology changed markedly over this period, as the virus evolved (lost virulence) and population immunity increased. Similarly, the 2009 pandemic virus, A(H1N1)pdm09, has remained in circulation, replacing the pre-pandemic A(H1N1) seasonal virus, and caused further severe illness during the 2010/11 northern hemisphere winter. In this regard, the interface between pandemic and seasonal influenza can be rather artificial, as is the counting of pandemic waves. For example, it could be argued that the UK experienced two pandemic waves during the 2009 pandemic (in summer and autumn 2009); but in fact the winter A(H1N1)-pdm09 activity in 2010/11 (after the pandemic was declared over) represented a third wave, from both an epidemiological and a virological perspective. A closer look at the incidence of seasonal influenza shows that in the years immediately following a pandemic, epidemics tend to be relatively severe and to affect younger age groups, compared with those that occur several decades later. Figure 1.1 illustrates the incidence of influenza-like illness (ILI) from 1966 to 2011 in English general practices; the epidemics in the 1970s soon after the 'Hong Kong' pandemic in 1969/70 are notably more severe than those in subsequent decades, although the one in 1989/90 was an outlier that may have been partially due to simultaneous respiratory syncytial virus (RSV) activity. Although

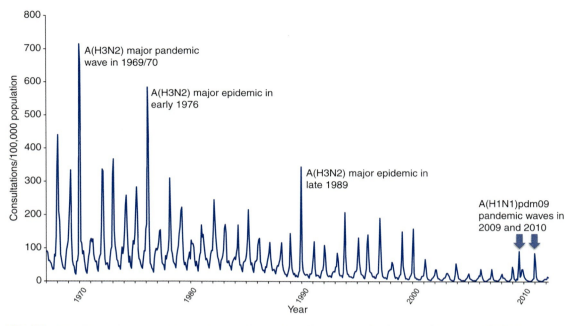

Fig. 1.1. General practice consultation rates for influenza-like illness (ILI) in England and Wales per 100,000 population (all ages) from 1968 to 2011, showing the 1968 and 2009 pandemics and major epidemics in 1976 and 1989. (Figure kindly provided by the Royal College of General Practitioners' (RCGP) sentinel primary care network – Weekly returns service.)

seasonal influenza epidemics produce lower level activity than pandemics, their repetitive annual nature means that cumulative morbidity and mortality probably exceed that associated with pandemic influenza and consequently seasonal influenza should not be underestimated as a major public health issue in its own right.

1.2 Influenza A and B

Although the influenza virus has been categorized into three types: A, B and C, influenza C is but one of several hundred viruses that together account for the 'common cold' and is not considered further in this text. Influenza A and B are considered to be the major human pathogens responsible for seasonal influenza. They are clinically indistinguishable, although influenza B attack rates tend to be far higher in children than in adults. This is undoubtedly related to the inherent antigenic stability of influenza B compared to A, and the likelihood that exposure in childhood will generate longer cross-protective immunity (Chapter 3). Nevertheless re-infection with both influenza A and B is well

recognized, and influenza A subtypes and influenza B co-circulate during the winter.

1.3 Clinical Features

Influenza in humans presents as an acute illness characterized predominantly by cough, malaise and feverishness, typically of rapid onset. Other common additional symptoms are: chills, headache, anorexia, coryza, myalgia and sore throat, which occur in 50–79% of recognized cases; sputum, dizziness, hoarseness, chest pain in <50% of cases; vomiting and diarrhoea are also described but occur in <10% of cases. These features are quite non-specific, making it difficult to distinguish individual cases of influenza from other respiratory virus infections, unless supported by laboratory testing or surveillance data indicating the presence of influenza in the community (Chapter 2). A typical illness lasts up to 5 days. In the vast majority of normal healthy individuals, influenza is miserable but self-limiting; however even in these groups occasional severe illness is described, resulting rarely in unexpected death.

An additional impact of seasonal influenza is felt through a range of associated secondary complications including: acute bronchitis, pneumonia, otitis media (in children), myocarditis, pericarditis myelitis, myositis, and neurological sequelae (febrile convulsions and Reye's syndrome in children; encephalitis in adults). The most common complication is acute bronchitis, but by far the most significant is bacterial pneumonia, where the common organisms described are *Streptococcus pneumoniae*, *Staphylococcus aureus* and *Haemophilus influenzae*. One of the least well-known facts about seasonal influenza is its strong association with minor cardiac rhythm abnormalities, even in healthy adults, which frequently go unrecognized. Recovery from influenza may be followed by a period of fatigue and lethargy lasting several weeks in a minority of individuals.

Seasonal influenza is associated with more severe illness and higher rates of death and hospitalization in neonates and children under 2 years of age; pregnant women; the elderly, especially those over 75 years; and people with underlying co-morbidities (e.g. asthma, diabetes, chronic obstructive pulmonary disease (COPD) and cardiac failure), in whom the acute infection may destabilize the underlying illness. With regard to possible differences between pandemic and seasonal influenza, it is not possible to predict in advance the clinical severity of the former compared with the latter as the different pandemics of the 20th century produced greatly contrasting disease severity (Chapter 5). Nevertheless it is reasonable to surmise that a novel virus against which humans have little or no immunity on balance might be expected to produce an illness of longer duration, associated with prolonged virus excretion (Chapter 8), compared with seasonal influenza. Even though the 2009 pandemic was extremely mild compared with those in 1918 and 1957, 15–20% of hospitalized cases required admission to an intensive care unit, emphasizing the virulence of even a mild pandemic virus.

1.4 Timing and Seasonality

The epidemiology of seasonal influenza is characterized in temperate zones of both the northern and southern hemispheres by epidemics of variable size which occur during the colder winter months, each one typically lasting 8 to 10 weeks. It is however important to note that influenza also occurs in tropical and subtropical zones; in these geographical areas where heat and humidity are year-round phenomena, there is an association of influenza activity with the rainy seasons. Thus influenza in the tropics is not strictly seasonal (in the winter/summer sense) and may occur in association with rainy periods. In the temperate zones where influenza activity is concentrated into the colder winter months various theories have been advanced to explain this pattern, including: improved virus survival in conditions of low temperature and low humidity; low levels of ultraviolet radiation; and close congregation of humans in domestic dwellings with low ventilation (windows closed). This concentration of disease activity makes epidemics rather more recognizable in temperate zones than in the tropics, because more acute pressure is generated on the healthcare system in a shorter period of time.

Usually one influenza A subtype (currently A(H3N2) or A(H1N1)) or influenza B will dominate during a winter season, but this is far from always the case and 'mixed epidemics' are possible. In the northern hemisphere the timing of influenza B activity tends to be later in the season (generally after Christmas) than influenza A, but this is not a fixed rule. Unlike other infections such as RSV, the timing of onset varies markedly from season to season. Influenza activity is documented year-round (at low levels in summer) and influenza outbreaks are well described 'out of season', suggesting that virus circulates constantly.

1.5 Burden of Illness and Clinical Attack Rates

In terms of its public health impact, seasonal influenza is often recognized as a disease of the elderly, the very young and people with high-risk chronic illnesses such as COPD and diabetes. Whilst this is true in relation to the likelihood of death and hospitalization, from another perspective it is totally incorrect. Large cohort studies of respiratory virus infection in families, which took place in the late 1960s and 1970s in the USA (Seattle, Washington; Tecumseh, Michigan; and Houston, Texas), have established that the highest annual attack rates for influenza occur in children and teenagers, and that these decline substantially with age; this is especially true for influenza B which affects adults far less frequently. Typical values for serological attack rates described in the major cohort studies of the 1970s are shown in Table 1.1. Roughly one half were associated with symptomatic illness.

Table 1.1. Summary of age-specific influenza A serological attack rates observed in major community studies in the USA (Seattle, Washington; Tecumseh, Michigan; and Houston, Texas) during the 1970s.

Age group (years)	Attack rate (%)
<1	20–30
1–9	15–45
10–19	17–40
20–29	16–21
30–39	17–21
≥40	12–20

The variability in attack rates reflects different populations, different seasons and different laboratory tests used between studies.

Of course whilst attack rates in the young are highest, infection generally carries fewer consequences in children over 2 years, teenagers and healthy adults with correspondingly low levels of morbidity, mortality and hospitalization. Thus, seasonal influenza is somewhat paradoxical with the highest attack rates in the young but the greatest public health impact in the elderly. It is especially noteworthy that in the region of 50–70% of influenza infections (as confirmed by serology) appear to be asymptomatic, a fact confirmed in the recent 2009 pandemic. This contradicts the popular myth that genuine influenza is always associated with prostration and debility, and that anything less severe could only be 'just a cold'. In fact, interesting data from healthcare workers in Glasgow, Scotland during an influenza A epidemic in 1993/94 revealed that of 518 workers (mainly nursing staff), 23% showed evidence of infection (based on serological findings) by the end of the season. However, 28% of those who had seroconverted could not recall any kind of respiratory illness that winter and 52% had not taken time off work. Thus clear opportunities for transmission within the hospital environment, along with evidence of asymptomatic infection, were revealed.

1.6 Influenza in Children

Until fairly recently, the impact of influenza in young children (aged less than 2 years) had been poorly appreciated; however it is now clear that the level of influenza-related hospitalizations in this age group is as high as in adults with high-risk underlying conditions. Children represent a special epidemiological phenomenon in relation to influenza, because they have poor respiratory etiquette and are known to excrete virus for longer and in higher titres than their adult counterparts; in addition their natural behaviour involves frequent close physical contact with both adults in the family home and other children through play. The risk of acquisition of influenza among adults is raised within households containing young children and there are epidemiological data which clearly indicate that during influenza epidemics, school sickness absence and paediatric admissions peak one to two weeks earlier than workplace absenteeism and hospital admissions in adults within the same community. These data strongly suggest that children act as sentinels for influenza activity within communities and play a major role in propagating transmission in households and communities. These points are highly relevant in relation to infection control practices and possible pandemic countermeasures such as school closures (Chapter 16) and the targeting of vaccination (Chapter 15).

1.7 Diagnostic Certainty

One of the biggest problems related to fully estimating the burden of seasonal influenza relates to case ascertainment. Until the advent of neuraminidase inhibitors (Chapter 14), there were few practical options for targeting the virus through treatment and instead general supportive care and simple treatments aimed at symptom suppression were the norm and there were no clear advantages in confirming the diagnosis using virological tests. Even with the availability of neuraminidase inhibitors from 1999 onwards, the cost, complexity and timeliness of diagnostic tests make it neither practical nor economic to confirm the illness before commencing treatment; instead therapy should generally be initiated on clinical suspicion combined with information from surveillance data. Influenza-related hospitalization frequently occurs due to disease complications; there is again little perceived clinical value in making a diagnosis of influenza at this late stage in the illness and indeed less chance of a positive test several days after the onset of symptoms because virus shedding is likely to have declined. Thus, in all probability, true disease burden remains significantly underestimated.

1.8 Excess Mortality and Morbidity

Despite the lack of established culture within healthcare systems for making a definitive diagnosis of influenza, severe epidemics have always achieved prominence through societal disruption and a phenomenon known as excess mortality; in essence a large number of unexpected deaths brought together in time and space by the occurrence of influenza – the ultimate example being pandemic influenza itself. This phenomenon was first noted by historical writers (usually ecclesiastical) who chronicled outbreaks of 'epidemic fevers' stretching back several centuries (Chapter 5) some of which will have been due to influenza. Modern epidemiological techniques, based on those pioneered by Selwyn Collins and substantially refined by Robert Serfling, have now been applied to the same basic observations in order to quantify the number of 'excess deaths' during a period of known influenza activity. Provided the source data are robust, this calculation can be performed retrospectively or in near real time (a few days behind). All methodologies are based around the calculation of a relevant 'baseline' for deaths (allowing for seasonal variations) and then calculating the surplus of deaths over and above baseline, coinciding with periods of known influenza activity. One of the main findings during influenza epidemics is that deaths which are actually ascribed to influenza at death certification represent a relatively small proportion

(about 10%) of the total excess deaths observed. The remainder are ascribed to secondary complications, e.g. pneumonia, and underlying chronic illnesses such as cardiac failure. Thus, it is now accepted convention that all-cause mortality should be considered when estimating the burden of mortality associated with influenza. The same techniques have also been applied more recently to hospital admission data, generating clear evidence of excess morbidity during periods of influenza activity, and illustrating the surge capacity required in healthcare systems to deal successfully with large epidemics and pandemics.

It is now clear that influenza epidemics frequently produce excess mortality which is mainly seen in the elderly. On occasions, the excess deaths noted during an epidemic are followed by a much smaller deficit in deaths over the next few weeks, suggesting that influenza kills some frail and elderly people whose deaths would have occurred soon in any case; whilst probably true, these still represent a minority of all excess deaths. During the last large influenza epidemic in the UK in 1989/90 it is estimated that 29,000 excess deaths occurred in a period of about 60 days, almost entirely in people age 75 years and over. Even after adjusting for a post-epidemic deficit, the excess death toll was still about 17,000 (Fig. 1.2).

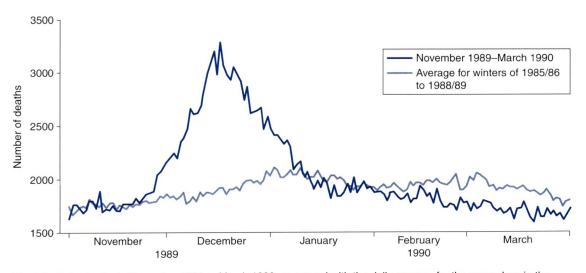

Fig. 1.2. Daily deaths in November 1989 to March 1990, compared with the daily average for the same days in the winters of 1985/86 to 1988/89, Great Britain. (Redrawn from Ashley *et al.*, *Population Trends* 65 (Autumn 1991) under the Open Government Licence and Framework (http://www.nationalarchives.gov.uk/doc/open-government-licence/open-government-licence.htm). Source: Office for National Statistics licensed under the Open Government Licence v.1.0.)

It is estimated that there were about 36,000 influenza-related deaths per annum in the USA during the relatively mild decade from 1990 to 1999. Excess deaths due to influenza do not occur to the same extent every season, indeed they are highly variable; however one remarkable consistency is in their age distribution. Longitudinal data suggest that at least 80% of seasonal influenza excess deaths occur in individuals aged 65 and over, even though excess mortality varies from year to year (Fig. 1.3).

1.9 High-risk Illnesses

The risk of seasonal influenza-related complications, hospitalization and death follows a U-shaped curve with an elevated risk that decreases over time from birth to 2 years of age, which then begins to increase sharply from the age of 50 years onwards. However, in public health and health system terms, the most noticeable impact can be seen from the age of 50 years but rates continue to rise sharply after this. In relation to hospital admissions, the extent of the problem in public health terms is disproportionately felt beyond 75 years of age, because lengths of hospital stay increase markedly at this point, reflecting in part the relative difficulty of discharging very elderly patients back into the community. Thus age on its own can be regarded as a major risk factor for complications and deaths due to seasonal influenza.

However, in addition to age per se, it is also well recognized that the rates of secondary complications, hospitalizations and deaths due to seasonal influenza infection are higher in individuals with certain underlying co-morbidities, compared to those who are healthy. Not only do these patients appear more vulnerable to influenza, the infection can also destabilize or decompensate underlying conditions such as diabetes, angina and cardiac failure. Similar observations have been made from multiple epidemiological studies and there is very solid agreement that 'high risk' groups can be defined as those with: chronic respiratory disease (asthma, COPD); chronic heart disease; diabetes; renal disease; significant immune suppression; and pregnant women. In turn, this explains the remarkable international consistency regarding the core groups recommended for annual influenza vaccination. However, up until the 2009 pandemic relatively few countries had actively targeted pregnant women; this seems likely to change. The clear observation that individuals who are immune suppressed are at greater risk from seasonal influenza clearly raises significant public health concerns about the potential impact of a novel, virulent pandemic virus in parts of the world affected by a high prevalence of HIV, most notably sub-Saharan Africa and parts of Asia. Although not a high-risk illness, smoking has also been identified as a relevant risk factor. In the Israeli military, clinical

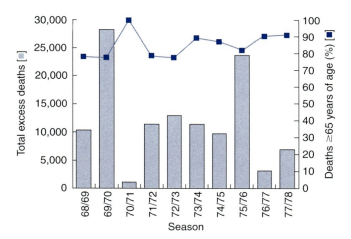

Fig. 1.3. Estimated excess deaths among adults attributable to influenza and the percentage in people ≥65 years, England & Wales (1968/69 to 1977/78 winter seasons). (Data from Tillet *et al.*, 1983; reproduced from an original by J.S. Nguyen-Van-Tam; first appeared in Nguyen-Van-Tam, J.S. (1998) Epidemiology of influenza. In: Nicholson, K.G., Webster, R.G. and Hay, A.J. (eds) *Textbook of Influenza*. Blackwell Science, Oxford, UK.)

attack rates during an epidemic were higher in the same unit among smokers compared to non-smokers, and other studies suggest that illness severity and sickness absence due to influenza are increased in smokers compared with non-smokers.

The identification of high-risk groups has driven annual demand for seasonal influenza vaccines around the world; in turn this drives not only the availability of manufacturing capacity for a future pandemic vaccine (Chapter 15), but also policy assumptions about the size and composition of high-risk groups that might be targeted for specific pandemic interventions. This is a difficult area of policy setting that illustrates the need for effective real-time surveillance during a pandemic. A repeat of the 1918 pandemic in the present day would most likely result in the targeting of young adults for universal vaccination; whilst the 2009 pandemic not only highlighted the risks to pregnant women but also drew attention to a new risk group defined by morbid obesity. However, the interrelationship between the latter and high levels of underlying chronic illnesses is difficult to disentangle.

1.10 Nosocomial Infection and Outbreaks in Semi-closed Communities

Outbreaks in hospitals, nursing homes and boarding schools are a notable and common feature of seasonal influenza. In a review of 41 nursing home outbreaks in the USA, an average attack rate of 43% was recorded during epidemic periods and 16% at other times. Attack rates in boarding school outbreaks appear highly variable, ranging from 20 to 90% in the published literature. These most often occur during periods of known community influenza activity but are also well described 'out of season', before and after periods of wider community activity. In general, they can be successfully interrupted by the application of cohorted care and strict droplet and contact precautions (Chapter 8). Outbreaks which occur prior to the onset of widespread seasonal activity often do so in boarding schools, which can act as sentinel institutions, giving early warning of more widespread community activity. Outbreaks which occur in nursing homes towards the end of the winter season have been attributed to drifted strains against which the annual vaccine (given some 6 months previously) is no longer a close match. On occasions, such outbreaks act as 'herald events' that

give an indication of which strains might predominate in the forthcoming winter season. Likewise, even when vaccine and wild viruses are considered to be still well matched at the end of the season, waning of antibodies in elderly vaccinees has been attributed as the cause of outbreaks; this points to a need for improved vaccines in the elderly. Risk factors for influenza outbreaks in closed institutions include: low influenza vaccine uptake; a large number of residents living in close proximity to each other; and allowing staff members to be employed part-time in other institutions (potential for nosocomial spread between sites). In long-term care establishments, there are persuasive data which suggest that vaccination of staff reduces mortality among residents (irrespective of the latter's vaccination status); yet influenza vaccine uptake among health and social care workers generally remains low. Mortality rates tend to be highest in institutions housing the frail elderly and the immune suppressed; for example mortality rates of up to 70% have been described due to influenza outbreaks in stem cell transplant units. These types of institutions will present critical infection control issues in the event of a future pandemic, as was the case in 2009.

1.11 Summary

A great deal is known about the epidemiology of interpandemic or 'seasonal' influenza; this provides essential background knowledge for an understanding of pandemic influenza. Seasonal influenza is characterized by periods of increased activity lasting 8 to 10 weeks that are unpredictable in their precise timing although always in winter in temperate zones. Morbidity and mortality are concentrated at the extremes of age, notably in children under 2 years and the elderly; however people of any age with certain chronic illnesses are also more severely affected. Excess mortality varies from year to year but is generally concentrated in the elderly. Annual vaccination is recommended for those at increased risk of complications and death; in most countries with active policies, this entails targeted vaccination of people aged 65 years and over, adults with high-risk conditions, pregnant women and sometimes younger children. In addition, health and social workers should be targeted in order to reduce opportunities for nosocomial spread, including the risk of outbreaks in co-located, vulnerable, hospitalized patients, e.g. on stem cell transplantation units; and to maintain adequate staffing levels during periods of influenza related surge.

Understanding the epidemiology of seasonal influenza teaches the pandemic planner the general principles of how influenza behaves in human populations and how this can be monitored. Similar data on the epidemiology of an emerging pandemic virus will be needed within a rapid timeframe in order to inform forecasting, severity assessment and the deployment of countermeasures.

- Because of its recurrent nature, and its occurrence in short but intense epidemics, the public health importance of interpandemic (or seasonal) influenza is considerable. It is estimated that in the relatively 'quiet' period between 1990 and 1999 in the USA, interpandemic influenza accounted for 36,000 deaths per annum. Short epidemic periods of intense activity also produce pressure on health services.
- Pandemic viruses are, by definition, novel in humans. However they go on to become 'normal' interpandemic or seasonal viruses. The A(H3N2) viruses in current circulation are in fact no more than distant evolved relatives of the A(H3N2) virus that caused the 1968 pandemic. Influenza A(H1N1)pdm09 was classified as a pandemic virus in winter 2009/10 but as a seasonal virus in winter 2010/11.
- Interpandemic influenza is characterized by distinct seasonality in the temperate zones of the world (winter activity), explosive epidemics typically lasting 6–8 weeks and serological attack rates of 5–15%, of whom perhaps one half become ill with symptoms.
- Paradoxically, interpandemic influenza is a disease of pre-school and school age children in whom the highest attack rates are recorded. However the burden of excess mortality and complications are concentrated in the very young (typically under 2 years of age), the elderly and people with underlying high-risk conditions such as diabetes, lung disease and heart disease

Further Reading

Dolan, G.P., Harris, R.C., Clarkson, M., Sokal, R., Morgan, G., Mukaigawara, M., Horiuchi, H., Hale, R., Stormont, L., Béchard-Evans, L., Chao, Y.S., Eremin, S., Martins, S., Tam, J.S., Peñalver, J., Zanuzadana, A. and Nguyen-Van-Tam, J.S. (2012) Vaccination of health care workers to protect patients at increased risk for acute respiratory disease. *Emerging Infectious Diseases* 18(8), 1225–1234.

Fleming, D.M. and Elliot, A.J. (2008) Lessons from 40 years' surveillance of influenza in England and Wales. *Epidemiology and Infection* 136(7), 866–875.

Fox, J.P., Cooney, M.K., Hall, C.E. and Foy, H.M. (1982) Influenzavirus infections in Seattle families, 1975–1979. II. Pattern of infection in invaded households and relation of age and prior antibody to occurrence of infection and related illness. *American Journal of Epidemiology* 116(2), 228–242.

Glezen, W.P. and Couch, R.B. (1978) Interpandemic influenza in the Houston area, 1974–76. *New England Journal of Medicine* 298(11), 587–592.

Hall, C.E., Cooney, M.K. and Fox, J.P. (1973) The Seattle Virus Watch: IV. Comparative epidemiologic observations of infections with influenza A and B viruses, 1965–69, in families with young children. *American Journal of Epidemiology* 98(5), 365–380.

Monto, A.S. and Kiouhmehr, F. (1975) The Tecumseh study of respiratory illness. IX. Occurrence of influenza in the community, 1966–1971. *American Journal of Epidemiology* 102(6), 553–563.

Nguyen-Van-Tam, J.S. (1998) Epidemiology of influenza. In: Nicholson, K.G., Webster, R.G. and Hay, A.J. (eds) *Textbook of influenza*. Blackwell Science, Oxford, UK, pp. 181–206.

Reichert, T.A., Simonsen, L., Sharma, A., Pardo, S.A., Fedson, D.S. and Miller, M.A. (2004) Influenza and the winter increase in mortality in the United States, 1959–1999. *American Journal of Epidemiology* 160(5), 492–502.

Teo, S.S., Nguyen-Van-Tam, J.S. and Booy, R. (2005) Influenza burden of illness, diagnosis, treatment and prevention: what is the evidence in children and where are the gaps? *Archives of Disease in Childhood* 90(5), 532–536.

Tillett, H.E., Smith, J.W. and Gooch, C.D. (1983) Excess deaths attributable to influenza in England and Wales: age at deaths and certified cause. *International Journal of Epidemiology* 12, 344–352.

2 Influenza Surveillance and Pandemic Requirements

JOHN M. WATSON AND RICHARD G. PEBODY

Health Protection Agency, London, UK

- What is the purpose of influenza surveillance?
- How is surveillance information used?
- What are the different types of surveillance information?
- What are the key elements of pandemic influenza surveillance?

2.1 Purpose of Influenza Surveillance and Use of the Information

Influenza is not only a miserable illness suffered by individuals, but also an infectious disease that is transmitted from person to person, characteristically occurring in epidemics affecting whole populations. Influenza surveillance is carried out in order to provide an early alert of impending activity in the population, to inform healthcare professionals and the wider community of the extent and severity of current and past activity, and to provide information for treating, preventing and controlling influenza. This chapter largely focuses on influenza surveillance in the UK but key international schemes are also mentioned, and the principles will apply to national influenza surveillance systems in place in other countries.

Early warning is a key purpose of surveillance. Information about the types and characteristics of influenza viruses that have been identified elsewhere in the world or detected in early sporadic cases within the UK, provides information about the potential threat to the population and the probable effectiveness of planned control measures such as immunization and the use of antiviral drugs. The potential for a mismatch between the current seasonal influenza vaccine and circulating strains of influenza virus may become apparent at this time. Information on the nature and range of clinical illness typically being observed in confirmed influenza infection cases, and of those being most affected (such as by age and clinical risk group),

gives an indication of the severity of the illness and the likely need for health service support. The extent of spread of the illness, including numbers and age groups within a population affected, and the rapidity with which different geographical areas are affected, provide further indication of the potential threat with the possibility of review and strengthening of control measures if appropriate (e.g. re-emphasis of the need for vaccination and of the importance of good respiratory and hand hygiene).

Both healthcare professionals and the wider public wish to know about the nature and extent of influenza activity once it begins within the UK, who is at greatest risk, how bad it is likely to get and when it might die down. Healthcare professionals will use this information in the management of individual patients who have illness that may be due to influenza infection and in the organization of health services to cope with large numbers of influenza cases occurring in the population. The wider public wish not only to have an understanding of how likely it is that they or their families, friends, colleagues, etc. will become ill, but also how likely it is that they will become seriously ill. Organizations from local businesses to national government need to be able to plan for absence from work as a result of illness. Surveillance information can provide a rapid and representative assessment of the extent of current activity. In addition, using data from influenza activity in previous years, information about the circulating strains of the influenza virus and data from parts of the world that have already seen activity with the same viruses, surveillance can be used to estimate when the peak of activity is likely to occur and when activity will subside.

During influenza epidemics, surveillance data can be used to estimate the impact of influenza on the population as a whole as well as on specific subgroups, including morbidity and mortality experienced and the use of healthcare. These data, combined with information about uptake of measures like vaccination, can be used to assess the effectiveness of control measures. Assessment of the impact of control measures is then used in review of treatment, prevention and control policies for strengthening the management of future epidemics.

2.2 Influenza Surveillance Pyramid and Challenges to Quantifying Influenza

Influenza virus infection may cause a symptomatic illness or no apparent illness at all (asymptomatic infection): 50% of infections may be asymptomatic. The typical symptoms among those who become ill are those of an 'influenza-like illness' or 'ILI' (sudden onset of fever, respiratory symptoms including cough, and systemic symptoms including tiredness and muscle aches). Some people, however, may experience little more than the symptoms of a cold while others may rapidly develop severe respiratory illness requiring hospital care. The clinical features and severity of the illness caused by influenza is dependent on a range of factors including the virulence of the virus, the age and extent of immunity in the individual and the existence of underlying chronic health conditions. In many individuals, the influenza illness itself may be unpleasant but the principal threat to their health is the exacerbation of an underlying chronic condition such as chronic respiratory or cardiovascular disease. Thus among those who become severely ill as a result of influenza, many will present for healthcare with pneumonia, heart failure, stroke or other complications of the initial influenza infection.

Influenza virus is not the only microorganism to cause an ILI. Many other respiratory viruses, such as respiratory syncytial virus (RSV) and the viruses causing the common cold, as well as a number of bacteria and other infections (such as *Mycoplasma pneumoniae*, *Legionella pneumophila*, *Chlamydophila pneumoniae*) may cause not only a typical respiratory illness but also an ILI, and may lead to exacerbation of underlying chronic diseases.

Most people with mild respiratory or ILI will take care of themselves without seeking advice or care from health professionals. Among those seen in primary care very few will be investigated as to the precise cause of their illness. Even among those ill enough to require hospital care, the initial infection leading to their illness may no longer be apparent and will not be looked for. Consequently, reports of confirmed influenza infections represent only a small and selected minority of all such infections occurring in the population. Surveillance of influenza activity has therefore been developed to combine a range of indicators of influenza activity, none of which, on its own, is sufficient to describe the occurrence of the infection but, when used in combination (and in comparison to similar data from previous years), provide a representative assessment of the activity of influenza virus infection in a population.

Information is collected for different segments of the population according to the severity of the illness caused by infection. This is represented in the 'influenza pyramid' (Fig. 2.1). This illustrates that, during influenza activity, many in the population will remain uninfected or may have infection without illness.

Age-specific serological surveys assessing the presence of influenza-specific antibodies occurring after infection are needed to assess the overall extent of infection (both symptomatic and asymptomatic) in a population. Measures to assess the occurrence of illness in the general population (including people who do and do not seek healthcare) have been recently developed using various survey methods. Well-established general practice (GP) surveillance systems are used to assess the numbers and characteristics of patients seeking primary care for illness likely to be due to influenza and the contribution of influenza virus infection in a representative subset of these individuals. More recently developed hospital-based surveillance systems are now being implemented to assess the number of people admitted for hospital care for influenza (at least among those with illness investigated and shown to be due to confirmed influenza infection) and to assess the number dying with confirmed influenza infection. Finally, population vital statistics on the numbers of people dying each week, and the broad causes of those deaths, are used to estimate the likely total number of people dying as a result

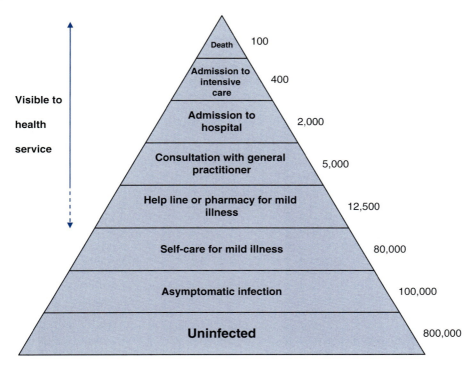

Fig. 2.1. Influenza pyramid in a substantial epidemic or pandemic wave. Based on a population of one million, with a 20% infection rate, a 10% clinical attack rate, a 2% case hospitalization rate and a 0.1% symptomatic case fatality ratio. Note that these percentages are illustrative; for example, case fatality ratio in 1918 was 2.5%, whereas in 2009 it was <0.05%.

of influenza virus activity in the population by comparison with previous seasons.

2.3 Sources of Influenza Surveillance Data in the UK

The principal types of surveillance data in the UK are shown in Table 2.1. While some of these data provide an indication of influenza activity in specific layers of the influenza pyramid, others (such as laboratory reports) include data derived from more than one of the layers.

2.4 Lessons for Surveillance from the 2009 Pandemic and Subsequent Influenza Activity

The 2009 influenza pandemic which was due to the A(H1N1)pdm09 virus presented a number of challenges to surveillance which had not been fully anticipated. The clinical illness associated with the infection was generally mild but, as a result of a propensity to cause infection and illness, particularly in young children and adults, was associated with a high number of severe illnesses in young people. It emerged in the Americas but spread quickly to the UK at a time when insufficient was known about the level of threat it posed. The initial response in the UK involved identifying all cases and offering them antiviral treatment and their close contacts prophylaxis. At the same time, cases were being counted and contacts traced so as to determine the transmission characteristics of the disease and whether it had reached the point of sustained community transmission. Little was known about the extent of very mild clinical infection or of asymptomatic infection, both of which would be expected to confer subsequent immunity. There was a suggestion from commentators in a number of parts of the world that the global response to the pandemic was excessive and inappropriate to what ultimately emerged as a generally mild disease. In the subsequent influenza seasons in the southern and northern hemispheres, the A(H1N1)pdm09 virus

Table 2.1. Seasonal influenza surveillance: sources, advantages and limitations.

Source	Advantages	Limitations
Consultations for influenza in sentinel networks of primary care general practice surgeries	• Estimates clinical incidence when linked to a registered population • Can be linked with virological testing to corroborate clinical diagnosis, and to vaccination records to estimate vaccine effectiveness • Provides age-specific data by time period and geographical area	• Based on clinical diagnosis of ILI, with or without formal case definition, and usually without virological confirmation • Cannot record ILI cases that do not consult with primary care practitioner (those 'below the radar')
Hospital admissions	• Useful to quantify extent of severe illness due to influenza • Virological information is more often available than in cases seen in primary care • Risk factors for severe disease can be assessed • Can provide clinical data on process of care, prognosis, dependency and case fatality	• Difficult to identify all hospital admissions due to influenza (many hidden under alternative diagnoses) • Difficult to obtain detailed information in real time • Once hospital system saturated, unable to measure further (unmet) need for hospital care
Calls to health help lines and Internet queries on influenza	• Provides potential indication of level of activity in community in people not consulting primary care or using pharmacies • Help lines can be linked to antiviral treatment allocation, providing information about demand • Can potentially be linked to virological self-sampling schemes	• Numbers of people seeking advice may be influenced by levels of public concern as much as levels of illness • Non-specific: based on self-diagnosis and patient reporting of symptoms
Deaths reported to be due to confirmed influenza, and estimates of excess mortality from population statistics	• Provides assessment of the impact of severe disease • Enables determination of groups most vulnerable to severe disease and complications • 'Nowcasting' can potentially adjust for reporting delays to allow for more real-time data	• Delay between date of illness onset, death and recording in official statistics • Only small proportion of total influenza-related deaths are ascribed to influenza as the primary cause of death • Shortage of physicians and large number of deaths may prevent accurate certification during a major epidemic/pandemic
Laboratory virology data	• Provides information on type, subtype and strain of influenza viruses circulating • Corroborates information about clinical activity in the community or in hospitalized patients • Testing for antiviral drug resistance is possible • Provides data on other respiratory virus pathogens mistaken for influenza • Denominator information on positive and negative results on respiratory swabs allows positivity rate to be monitored	• Specimens taken from selected subset of patients – may not be representative of population • Data yield highly dependent on quality and timing of both clinical specimen and receiving laboratory • Cannot be used to determine incidence (due to lack of denominators) other than in directed schemes

Continued

J.M. Watson and R.G. Pebody

Table 2.1. Continued.

Source	Advantages	Limitations
Sickness absence data	• Where obtained, can provide indicator of impact of influenza epidemics in the workplace and schools • May help in assessment of economic cost of lost productivity and wider societal impact	• Cause of sickness absence not usually recorded • Scope for significant misdiagnosis if data based on self-certification are used • Schools data disrupted during holiday periods • During epidemics, workplace absence may be due to illness, care of ill dependants or fear of infection through attending work
Sales of over-the-counter cough/cold/flu remedies	• Captures data on cases not seeking formal healthcare	• Non-specific • Availability may be limited due to commercial sensitivity • Fails to capture those who self-medicate with widely available over-the-counter medicines (e.g. paracetamol) or who take nothing

was associated with considerably elevated morbidity and mortality in young adults including many without recognized risks factors for severe disease.

As a result of these challenges, new surveillance systems were developed rapidly during the pandemic and further developed in the period following. The aim of these developments has been to obtain earlier and more accurate assessment of the severity of an impending influenza pandemic and to determine the full extent of infection and illness in the whole population.

Specific objectives of the surveillance developments since the 2009 pandemic have been to:

- provide more robust systems for identifying and collating information on all cases in the early part of a pandemic to provide a more accurate case count;
- establish systems to collect detailed information on early confirmed cases and their close contacts to provide information on clinical and transmission characteristics;
- develop methods to gather information rapidly from early outbreaks to assess impact in the population;
- establish surveillance of confirmed influenza cases in patients admitted to hospital, and those dying, in order to assess the occurrence of severe disease and the groups at increased risk of severe disease; and

- develop systems to assess the level of clinical illness occurring in the community and to monitor healthcare seeking behaviour (including people not seeking formal healthcare) which, combined with surveys using collection of serological samples, enable an estimation of the proportion of the population infected and how that varies in different age groups.

2.5 Systems Existing in the UK Including Links to International Systems

The UK has a range of surveillance systems in operation which aim to provide a rapid understanding of the epidemiology of influenza at all the levels of the seasonal influenza disease pyramid. In particular, surveillance aims to describe the onset, intensity and spread of influenza at each of these levels.

Community surveillance systems aim to provide an indication of influenza in the general population. In the UK, the information from two telephone help lines (NHS Direct in England and NHS-24 in Scotland) has been utilized in a syndromic surveillance system. Two particular indicators have been shown to be highly predictive of influenza activity (cold/flu calls and fever calls in children). This syndromic system is often one of the first to provide a signal of influenza transmission and thus the start of the influenza season.

Each of the UK countries has developed primary care sentinel surveillance schemes. In England, the Royal College of General Practitioners (RCGP) Birmingham Research Unit has recruited a network of more than 100 GPs across the country to create a sentinel surveillance scheme that has been in operation for more than four decades. The long-standing nature of the scheme means that GPs are well practised in accurate recording of the patient's illness. The weekly ILI consultation rate is one of the key indicators to demonstrate the onset of seasonal influenza activity, which age group is being mainly affected and when activity is peaking. In addition, the scheme has a linked virological swabbing system, whereby GPs take a respiratory swab from a sample of patients presenting with acute ILI. This provides information on the characteristics of the influenza viruses that are circulating in primary care during the season. Similar schemes operate in Wales, Northern Ireland and Scotland.

In recent years, all UK GPs have started to use patient information management systems. These have been developed by a number of software companies. This has provided opportunities for development of new surveillance systems with little or no reporting burden on the GP, as information is automatically extracted from the GP information system. The RCGP has now developed such a system. In addition, a primary care syndromic surveillance system has been developed based on one GP software supplier with extensive coverage across the UK (Health Protection Agency (HPA)/ Q-Surveillance). This syndromic surveillance system has a range of indicators including ILI. In addition to providing information about the onset, spread and peak of influenza activity, the extensive coverage means that indicators are available down to the local level.

Virological surveillance complements these epidemiological surveillance systems and provides an understanding of the characteristics of the circulating influenza viruses. For example, antigenic and genetic characterization of influenza isolates determines the predominant circulating strain in any season and how well it matches that season's vaccine strain. Sampling and testing of fatal cases identifies whether a particular strain is associated with severe cases; and the collation of information from samples of cases from primary and secondary care determines whether antiviral drug resistance is an emerging issue.

Each season, it is important to gain a rapid understanding of the population-level impact of influenza. The UK has a long-standing excess mortality monitoring system based upon weekly all-cause all-age death registrations from the Office for National Statistics (ONS). This is analysed each week, where the current week's number of death registrations are compared to what is expected from historical data (when influenza was not circulating). This provides an indication of whether there are more deaths than expected using a Serfling modelling approach. A newly implemented system has recently been established as part of an EU-funded project (Euro-MoMo) which provides some refinements with age- and region-specific excess mortality monitoring.

The HPA and the UK Departments of Health also monitor the roll-out of the annual seasonal influenza vaccine programme. Immunization is administered through primary care to those from 6 months to 64 years of age in specific clinical groups, all pregnant women, and those aged 65 years and over. In addition, a healthcare worker programme is delivered by the UK national health service (NHS) to health professionals who are in direct contact with patients. The influenza vaccine uptake in both programmes is monitored closely. Information on vaccine uptake in primary care overall, by age group and by risk group is collected each week during the influenza season at local, regional and national level through a bespoke system known as 'ImmForm'. This allows preemptive action to be taken if there is evidence that certain groups (e.g. by risk group or geographical area) have a lower than expected uptake. A similar reporting system through ImmForm operates to monitor uptake amongst healthcare workers during the season. An end-of-season report is produced for both systems which allows lessons to be learnt for the forthcoming season.

Influenza vaccine effectiveness (V_E) monitoring has been introduced in the UK in recent influenza seasons. This is based on the influenza surveillance systems in primary care. Patients who present with ILI in these schemes are swabbed and information is collected on the patients' vaccination status together with data on key confounding factors such as age and time of onset. A case–control study, using the swab-negative case–control approach, is used to estimate V_E and is being utilized increasingly internationally.

The information from these UK schemes is reported during the influenza season every week in the weekly HPA Influenza Report, which is sent to key stakeholders in the UK and internationally and is publically available on the HPA website. In addition, each week the HPA reports key influenza activity indicators to the European Centre for Disease Prevention and Control (ECDC) – these are summarized in the ECDC Weekly Influenza Surveillance Overview (WISO) and also shared with the World Health Organization (WHO) Regional Office for Europe. Finally at the end of the season, a full analysis is published in the HPA Annual Influenza Report.

2.6 Pandemic Surveillance: Additional Requirements and Overlap with Seasonal Surveillance

With the emergence of A(H1N1)pdm09 in spring 2009 (Fig. 2.2), it was necessary to gain a rapid understanding of the clinical, epidemiological and virological characteristics of this novel virus. Key epidemiological parameters included the severity of the infection (as measured by the case severity ratio such as the case fatality rate) and the infectiousness of the new virus (as measured by clinical attack rates). Table 2.2 summarizes the key elements of pandemic influenza surveillance.

This information in the UK was rapidly collected through a series of new and existing surveillance systems. The First Few Hundred system (FF100), one of the key new surveillance systems established, captured information on the first few hundred laboratory-confirmed cases of A(H1N1)pdm09 and their close contacts. Although the index cases were mainly imported from Mexico and North America, they provided important information on the clinical features of the novel virus infection, household secondary attack rates and evidence of effectiveness of antivirals in reducing disease severity and preventing household transmission. Furthermore, no deaths were observed among these initial FF100 cases suggesting the virus did not have the severity profile of the 1918 pandemic.

One of the key policy questions that arose in the UK during the summer of 2009 was when community transmission of this novel virus had become established. This required use of the existing syndromic surveillance systems – in particular Q-Surveillance and NHS Direct – which were able to provide detailed daily localized epidemiological information. This was important to detect early signs of possible community activity. The NHS Direct telephone surveillance scheme was further enhanced through the addition of self-swabbing of callers with acute respiratory symptoms. This, together with other surveillance sources, provided

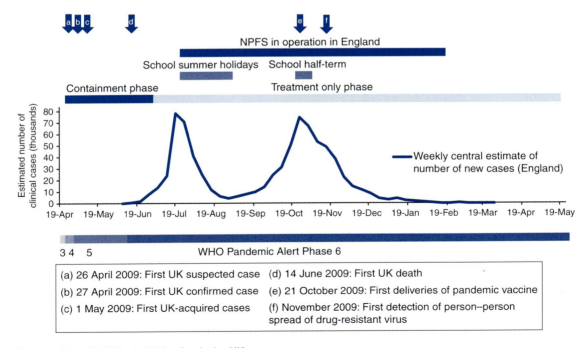

Fig. 2.2. The A(H1N1)pdm09 timeline in the UK.

Table 2.2. Key elements of pandemic influenza surveillance.

Early identification of new influenza virus activity in a country	• Intelligence about activity of new virus in neighbouring and other countries • Identification of clinically suspected cases (e.g. in travellers from affected countries) and testing for influenza virus infection • Characterization of influenza virus in those infected
Assessment of the characteristics of early cases of confirmed pandemic influenza in a country	• Collection of clinical, epidemiological and virological data on early cases and their contacts • Identification of early severe (hospitalized and/or fatal) cases and collection of risk factor information • Determination of overall severity of illness among those who have been infected
Monitoring of the spread and impact of the pandemic in the population	• Use of routine community and hospital-based surveillance systems to determine spread of influenza in different segments of the population (Fig. 2.1) • Identification of deaths due to confirmed influenza infection and excess mortality in the population
Monitoring of pandemic response measures	• Assessment of uptake, effectiveness and safety of pandemic influenza vaccines (when available) in the population groups targeted • Assessment of the effectiveness of antiviral drugs for both treatment and prophylaxis, and occurrence of side effects and drug resistance

key information to determine that community transmission had started in June 2009 in the West Midlands and London.

In autumn 2009, a telephone line service was implemented in England to distribute antivirals to people calling with influenza-like symptoms and to reduce pressure on primary care (Focus Box 9.1). This service (the National Pandemic Flu Service (NPFS)) also provided important surveillance data on the spread and intensity of the pandemic during the second wave in late 2009. As a result of the diversion of patients to the NPFS, rates of consultation for influenza in the GP sentinel surveillance schemes needed to be interpreted with considerable caution. A self-swabbing scheme (as implemented in NHS Direct) was undertaken through the NPFS to provide virological data to support information on the occurrence of pandemic influenza in the general population.

Two of the key questions that arose during the pandemic were what the population immunity to this novel virus was, and how many infections had occurred. This was vital information (together with the hospitalization and mortality data) to understand the severity of the pandemic – as measured by parameters such as case hospitalization and case fatality rates. The age-specific susceptibility profile and infection attack rate was measured through the implementation of population based sero-epidemiological surveys that measured the age-specific distribution of A(H1N1)pdm09 specific antibody before, during and after the pandemic waves.

Hospital surveillance of influenza has traditionally been a blind-spot in many national surveillance systems. During the 2009 pandemic many countries, including the UK, established reporting systems for hospitalized cases of pandemic influenza. These systems provided important information on the clinical presentation of more severe cases, underlying risk factors for severe disease, the complications observed and case management.

New individual reporting systems for fatal influenza cases were also implemented in many countries. These systems provided important epidemiological information on the people dying with confirmed pandemic influenza infection and, in particular, specific underlying risk factors for severe disease (Fig. 2.3). These surveillance systems provided valuable complementary information to the excess mortality monitoring systems that utilized routine vital statistics to estimate the impact of pandemic influenza at the population level.

One of the key information demands during the pandemic was to understand what the impact was on the healthcare system. Inherent delays in reporting of cases presented a challenge, which was overcome through employing 'nowcasting' approaches,

J.M. Watson and R.G. Pebody

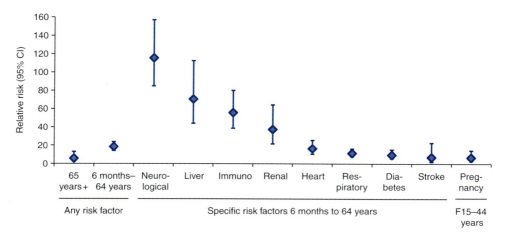

Fig. 2.3. Laboratory-confirmed A(H1N1)pdm09 deaths and risk factors for death, 2009/10, England. (Based on data available from http://www.eurosurveillance.org/images/dynamic/EE/V15N20/art19571.pdf.)

whereby reporting delays are adjusted for to estimate the current number of severe cases based on observed data. Real-time modelling attempts to forecast the future trends in the pandemic: a challenging endeavour particularly as many of the key parameters, e.g. population contact rates, will change in response to the pandemic (Chapter 13).

2.7 Influenza from Animals

Influenza in animals (including avian influenza), its surveillance in animal populations, and its impact in humans, are covered elsewhere (Chapter 4). In humans, most influenza is contracted as a result of human-to-human transmission. Influenza in humans may, however, result from contact with animals that are infected with influenza viruses. In most circumstances, these infections are with viruses that are adapted to survive and transmit in animals (particularly in birds and pigs, but many other animal species are susceptible to influenza viruses). The infection occurring in human contacts is often mild or inapparent but may, as in the case of avian influenza A(H5N1) infection, cause very severe illness in the human host.

Surveillance for such cases of illness in humans is important. In many instances, the infection will spread no further but identification and characterization of the animal virus that has caused illness in humans enables an understanding of the viruses with human disease potential, the animal groups in which they occur, their geographic spread and changes in their genetic constitution.

In some instances, however, such cases may indicate the occurrence of viruses with pandemic potential such as the swine influenza viruses in Mexico and the USA in early 2009 that went on to cause the 2009 pandemic.

Vigilance for these influenza viruses, through surveillance, requires a combination of clinical and public health awareness and microbiological investigation. The occurrence of severe influenza, particularly in otherwise fit children and adults, and the occurrence of unusual features in severe influenza, should alert clinicians to the possibility of novel influenza viruses and prompt investigation including enquiry about animal contact. Similarly, the occurrence of unusual outbreaks of respiratory or ILI, particularly out of the traditional influenza season, should prompt epidemiological and microbiological investigation including the potential role of transmission from animals.

2.8 Developments and 'Non-standard' Approaches to Influenza Surveillance

Following the 2009 pandemic, a number of priority areas for surveillance strengthening have been identified as part of a series of high-level reviews.

Firstly, the importance of having systems able to monitor the incidence of infection in the general population and to track changes in healthcare seeking behaviour. A series of approaches have been tried, or are planned, including use of web-based surveys of the population that follow recruits through the season (FluSurvey, http://flusurvey.org.uk/);

recruiting and following prospective household cohorts (FluWatch, http://www.fluwatch.co.uk/); and undertaking random digit dialling telephone surveys to question members of the general public.

Another key unknown is the number and distribution of people within the population who have been infected (for both pandemic and seasonal influenza). Serial population-based sero-prevalence surveys provide an opportunity to measure the age-specific infection attack rate in the general population. These data can be used to estimate the proportion of infections that are asymptomatic and to assess the case severity ratio for both seasonal and pandemic influenza.

The other area which has been recognized to require strengthening post-pandemic is severe disease surveillance. Many countries, including the UK, are now setting up hospital-based severe disease surveillance systems. Establishing routine reporting systems for seasonal influenza in hospital means that baselines and thresholds can be established. This will strengthen considerably the early assessment of the severity and impact of any future pandemic.

- Influenza surveillance provides an early warning of increasing disease activity in the population; it informs government, healthcare professionals and the wider community of the extent and severity of current and past activity, and provides information for treating, preventing and controlling influenza.
- Information from coordinated international epidemiological and virological surveillance provides information about the potential threat to populations and the probable effectiveness of control measures. Healthcare professionals use surveillance information for individual patient management, and to organize health services to cope with epidemic periods. Surveillance gives the wider public an understanding of how likely it is that they will become ill, and businesses use the information to plan for work absences due to illness. During epidemics, surveillance data are used to estimate the impact of influenza on the whole population as well as on specific subgroups and measure the effectiveness of interventions – in particular influenza vaccine.
- There are many sources of influenza surveillance data including: consultations in primary care, hospital admissions, virological data, death registrations, laboratory virology data, sickness absence data, calls to health help lines and Internet queries on influenza, and sales of over-the-counter cough, cold and flu remedies.
- The key elements of pandemic surveillance are early identification of novel influenza virus activity, assessment of the epidemiological and virological characteristics of early cases of confirmed pandemic influenza, monitoring spread and impact, assessing severity and monitoring of countermeasures.

Further Reading

Department of Health (2011) Seasonal Flu Plan. Winter 2011/12. Available at: http://www.dh.gov.uk/en/Publicationsandstatistics/Publications/Publications-PolicyAndGuidance/DH_127051 (accessed 1 April 2012).

Department of Health (2011) UK Influenza Pandemic Preparedness Strategy 2011. Available at: http://www.dh.gov.uk/en/Publicationsandstatistics/Publications/PublicationsPolicyAndGuidance/DH_130903 (accessed 1 April 2012).

Health Protection Agency (2010) Epidemiological report of pandemic (H1N1) 2009 in the UK. Available at: http://www.hpa.org.uk/Publications/Infectious Diseases/Influenza/1010EpidemiologicalreportofpandemicH1N1 2009inUK (accessed 1 April 2012).

Health Protection Agency (2010) Surveillance of influenza and other respiratory viruses in the UK: 2010–2011 report. Available at: http://www.hpa.org.uk/web/HPAweb&HPAwebStandard/HPAweb_C/1296687412376 (accessed 1 April 2012).

Nicoll, A., Ammon, A., Amato Gauci, A., Ciancio, B., Zucs, P., Devaux, I., Plata, F., Mazick, A., Mølbak, K., Asikainen, T. and Kramarz, P. (2010) Experience and lessons from surveillance and studies of the 2009 pandemic in Europe. *Public Health* 124(1), 14–23.

World Health Organization (2012) Influenza surveillance and monitoring. Available at: http://www.who.int/influenza/surveillance_monitoring/en/ (accessed 1 April 2012).

3 Basic Influenza Virology and Immunology

Lars R. Haaheim[1] and John S. Oxford[2]

[1]Formerly University of Bergen, Bergen, Norway, Retired; [2]Queen Mary College, and Retroscreen Virology Ltd, London, UK

- How do antibodies against haemagglutinin and neuraminidase differ in the way they interfere with the viral replication cycle?
- How do the adamantane and neuraminidase-inhibitor drugs work?
- What role does cell-mediated immunity play in combating influenza infection?
- What is immunological memory?

3.1 Introduction

Influenza virology and immunology are both immensely complex subjects. Nevertheless, the non-specialist requires a certain knowledge of each to understand the origins of past influenza pandemics (Chapter 5), the threat posed by novel avian influenza viruses (Chapter 4) and the role of possible response measures such as vaccines (Chapter 15) and antiviral drugs (Chapter 14). It is important to understand that all viruses are intracellular obligate parasites. This is just another way of saying that the virus cannot replicate unless it gets inside a host cell. Briefly, a virus is a piece of genetic material, protected by proteins and in some cases also by a membrane, on the look-out for a cell to invade so that it can re-programme it to make copies of itself.

3.2 The Virus

The exotic names given to influenza viruses denote their geographical origin. There are three types of influenza virus, namely A, B and C, the former of which can be divided into a range of subtypes (Table 3.1). They all belong to the *Orthomyxoviridae* family of viruses (from the Greek *myxo* meaning 'mucus'). However, this chapter will focus on influenza type A, which is the only type of influenza associated with pandemic influenza and which is able to infect birds, pigs, horses, humans and some

aquatic mammals. Type B is mainly a human pathogen and causes occasional winter outbreaks and epidemics, whereas type C gives only mild or unapparent disease and is considered to be one of the several hundred unrelated viruses which together cause the syndrome known as the 'common cold'.

The influenza virus is a medium-sized enveloped virus with a segmented negative sense RNA as its nucleic acid. This means that the viral RNA (vRNA) cannot function as a messenger RNA (mRNA) to translate the genetic information to viral proteins. It has first to be transcribed into a mirror image copy (the positive strand) by an enzyme carried in the virus (RNA transcriptase). The influenza genome has eight separate segments coding for ten different proteins, of which eight make up the structure of the virus itself and two remain inside the cell and help direct virus synthesis and inhibit host defences (Table 3.2, Fig. 3.1).

One can visualize spikes on the viral surface by electron microscopy, and these are the surface proteins haemagglutinin (HA) and neuraminidase (NA). Sometimes one can discern the internal components as bundles of segmented striped filaments. These are the nucleoproteins and P1, P2 and PA proteins surrounding the viral RNA (Figs 3.1 and 3.2).

Birds, particularly large migratory aquatic birds, form the natural animal reservoir for all known influenza A subtypes (Table 3.1). The current list of 17 HA subtypes and nine NA subtypes may well expand with time. This vast pool of influenza genes

Table 3.1. Distribution of influenza A subtypes among some animal species.[a,b]

HA subtype	Found in	NA subtype	Found in
H1	Humans, pigs, birds	N1	Humans, pigs, birds
H2	Humans, birds	N2	Humans, pigs, birds
H3	Humans, pigs, horses, birds	N3	Birds
H4	Birds	N4	Birds
H5	Birds	N5	Birds
H6	Birds	N6	Birds
H7	Horses, birds	N7	Horses, birds
H8	Birds	N8	Horses, birds
H9	Birds	N9	Birds
H10	Birds		
H11	Birds		
H12	Birds		
H13	Birds		
H14	Birds		
H15	Birds		
H16	Birds		
H17[c]	Bats		

[a]Avian A(H5), A(H7) and A(H9) strains have sporadically infected humans to give systemic disease.
[b]The commonly referred to 'bird flu' from South-east Asia and Egypt belongs to the A(H5N1) subtype.
[c]The neuraminidase (N) of the H17 influenza A virus found in little yellow-shouldered bats is also extraordinarily different from the nine neuraminidases of the other known influenza viruses.

Table 3.2. Gene segments of influenza A virus, in decreasing size order.

Segment	Name	Function
1 2 3	PB2 PB1(-F2) PA	Polymerase complex. Involved in viral replication. New drugs can block vital stages of RNA transcription
4	HA	Haemagglutinin, a glycosylated surface protein shaped like a Toblerone® chocolate bar. Initiates infection by binding to cellular receptors. Antigenically highly variable, 17 subtypes. Vaccines induce immunity to HA
5	NP	Nucleoprotein, encapsidates the RNA segments. The RNA–NP complex is designated RNP. Antigenically very stable but type specific (A, B, C)
6	NA	Neuraminidase, a glycosylated surface protein that looks like a mushroom. Enzymatically splits off newly made virus from the host cell. Antigenically variable, nine subtypes. Blocked by neuraminidase inhibitor drugs[a]
7	M1	Matrix protein. Located under the surface lipid layer and provides physical stability to the virus. Antigenically very stable, but type specific (A, B, C)
	M2	Ion channel, just a few copies in the viral membrane. Antigenically very stable. Physically blocked by the adamantane drugs[b]
8	NS1 NS2 (NEP)	Non-structural proteins: NS1 inhibits the host's interferon synthesis. NS2 helps exporting the viral RNA (complexed with NP) to the cytoplasm

[a]Oseltamivir, zanamivir, laninamivir and peramivir.
[b]Amantadine and rimantadine.

represents a potential contagious threat to humans, as there is today only some varying degree of pre-existing population immunity to the H1, H2 and H3 haemagglutinins and to the N1 and N2 neuraminidases and none to the remaining subtypes such as H5. On rare occasions such as 1918, 1957, 1968 and 2009, novel influenza viruses may cross the species barrier and infect people and then further mutate to allow person-to-person spread, hence becoming pandemic viruses (Chapter 4).

L.R. Haaheim and J.S. Oxford

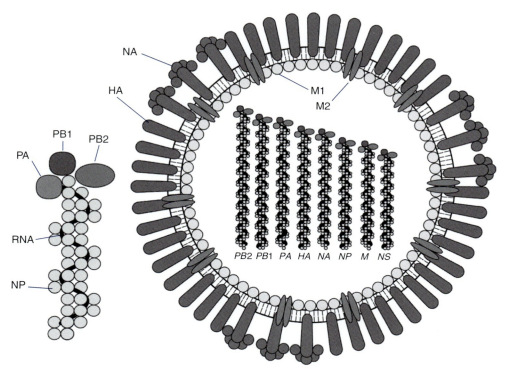

Fig. 3.1. The influenza virus. (Courtesy of Karl Albert Brokstad, University of Bergen.)

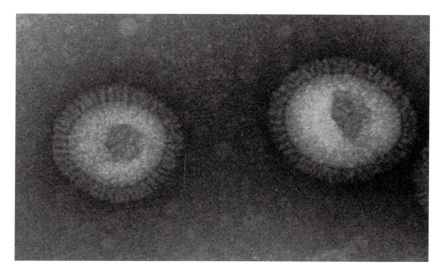

Fig. 3.2. Electron micrograph showing two virus particles, approximate diameter is 100–150 nm. The surface proteins haemagglutinin and neuraminidase can be seen as spikes, and the nucleoprotein can be seen through the damaged viral membrane (although the different shapes of the HA and NA spikes cannot be seen in this image). (Courtesy of WHO Collaborating Centre for Reference and Research on Influenza, Melbourne, Australia; micrograph prepared by Ross Hamilton.)

3.3 Nomenclature

The current system of nomenclature designates the type/animal host (if non-human)/geographical place of isolation/strain number/year of isolation (two or four digits) and, if type A, followed by a bracket with H and N subtype designation. This system was initially based on antigenic differences and similarities between viruses, mostly based on the haemagglutination-inhibition test (see later). In recent years, advances in rapid genetic characterization of the viruses by deep nucleotide sequencing has enabled the construction of phylogenetic (family) trees that offer a much more detailed picture of the relationship between viruses. It is in this context that the term 'clade' is used to cluster genetically related strains into smaller groups.

For example, the human isolate A/Anhui/1/2005 (H5N1) was from a zoonotic case in 2005 where a person in the Anhui province of China was infected with an avian A(H5N1) influenza strain.

Typically, the nomenclature of human influenza strains is most frequently encountered by the non-virologist in relation to the World Health Organization (WHO) recommendations for seasonal influenza vaccine antigen composition, e.g. for the northern hemisphere for 2010/11:

- A/California/7/2009 (H1N1);
- A/Perth/16/2009 (H3N2);
- B/Brisbane/60/2008.

A much-used classical human influenza virus strain, the so-called PR8 virus which we will meet again below, has the formulation A/Puerto Rico/8/34 (H1N1). The PR8 strain is a frequently used partner when high-yielding virus seed strains are prepared for vaccine purposes (Chapter 15). The 1918 Spanish flu virus is exemplified by the strain A/Brevig Mission/1/1918 (H1N1), the Asian flu pandemic in 1957 by A/Singapore/1/1957 (H2N2), the Hong Kong pandemic of 1968 by A/Hong Kong/1/1968 (H3N2) and the pandemic of 2009 by A/California/7/2009 (H1N1) – later abbreviated by WHO to 'A(H1N1)pdm09' and used extensively throughout this text.

3.4 Replication

Step 1: The virus hooks on to the host cells

The virus must first attach somewhere on the host cell surface, usually in the respiratory tree such as the nose, throat or trachea. This can be visualized much as a space rocket docking on to an orbiting space station. This is the first step in a 7-hour-long complicated process of making more identical copies of itself. Viruses often make use of existing host cell receptors that have beneficial primary purposes other than serving as attachment points for pathogens!

The haemagglutinin spikes on the influenza virus attach to human cells at an N-acetyl-neuraminic acid (sialic acid) residue attached to a sugar molecule (N-glucosamine); these are abundant on epithelial cells in the human airways. The precise chemical bond between the sialic acid and the sugar molecule determines whether human influenza viruses or avian influenza viruses can bind to the respiratory epithelial cells. Human influenza strains preferentially bind to so-called α-2,6 linked receptors, whereas avian virus strains prefer an α-2,3 linkage. This distinction is not absolute. In humans most of the receptors are of the α-2,6 type, but α-2,3 structures are also present in the lower airways.

Step 2: The virus enters the cell and starts replicating

The next and important step for the influenza virus is to enter the host cell. This is done by a process called receptor-mediated endocytosis where the cellular membrane invaginates and encloses the virus particle, thus creating an endosome (a vesicle) inside the cell. More than 25 human genes are involved in this process. The virus is still separated from the cell's machinery and will still need to enter the cytoplasm by a two-step process. First the endosome allows protons to enter, so creating an acid environment which produces a conformational change in the HA molecule, exposing a fusion motif of five hydrophobic amino acids which catalyse a fusion event with the endosomal membrane. Simultaneously, protons are also pumped inside the virus particle dissociating the M1 protein and RNA–nucleoprotein complex (RNP), thus allowing the latter to enter the cytoplasm and migrate to the host cell nucleus. The M2 protein in the viral membrane performs this ion-channel function. The older anti-influenza A drugs amantadine and rimantadine physically block the open channel in the M2 and thus abort the replication process.

The subsequent steps in the replication cycle are many and rather complicated, but after the viral nucleic acid has migrated to the nucleus two processes take place: one uses the virus's own enzymes to make copies of the incoming viral RNA to act as messenger RNA, whilst the other transcribes these positive strands to make negative strands for new viruses. The net effect is to take over the host cell and produce virus proteins and RNA. This is not a 'walkover victory' for the virus. It is clear now that as many as 5000 human cell genes of eight classes are involved in these replicative steps and the subsequent fight back that begins within hours of initial infection. Some of these host genes will become targets for a new generation of virus inhibitor drugs.

Step 3: New viruses are released and ready to infect new cells

When the newly made influenza proteins and genetic material have been produced over a period of 7h or so, the viral surface proteins (HA, NA and M2) assemble on the cellular membrane and the other viral proteins locate themselves just beneath. Through a budding process around 10,000 new virus-like spheres are ready to be set free. Each haemagglutinin spike on the viral surface is a trimer consisting of three identical HA proteins held together by non-covalent bonds. For an influenza virus particle to be infectious the HA monomers must undergo cleavage by a trypsin-like enzyme from the host organism. This is essential, as the influenza virus does not code for its own proteolytic enzymes. In most cases with human influenza strains, a very particular enzyme in the respiratory airways, either secreted by certain epithelial cells or from resident bacteria, is required. In contrast the HA molecule in highly pathogenic avian viruses is slightly modified, making it sensitive to cleavage by a wide range of intracellular host enzymes in a range of tissues, thus allowing viral spread to multiple organs. In birds influenza is pantropic causing disease in the brain, liver and intestine.

The final release of newly made virus is aided by the viral NA enzyme splitting off sialic acid, which holds the HA of the new virus bound to the host cell. The NA acts like a midwife facilitating the release (birth) of new viruses. This is the mechanism that is blocked by important anti-influenza drugs – the neuraminidase inhibitors (oseltamivir: Tamiflu®; zanamivir: Relenza®; peramivir: Rapiacta®/Peramiflu®; and laninamivir: Inavir® (Chapter 14)). These drugs do not stop the virus from infecting the cell, but rather interfere with the release of newly made viruses from cells already infected. Once the newly made viruses are detached they will attempt to infect a new cell. The cycle continues, leaving in its wake dead epithelial cells, until stopped by the host's immune system. But as long as new viruses are produced, the host may be contagious to others if the concentration of virus in sputum, nasal discharges or cough droplets is sufficient. Importantly, there are some indications that an infected person may be contagious for a short period (one day or so) before the onset of clinical illness, but this is not adequately known at the present time (Chapter 8).

3.5   The Immune Response

The innate response

The innate response is the first line of defence, sometimes called 'natural immunity'. Having negotiated the formidable physical barriers such as the mucus lining and cilia in the airways, the main defence players are a range of white blood cells such as the natural killer cells, macrophages and granulocytes in the invaded tissue, as well as a special set of cells called dendritic cells. The latter have long projections from their surfaces (dendrites) allowing efficient scanning and uptake of foreign material; they are particularly active in recognizing certain pre-defined structures from external sources (e.g. infectious agents). They and other cells like macrophages and granulocytes will take up, destroy and process the foreign material and initiate the adaptive immune system (see below). They are therefore also called antigen-presenting cells (APCs).

It is particularly important to know that the innate immune system has no ability to adapt to (i.e. learn from) its previous experience. The innate response is the first line of defence and is able to react immediately before the adaptive response is ready, which could take 3 to 4 days. Without the innate immune system, we would have serious problems combating even the most insignificant of infections. To give some idea of its power, a recent study using volunteers deliberately infected with influenza virus in a quarantine unit discovered many host genes in action. In individuals who were infected but showed no clinical signs, there was stronger evidence of cell-mediated innate immune responses as well as active antioxidant responses. These volunteers responded by inducing a leucocyte response with enhanced cellular protein biosynthesis. Over 5000 genes were detected whose temporal expression differed between asymptomatic and symptomatic volunteers.

The adaptive immune response

The humoral response

The B-lymphocytes have pre-formed antibodies on their surfaces acting like receptors for foreign material. After an intricate sequence of antigenic stimulation and re-shuffling of the gene complexes coding for the various parts of the immunoglobulin proteins, they end up as antibody-secreting cells, the final stage being the plasma cells secreting fine-tuned antibodies. These cells can be described as specialized factories secreting large quantities of antibodies that are tailor-made to the antigen in question. Not all antibodies are equally well adapted to bind to the antigen, they differ in affinity (binding strength) to the antigen. Some antibodies have the capacity to recognize a wider range of different antigenic structures; they are cross-reactive. Another arm of the B-cell activation process is to generate memory cells. They will home to and reside in the bone marrow. At random intervals perhaps extending a lifetime they will leave and be on the look-out for recognizable antigenic material and, if this is found, be reactivated to form new plasma cells. As a bonus, new and fresh memory cells will be generated as well. Additionally, it is also recognized that the bone marrow may harbour certain long-lived plasma cells continuously secreting antibodies for years, if not life.

The cellular response

Although antibodies are particularly good at neutralizing free virus and recognizing viral proteins on infected cells, an equally significant arm of the immune response is the generation of helper and cytotoxic T-lymphocytes. The latter will find and destroy host cells exhibiting foreign material (e.g. fragments of viral structures) on their surface. T-cells, like B-cells, have specialized receptors on their surface able to recognize foreign material. A requirement for binding to a foreign structure of an infected cell is that the fragment is presented, or literally 'served', on a class 1 major histocompatibility complex (MHC) on the surface of the host cell,

signalling that an infection is in progress. Most cells in our body have such MHC class 1 molecules. Therefore in an infected cell the scene is set for a killer cell attack.

The antibody response, on the other hand, requires the assistance of T-helper cells. For these cells to recognize foreign material, the fragments must be presented on a class 2 histocompatibility complex. The MHC class 2 complex is only found on APCs such as macrophages, B-lymphocytes and dendritic cells.

There is a large degree of cooperation between the initial innate response and the two subsequent arms of the adaptive response, sending chemical messages (lymphokines and cytokines) between them to refine and direct the appropriate immune reaction. Understandably this is at the sharp end of current research and surely will bring huge medical dividends when we wish to upgrade or even downgrade the immune response.

3.6   The Variable Virus

Antigenic drift

Most RNA viruses have no proof-reading mechanism, leading to errors and mistakes during the replication cycles involving multiple copying of the 13,000 nucleotides in the influenza virus genome. As much as 10% of the virus population can be mutants. The influenza viruses in particular seem to be promiscuous and to a large extent accept these 'mistakes' without compromising the required three-dimensional structures of the viral proteins, in particular the HA and NA on the viral surface. The mutational changes are mainly on the outer heads of both HA and NA where antibodies can interact with the proteins. These subtle changes are called 'antigenic drift' and are minor differences in the antigenic make-up that may manifest themselves as new field variants ('strains', 'isolates') that could cause winter outbreaks and epidemics. For the human population previous immunological experience against viruses of previous seasons will to some extent protect an individual, at least against serious infections. At the same time, herd immunity in the population is likely to facilitate the emergence of new and antigenically 'drifted' strains by exerting immune selection pressure on the existing viruses and therefore giving 'new' variants a selective advantage. Essentially the virus is Darwinian in its nature whereby only the fittest mutants survive and may become dominant. It is assumed that subclinical infections occur frequently. This should be considered as an advantage to humans, as it may allow boosting and refreshing of pre-existing cross-reactive immunological memory. Such minor antigenic changes in the HA and NA are seen almost every winter. It is therefore important for the efficacy of trivalent seasonal influenza vaccines that they keep abreast with the changing viruses in the field. This is the reason why the WHO updates its vaccine strain recommendation twice yearly, once per hemisphere, inserting new drift mutants with changed HA and NA.

Antigenic shift and reassortment

More fundamental changes than just a single amino acid change in HA are necessary for a pandemic to take place. This is designated 'antigenic shift' and is seen when a novel influenza A virus strain or subtype is introduced into the human population. 'Novel' in this context is to be understood as a virus that mankind has little or no pre-existing immunity against. It has to be admitted that this definition was challenged by the emergence in 2009 of A(H1N1)pmd09, where the older population had some immunity from previous encounters with influenza A(H1N1) in the 1940s and 1950s. So the definition of a novel pandemic virus is now recognized as being wider than simply new HA and NA and, rather, as having a novel combination of genes that can allow it to be virulent and spread widely. Obviously a significant proportion of the population, as in 2009, would have no antibody otherwise the new virus would be unable to find victims.

If a human or an animal is simultaneously infected by strains of different virus subtypes, this provides a chance for reassortment of the eight gene segments from each virus. In theory, this could generate 256 combinations of new viruses. During the process of genetic reassortment, the HA gene, and also occasionally the NA gene, can be replaced, with or without the introduction of one or more of the other six gene segments from the other virus. If one of the 'parent' viruses is of a subtype to which humans have no prior immunity such as avian influenza A(H5N1), we may face a situation where a 'new' virus with one or two novel surface antigens could be seeded into the human population and cause an explosive outbreak. Pigs, as noted below, are an important component in the evolution of pandemics. They have both types of receptors throughout their airways, allowing them to be infected by human and avian viruses simultaneously and are believed to be a likely mixing vessel to generate new gene constellations and, potentially, novel viruses. It is possible that the pandemics of 1957, 1968 and 2009 arose because pigs served as a mixing vessel for an avian and a circulating human strain to generate a new human pandemic virus (Fig. 3.3).

Experimentally, the reassortment mechanism has been used for a long time in the laboratory for generating 'seed' virus for vaccine production by doubly infecting embryonated eggs with a field strain and at the same time a well-characterized laboratory strain with good growth potential (typically the PR8 virus). From the resulting mixture of viruses it is possible to isolate a new virus with surface HA and NA antigens of the field strain and the other 'good growth' genes from the laboratory strain. Also, for live-attenuated influenza vaccines strains reassortment is performed between the HA and NA of a selected field isolate and a well-characterized attenuated laboratory master strain, to generate an attenuated or weakened vaccine virus with surface proteins from the field isolate (Chapter 15).

Whether reassortment is a frequent occurrence in the field is uncertain. As an example, two human strains of the A(H3N2) and A(H1N1) subtypes must have reassorted around 2001 to generate an A(H1N2) subtype, which now is detected widely across the globe. The 2009 pandemic virus took 18 years to achieve take-off in humans, quickly mixing genes in South-east Asia. However, it should be noted that other cases of human–human reassortment may have occurred previously but may have gone undetected, not being able to spread widely. In fact, the A(H1N2) subtype was detected sporadically in humans in China in 1988 but did not seem to spread further.

Reverse genetics

Over the last decade or so a new biotechnology process called 'reverse genetics' has been developed for negative stranded RNA viruses that can be used quickly, and in a controlled fashion, to generate vaccine 'seed' viruses, e.g. from highly pathogenic avian viruses, which can be safely used in the laboratory or production unit. Briefly, the two genes coding for the HA and NA surface antigens from the avian virus (e.g. A(H5N1)) are added to the

Pandemic mode 1

Pigs have receptors for both avian and human influenza viruses. A doubly infected pig may select a reassortant (mixed gene) virus that could infect and spread among people (as probably happened in 1957, 1968 and 2009).

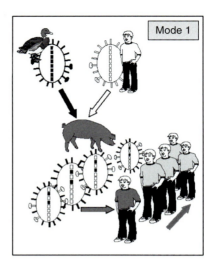

Pandemic mode 2

Humans could be infected with an avian influenza virus. Through accumulations of point mutations (genetic adaptation) a variant could arise that could spread efficiently from person to person. This mode was probably the mechanism behind the appearance of the A(H1N1) Spanish influenza in 1918.

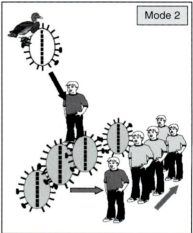

Pandemic mode 3

Humans could simultaneously be infected with both avian human influenza viruses. A reassortant virus could be selected that could infect and spread among people. So far not a documented pandemic mode, but human–human reassortants have been documented (e.g. A(H3N2) + A(H1N1) to give A(H1N2)).

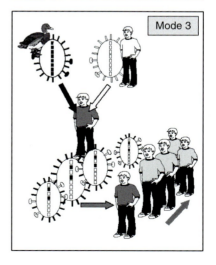

Fig. 3.3. Pandemic modes.

L.R. Haaheim and J.S. Oxford

remaining six genes from a laboratory strain, such as the PR8 virus, to create a replication-competent virus in an approved cell line. Point mutations, for example in the HA gene, are engineered at certain critical sites at the same time, such as the critical hydrophobic sequence by manipulating a DNA transcript of the RNA, creating a 'designer virus' suitable and safe for vaccine use. This procedure can speed up the modification of a dangerous field virus into a licensed vaccine and safe strain within a few weeks. The method is used widely in research laboratories to alter other influenza virus genes and correlate such mutations with changes in virulence. Thus, we try to answer the biggest question of all: what is the genetic nature of a fully virulent flu virus?

Consequences for the immune response

The various types of cross-immunity should be remembered as being extremely useful for the immune response, allowing earlier immunity to assist in neutralizing virus and clearing virus-infected cells (see 'Antigenic drift', above). If cross-reactions are within the same subtype, it is occasionally called *homosubtypic* immunity, recalling that the genetic and immunological ('antigenic') differences between the HAs from various subtypes (Tables 3.1 and 3.2) are quite substantial. We benefit frequently from cross-immunity between strains within a subtype. Previous winters' exposure to strains within the same subtype will to some extent modify and lessen the clinical impact once infected with the same or a closely related strain, thereby reducing the viral load in the airways and infectiousness to others in terms of virus quantity and duration of shedding. Thus, widespread cross-reactive herd immunity in the population will lessen the epidemiological impact in the community.

Heterosubtypic immunity is defined as immunity that transcends the subtype barrier. Such immunity could be mediated by unrecognized and yet similar antigenic stretches in the HA molecules of the two subtypes, possibly in shared regions deep in the stem of the HA, or, more likely, by immunity mediated by the more antigenically stable M1, M2e and NP proteins which are the main targets for the cytotoxic cellular immune response. This wide immunity is at the centre of development of 'universal influenza vaccines' that transcend the sub-types and would be effective year on year.

Should these vaccines become reality, then vaccine could be stockpiled to mitigate the first wave of any pandemic, regardless of subtype.

Measuring the antibody response

It was observed in the 1940s that influenza viruses had the capacity to bind to red blood cells from birds, humans and animals and make them clump together. This phenomenon is used in a laboratory test called the haemagglutination test to quantify amounts of virus or as a haemagglutination-inhibition test (HI test) to measure blocking antibodies. In simple terms, one takes serial dilutions of a serum from a patient who has had an influenza infection or been vaccinated, and mixes these with a standardized quantity of virus, letting the virus and serum dilutions react for a certain time; into this mixture is then added a suspension of red blood cells (e.g. from turkey or horse). If the serum sample contains antibodies able to bind to the virus particles, its ability to clump the red cells (haemagglutinate) will be blocked and can be measured as a titre, i.e. how many times a serum sample can be diluted before the virus can again haemagglutinate the red cells.

This test is still considered to be the 'gold standard' procedure for measuring the efficacy of influenza vaccines. A certain percentage of the vaccinees must have obtained a particular pre-defined level of HI antibodies in order for the vaccine to be licensed. A similar general procedure is used for virus-neutralization tests. Here one uses live virus, and the red cells are replaced by a laboratory cell line (frequently dog or monkey kidney cells). Again, non-neutralized virus will infect the cells and presence of newly made virus can be measured and the neutralizing antibody titre calculated.

The HI titre is used by the vaccine licensing authorities as a surrogate marker or correlate of immunity. The neutralizing antibodies are more relevant as they are measuring biological activity using live virus. However, the latter test is a complicated and time-consuming procedure and is therefore mostly used in research settings. Also, the particular requirement for some avian HA subtypes that prefer the α-2,3 cellular receptor has been a particular challenge for both the HI test and the neutralization assays. The 'magic HI titre' of ≥1:40 is generally accepted to indicate immunity.

3.7   Pandemics

As we have seen (and is covered in more detail in Chapter 4), occasional transfer of avian influenza to humans and even human-to-human transmission have happened many times, but in order to cause a pandemic there are more conditions to be met. In brief, the novel virus must be able to cause disease and spread efficiently from person to person (Fig. 3.4).

The most devastating pandemic in recent history was the Spanish influenza of 1918. At that time the precise infectious agent was unknown and Pfeiffer's bacillus was the suspect. It took another 13 years before influenza virus was identified and could be grown experimentally in a laboratory, namely in 1931 (isolates from pigs) and 1933 (isolates from humans). Several decades later and based on subsequent studies of sera from elderly people who had survived the pandemic, it was concluded that the 1918 virus must have belonged to the subtype A(H1N1). The specific genetic make-up of the virus was unknown until recently when lung material from a 1918 victim found in a permafrost grave in Alaska, as well as archived formalin-preserved sections of lung tissue from young soldiers who died of Spanish flu, were analysed and the complete nucleotide sequence of the HA gene was constructed from RNA fragments. This was an impressive and highly significant scientific breakthrough.

The 1918 virus most likely had an avian origin and reassortment in a non-human host such as a pig may not have been involved in the process. In other words, an avian virus may have adapted directly to humans without the need for reassortment in an intermediate host such as the pig. These features make the virological origins of the 1918 pandemic very different from those in 1957, 1968 and 2009 and may in turn explain the quantum difference in severity between 1918 on the one hand and the subsequent pandemics on the other. This finding defines the serious pandemic threat currently posed by A(H5N1) 'bird flu' (Chapters 4 and 5).

Knowledge of the genetic sequence of the 1918 flu has allowed the virus itself to be reconstructed by 'reverse genetics' and tested in animal models. These studies confirmed what the doctors in the field had seen, namely that the virus was highly lethal, replicated rapidly in the patients' lungs and also more rarely spread to other organs such as the brain. Figure 3.3 shows the various modes of generating pandemic strains. What specific properties of the virus made the 1918 virus so lethal to people? We still do not know. The scientific consensus is, however, that influenza virus pathogenicity is a multigenetic phenomenon involving many or perhaps all of the ten virus-coded proteins.

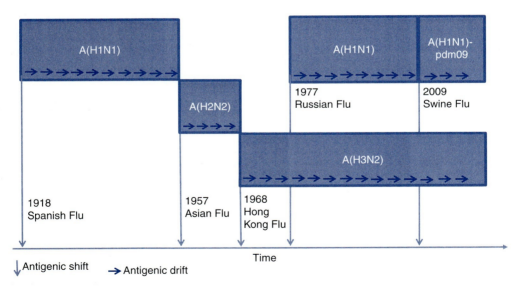

Fig. 3.4. Influenza A antigenic shifts and pandemics in the 20th century and early 2000s (note 1977 is not generally regarded as a pandemic).

L.R. Haaheim and J.S. Oxford

3.8 The First Pandemic of the 21st Century and Future Threats

The isolation of a swine influenza A(H1N1) virus from two children who had not been in contact with pigs in Orange County, California in April 2009 and the coincident outbreak of cases of community-acquired pneumonia in Mexico City alerted WHO to a virus sufficiently novel to be designated the first pandemic of the 21st century. Virologically we have learnt that the virus had evolved over 18 years, probably in the subtropical equatorial regions of South-east Asia, recognized by molecular geneticists as the incubator of new influenza viruses. It was a multiple reassortant having genes from avian, human and pig influenza viruses. Immunologically we learnt that immunity to a pandemic can be long lived: only a minuscule number of persons over 60 years of age were infected by the 2009 virus because of residual immunity from 50 or so years before.

The 2009 pandemic has been viewed as a dress rehearsal for possibly more virulent influenza A viruses to come. Sporadic cases of avian influenza A(H5N1) in humans, since 1997 frequently associated with an extremely high mortality, have raised the global awareness that a pandemic threat remains from this virus. But antigenic novelty per se is not enough; the virus must also undergo other changes so it can spread easily from one person to the next. Only very few cases of human-to-human spread of A(H5N1) have so far been documented. Some say this is sheer luck, and that the virus will eventually become pandemic, whereas others say that it shows that the A(H5N1) virus, having sporadically infected people since 1997, will never acquire such a capacity. We do not know, of course, but it is prudent to prepare for such a situation.

- Antibodies against HA will bind to the virus and prevent it binding to the host cell, i.e. the antibodies are neutralizing. Antibodies to NA will typically block or reduce the release of newly made virus particles from an already infected cell, i.e. these antibodies will dampen the replication of virus and thus reduce the clinical symptoms and how contagious an infected individual is to others.
- The adamantane drugs interfere with the proton transport function of the M2 protein (the ion channel) located in the viral membrane (hence are known as M2-channel blockers). As a consequence, genetic material from the virus cannot enter the cell and take advantage of the cellular machinery, and the replication cycle comes to a halt. The neuraminidase-inhibitor drugs block the function of the viral NA enzyme and thus inhibit the release of newly made virus particles from an already infected cell.
- Cell-mediated immunity will not block the initial infection but rather destroy virus-infected cells. This is a reciprocal cooperation between the humoral (antibody-generating) and cellular (cytotoxic T-cells) arms of the immune response, thus strengthening and modifying both.
- Immunological memory is the adaptive immunity's ability to respond quicker and stronger to a subsequent stimulation of foreign material. This foreign material can be a new infection with an identical or related virus. When we are 'primed', i.e. have experienced an earlier encounter with an infectious agent or a vaccine, the memory so generated will help us combat a subsequent infection much more efficiently.

Dedication

Lars Haaheim (1945–2011), my friend and virology colleague for 40 years, died in an accident on a fishing boat off the Norwegian Coast which he loved so much, in the summer of 2011. The Editors asked me to update this chapter and I am both honoured and sad to do this. Professor Haaheim performed precise laboratory work for his entire career, in Bergen, NIMR London, CDC in Atlanta and CSL in Australia. He analysed antigenic drift in virus HA and NA using monoclonal antibodies and human polyclonal sera. He bridged a gap between the laboratory and clinic and developed precise technologies to count antibody-producing plasma cells. Teaching was central to Lars's career and his student book is ever popular with its cartoon viruses and characters.

JSO

Further Reading

Collier, L., Kellam, P. and Oxford, J.S. (2011) *Human Virology*, 4th edn. Oxford University Press, Oxford, UK.

Eckert, D.M. and Kay, M.S. (2010) Stalking influenza. *Proceedings of the National Academy of Sciences USA* 107, 13563–13564.

Fraser, C., Donnelly, C.A., Cauchemez, S., Hanage, W.P., Van Kerkhove, M.D., Hollingsworth, T.D., Griffin, J., Baggaley, R.F., Jenkins, H.E., Lyons, E.J., Jombart, T., Hinsley, W.R., Grassly, N.C., Balloux, F., Ghani, A.C., Ferguson, N.M., Rambaut, A., Pybus, O.G., Lopez-Gatell, H., Alpuche-Aranda, C.M., Chapela, I.B., Zavala, E.P., Guevara, D.M., Checchi, F., Garcia, E., Hugonnet, S. and Roth, C., WHO Rapid Pandemic Assessment Collaboration (2009) Pandemic potential of a strain of influenza A (H1N1): early findings. *Science* 324, 1557–1561.

Huang, Y., Zaas, A.K., Rao, A., Dobigeon, N., Woolf, P.J., Veldman, T., Øien, N.C., McClain, M.T., Varkey, J.B., Nicholson, B., Carin, L., Kingsmore, S., Woods, C.W., Ginsburg, G.S. and Hero, A.O. III (2011) Temporal dynamics of host molecular responses differentiate symptomatic and asymptomatic influenza A infection. *PLoS Genetics* 7, e1002234.

Itoh, Y., Shinya, K., Kiso, M., Watanabe, T., Sakoda, Y., Hatta, M., Muramoto, Y., Tamura, D., Sakai-Tagawa, Y., Noda, T., Sakabe, S., Imai, M., Hatta, Y., Watanabe, S., Li, C., Yamada, S., Fujii, K., Murakami, S., Imai, H., Kakugawa, S., Ito, M., Takano, R., Iwatsuki-Horimoto, K., Shimojima, M., Horimoto, T., Goto, H., Takahashi, K., Makino, A., Ishigaki, H., Nakayama, M., Okamatsu, M., Takahashi, K., Warshauer, D., Shult, P.A., Saito, R., Suzuki, H., Furuta, Y., Yamashita, M., Mitamura, K., Nakano, K., Nakamura, M., Brockman-Schneider, R., Mitamura, H., Yamazaki, M., Sugaya, N., Suresh, M., Ozawa, M., Neumann, G., Gern, J., Kida, H., Ogasawara, K. and Kawaoka, Y. (2009) *In vitro* and *in vivo* characterization of new swine origin H1N1 influenza viruses. *Nature* 460, 1021–1025.

National Institute of Allergy and Infectious Diseases (continuously updated) Understanding the Immune System. Available at: http://www.niaid.nih.gov/topics/immuneSystem/Pages/default.aspx (accessed 30 March 2012).

Taubenberger, J.K., Hultin, J.V. and Morens, D.M. (2007) Discovery and characterization of the 1918 pandemic influenza virus in historical context. *Antiviral Therapy* 12(4 Pt B), 581–591.

University of South Carolina, School of Medicine (continuously updated) *Microbiology and Immunology On-line.* Available at: http://pathmicro.med.sc.edu/book/immunol-sta.htm (accessed 30 March 2012).

4 Influenza in Birds and Mammals

LESLIE A. REPERANT AND ALBERT D.M.E. OSTERHAUS

Erasmus Medical Centre, Rotterdam, The Netherlands

- What is the significance of influenza in wild and domestic birds?
- Why is influenza in the pig considered important?
- Is avian influenza A(H5N1) still a threat to humans?
- What are the major risk factors for zoonotic influenza transmission?

4.1 Introduction

Influenza A viruses may cause influenza in birds and other animal species. Wild waterbirds (such as ducks, geese, gulls and waders) are the natural reservoirs of avian influenza A viruses. In these species, the viruses typically cause an intestinal tract infection without apparent clinical signs. A wide diversity of avian influenza A viruses circulate in wild waterbirds. They are the ancestral precursors of all influenza A viruses found in other animal species, including humans. Wild waterbirds may transmit avian influenza viruses to poultry, resulting in sporadic disease outbreaks. A few subtypes have become established in poultry and circulate independently of wild birds. In poultry, avian influenza viruses typically cause a respiratory tract infection associated with mild clinical signs. For this reason, they are called low pathogenic avian influenza viruses (LPAIV). In terrestrial poultry, such as chickens and turkeys, LPAIV of the A(H5) and A(H7) subtypes can evolve into highly pathogenic avian influenza viruses (HPAIV). The latter cause systemic infection of multiple organs and rapid and high mortality in these species. HPAIV are not usually transmitted from poultry back to wild birds but HPAIV A(H5N1) that emerged and has circulated since 1997 is an exception. Avian influenza viruses of wild or domestic birds may be transmitted to mammals. They can cause isolated cases of infection, self-limiting outbreaks or large sustained epidemics.

The latter are eventually followed by the establishment and continued circulation of adapted variants in these new host species; this has occurred in domestic pigs, horses and dogs, in which a few subtypes are circulating independently of birds, but not so far in humans.

Although it has been suggested that the virus that triggered the 1918 pandemic influenza may have been transmitted directly from birds to humans, it is likely that the influenza viruses that caused past pandemics were transmitted from birds to an intermediary mammalian host, such as the pig, before further transmission to humans. In mammals, influenza A viruses typically cause a respiratory tract infection associated with mild to severe clinical signs. HPAIV A(H5N1) are unusual because they can cause a severe systemic infection in many mammalian species. Cross-species transmission of influenza viruses among mammals also occurs. Equine influenza virus of the A(H3N8) subtype has been transmitted from horses to domestic dogs, in which it has adapted and become established. Swine influenza viruses are occasionally transmitted from pigs to humans. They typically result in either isolated cases of infection or limited outbreaks. A remarkable exception is the A(H1N1)pdm09 virus at the origin of the 2009 influenza pandemic. This chapter discusses influenza viruses in birds and other animal species, their reported transmission to humans and their role in the onset of influenza pandemics.

4.2 Avian Influenza in Wild and Domestic Birds

Avian influenza in wild birds

Avian influenza viruses of virtually all possible combinations of the 17 haemagglutinins (HA) and nine neuraminidases (NA) described to date have been isolated in wild waterbirds. A high rate of influenza virus reassortment is described in wild waterbirds, resulting in the circulation of a wide diversity of subtypes and lineages. Their prevalence is typically highest in juvenile birds in autumn when they congregate prior to migration. They may be maintained from year to year by continuous yet possibly low circulation in wild birds during the other seasons, or may persist in aquatic environmental reservoirs. Avian influenza viruses can remain infectious in water for up to several months under adequate environmental conditions, such as low temperatures and low salinity levels. In wild waterbirds, they are transmitted via the faecal–oral route of transmission, which is likely facilitated by aquatic habitats, and cause intestinal tract infection without apparent lesions or clinical signs. Infection typically lasts 1 week, yet may be prolonged for up to several weeks, and results in massive shedding of the virus in birds' faeces.

HPAIV A(H5N1) are unusual because they can infect and cause a wide range of diseases in wild waterbirds. These viruses emerged in terrestrial poultry in South-east Asia in 1997 (see below) and spilled back in wild bird populations. They can infect a wide range of bird species, including non-aquatic birds and migratory species. They may cause subclinical infection, severe infection of the respiratory tract or fatal systemic infection in multiple organs in different species. Clinical signs of infection in birds include prostration, laboured breathing and neurological signs. These are associated with lesions of necrosis, inflammation and occasionally haemorrhage in the respiratory tract and potentially other organs (notably the brain). There is increasing evidence that wild migratory birds have played a role in the geographical spread of HPAIV A(H5N1) from South-east Asia to the Middle East, Europe and Africa. It remains unknown whether these viruses continue to circulate in wild birds independently of poultry or have reassorted with other avian influenza viruses in wild birds.

Avian influenza in domestic birds

Wild birds may transmit avian influenza viruses to poultry, resulting in sporadic outbreaks of usually mild disease. These cross-species transmission events may follow shared use of habitats or of drinking water between wild and domestic birds. A few subtypes of LPAIV have become established in aquatic and terrestrial poultry, and circulate in these species endemically, independently of wild birds. These include LPAIV of the A(H9N2) subtype circulating in a wide range of poultry species in South-east Asia; they have also caused infection in humans (see below). In poultry, LPAIV typically cause infection of the respiratory tract associated with mild clinical signs. These include nasal discharge and drop in egg production, in association with lesions of necrosis and inflammation in the respiratory tract. LPAIV in poultry may not easily be detected because the clinical signs associated with infection are usually mild and non-specific.

LPAIV of the A(H5) and A(H7) subtypes may evolve towards HPAIV in terrestrial poultry, such as chickens and turkeys. While the HA cleavage site of LPAIV has a single arginine residue, that of HPAIV has multiple basic amino acids that correlate with their virulence in poultry. Highly pathogenic avian influenza (HPAI) has been described in poultry since the late 19th century, yet the causative agent of the disease was identified in the 1950s. Since then, outbreaks of HPAIV infection in poultry appear to have been on the rise (Fig. 4.1a). Thirteen of the 24 HPAI outbreaks reported since 1959 have occurred since 1990. This may be due to the massive increase in domestic or industrially kept poultry populations worldwide over the past few decades. HPAIV cause severe systemic infection and massive infection of cells lining blood vessels, typically resulting in multi-organ and coagulation failure, and death within 2 days. Infected birds may show no clinical signs at the time of death, and/or present with internal haemorrhages and cyanosis, with oedema and discoloration of the legs, comb and wattle. These are associated with severe lesions of necrosis, inflammation and haemorrhage in multiple organs. Sudden onset of disease, explosive spread of the infection and rapid death characterize HPAIV infection in terrestrial poultry. Such viruses can emerge and circulate in these species probably because they are kept at high densities facilitating transmission despite high morbidity and mortality.

Containment and stamping out strategies (see below) are usually efficient measures for eradicating HPAIV from poultry populations. HPAIV A(H5N1) are an exception in that they emerged in 1997 in poultry in South-east Asia and have continued to circulate endemically in these species to date. It has been suggested that domestic ducks, which may become subclinically infected, play an essential role in maintaining these viruses. Also, trade, live markets and the absence of rigorous biosecurity measures in many parts of the world likely facilitate their continued circulation in industrially kept poultry. The circulation of these viruses in a range of poultry species has probably led to high reassortment rates and the evolution of various co-circulating lineages. Viruses from at least one of these lineages have spilled back from poultry to wild bird populations and spread geographically from South-east Asia to the Middle East, Europe and Africa in 2005. To date, HPAIV A(H5N1) circulates endemically in poultry in South-east Asia, the Middle East and West Africa.

4.3 Influenza in Other Animal Species

Avian influenza viruses and adapted variants have been isolated in animal species other than birds, in association with sporadic cases of infection, self-limiting outbreaks or sustained epidemics and continued circulation. The latter includes swine influenza viruses in pigs, equine influenza viruses in horses and canine influenza viruses in dogs. Self-limiting outbreaks of influenza virus infection have been reported in farmed American mink and harbour seals. Sporadic cases of infection with influenza virus have been described in whales and striped skunks. In addition, serological evidence of influenza A virus infection has occasionally been obtained in racoons, cattle, sheep, goat, yak, water buffalo, reindeer, fallow deer, as well as in some species of reptiles and amphibians. In mammals, influenza A viruses typically are transmitted via the respiratory route and cause a respiratory tract infection. This is characterized by lesions of necrosis and inflammation along the respiratory tract. Associated clinical signs include fever, weight loss, nasal and ocular discharge, coughing and laboured breathing. Morbidity is high but mortality is usually low in species where adapted variants have become established, unless bacterial infection complicates the course of infection. Mortality may be high upon cross-species transmission of influenza viruses. HPAIV A(H5N1) are unusual in that they can cause systemic infection and disease in a wide range of animal species.

Influenza in pigs

Wild or domestic birds may transmit avian influenza viruses to domestic pigs, resulting in isolated cases of infection, limited outbreaks, or the establishment and continued circulation of adapted variants (i.e. swine influenza viruses). There is also serological evidence of infection of wild boars with swine influenza viruses. These cross-species transmission events may follow shared use of habitats or of drinking water between birds and pigs, or introduction by humans via contaminated utensils or vehicles. A growing number of swine influenza virus subtypes are reported in pig populations worldwide, where they cause epidemics or circulate endemically (Fig. 4.1b). This increase in the diversity of swine influenza viruses may be associated with the massive increase in swine populations worldwide. Domestic pigs are susceptible to infection with avian and human influenza A viruses. In particular, some lineages of swine influenza viruses of the A(H1N1) and A(H3N2) subtypes have their origin in human influenza viruses. Cross-species transmission of the latest pandemic influenza virus A(H1N1)pdm09 has also been reported in pigs. These cross-species transmission events likely followed close contacts between humans and domestic pigs, during rearing and care giving. Frequent reassortment between swine, human and avian influenza viruses contributes to the large diversity of lineages found in pigs. Domestic pigs often are referred to as 'mixing vessels' because the cells along their respiratory tract harbour cellular receptors for both avian and human influenza viruses. This explains their susceptibility to both types of virus. Swine thus may facilitate the generation of influenza viruses that may productively infect humans, in particular through reassortment. Pigs may also transmit swine influenza viruses back to poultry.

HPAIV A(H5N1) have rarely been reported in domestic pigs. Upon experimental infection, they develop mild disease associated with low levels of viral replication and spread.

Influenza in equids

Wild or domestic birds may transmit avian influenza viruses to domestic horses. These cross-species transmission events may follow shared use of habitats or of drinking water between birds and horses, or introduction by humans via contaminated utensils or vehicles. They have resulted in the establishment of two lineages of equine influenza viruses of the A(H7N7) and A(H3N8) subtypes. Equine influenza A(H7N7) virus was last isolated in Egypt in 1989, but may circulate at low levels in some regions of the world, while the equine influenza

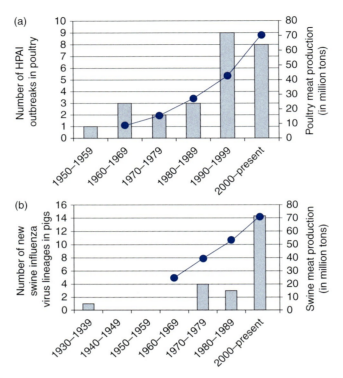

Fig. 4.1. (a) Number of highly pathogenic avian influenza outbreaks in poultry since the 1950s (light blue bars) and trends in global poultry meat production (dark blue points). (b) Number of new swine influenza virus lineages detected in pig populations since 1930 (light blue bars) and trends in global swine meat production (dark blue points).

A(H3N8) virus is endemic in the global horse population. In 1989, the transmission of avian influenza viruses of the A(H3N8) subtype in horses in China resulted in severe disease, associated with 20% mortality. These viruses were genetically and antigenically distinct from previously identified equine influenza viruses. The absence of cross-immunity between equine and avian influenza A(H3N8) viruses may have contributed to the high morbidity and mortality that was observed.

HPAIV A(H5N1) have not been reported in horses. However, they have been reported in donkeys in Egypt. Infected animals presented with mild respiratory tract disease.

Influenza in carnivores

Wild birds have transmitted LPAIV of the A(H10N4) subtype to farmed American mink in Sweden, resulting in epidemics of respiratory tract disease with 3% mortality. These cross-species transmission events likely followed the contamination of

mink food by foraging birds. Recently, transmission of swine influenza viruses of the A(H3N2) and A(H1N2) subtypes was reported in farmed American mink in North America. In one instance, consumption of infected swine meat was considered a potential route of transmission.

Historically, canids and felids were considered poor hosts for influenza A viruses. Serologic surveys of domestic dogs and cats detected only scarce and limited exposure to human influenza viruses, and natural infection with avian influenza viruses had not been reported in these species. The situation appears to be changing. Equine influenza viruses of the A(H3N8) subtype were recently transmitted to domestic dogs, possibly via the consumption of infected horse meat. These viruses now circulate in dog populations independently of horses and cause canine influenza. Infections are characterized by moderate to severe and potentially fatal respiratory tract disease. Since 2007, domestic dogs have been repeatedly reported infected with avian influenza viruses of the A(H3N2) subtype in

South Korea. These viruses cause severe respiratory tract disease with high mortality. They are transmitted among dogs, suggesting that they may circulate in this species independently of birds and become established in dog populations in this region of the world. Lastly, accounts of cross-species transmission of A(H1N1)pdm09 are increasingly reported from humans to domestic carnivores, including dogs, cats and ferrets. In addition, A(H1N1)pdm09 infection has also been reported in captive cheetahs, as well as in free-living striped skunks present on a mink farm potentially experiencing an outbreak. It is likely that other species will be shown susceptible to infection with this virus in the future. In carnivores, A(H1N1)pdm09 causes moderate to severe and potentially fatal respiratory tract disease. These cross-transmission events likely followed close contacts between infected humans and pet or captive animals.

Since 2004, HPAIV A(H5N1) have reportedly infected a wide range of carnivore species, including tigers, leopards, Owston's palm civets, domestic cats, domestic dogs, raccoon dogs, racoons, red foxes, stone martens and American mink. In these species, HPAIV A(H5N1) typically result in fatal systemic infection of multiple organs, including the respiratory tract, brain and liver, associated with severe respiratory and neurological clinical signs. HPAIV A(H5N1) were most likely transmitted to carnivores following consumption of infected birds.

Influenza viruses in other species

Wild or domestic birds may transmit avian influenza viruses to other species that share habitats or drinking water with birds, or that consume birds. Occasional outbreaks of avian influenza virus infection have been reported in harbour seals. These viruses may result in severe respiratory tract disease associated with high mortality. The epidemics typically fade out and it seems that these viruses have not become established in harbour seal populations. These repeated cross-species transmission events may have followed shared use of habitats, notably at haul-out sites, or consumption of infected wild birds by harbour seals. Avian influenza viruses have occasionally been isolated from whales, yet have not been associated with outbreaks of respiratory disease in these species.

Recently a novel influenza A virus containing a novel haemagglutinin, H17, has been discovered in Guatemala in little yellow-shouldered bats, a frugivorous bat species, widely distributed across Central and South America. The neuraminidase is also markedly different, suggesting ancient divergence from other influenza A viruses. At present there is no evidence of further interspecies transmission of this H17 virus but reassortment with existing influenza A subtypes is a possibility.

4.4 Zoonotic Influenza in Humans

Risk factors for zoonotic influenza virus transmission

Influenza A viruses infecting animal species have sporadically been transmitted to humans. To date, these include avian influenza virus from domestic or wild birds, avian influenza virus from infected harbour seals, and swine influenza viruses from pigs. There are no reports of human infection with equine or canine influenza viruses. Cross-species transmission of influenza viruses to humans generally follows close contacts between humans and infected animals or their products. There is limited serological evidence of avian influenza virus infection in waterbird hunters and in individuals involved in wild bird banding activities. De-feathering of infected wild swans resulted in two clusters of human infection with HPAIV A(H5N1) and six human deaths in Azerbaijan. Likewise, transmission of avian influenza virus from harbour seals to humans occurred upon necropsy of infected animals. Bathing or swimming in waters contaminated with HPAIV A(H5N1) may have led to human infection via inhalation or ingestion of water or self-inoculation of the upper respiratory tract or conjunctiva. Nevertheless, most human cases of infection with zoonotic influenza viruses result from close direct contact with poultry, swine or their products, and occupational exposure to poultry or swine greatly increases the risk of zoonotic influenza virus infection. At-risk activities include care giving, slaughtering, de-feathering, butchering and preparation of meat for consumption, leading to inhalation of infectious fomites, droplets or aerosols, or self-inoculation of the upper respiratory tract or conjunctiva. Nevertheless given the intensive contact between humans and their livestock worldwide, cross-species transmission of zoonotic influenza virus to humans remains a relatively rare event. However, these events appeared to be more frequent over the past decade possibly due to increased awareness, or in association with more frequent outbreaks in poultry and increasing virus diversity in pigs (Fig. 4.2).

Avian influenza in humans

Avian influenza viruses of the A(H5), A(H7 and A(H9) subtypes have caused human infection. Most sources of infection were poultry, with the exception of one strain of LPAIV A(H7N7), which was transmitted from infected harbour seals upon necropsy. Both LPAIV and HPAIV have been transmitted from poultry to humans; the virus pathotype in birds does not correlate with pathogenicity in humans. Reports of avian influenza virus infection in humans have increased in the past decades. Since 1999, LPAIV A(H9N2) infections have repeatedly been reported in humans in South-east Asia, mostly in children. They typically caused mild influenza-like illness. It is possible that a number of LPAIV A(H9N2) infections in humans went undetected. LPAIV and HPAIV of the A(H7) subtype have been reported in humans in North America and Europe mainly since the mid-1990s, in association with outbreaks in poultry. They typically caused mild ocular or respiratory tract infection, or both. Clinical symptoms include conjunctivitis and influenza-like symptoms, such as fever, nasal discharge and coughing. The disease typically recedes within 1 to 2 weeks. However, there has been one reported fatal case of severe respiratory tract infection with HPAIV A(H7N7), during a massive outbreak in poultry in 2003 in the Netherlands. The patient presented with pneumonia and acute respiratory distress syndrome and died of the infection. There were over 80 other human cases with mild respiratory or conjunctivitis symptoms.

HPAIV A(H5N1) first caused human infection in 1997 in Hong Kong, resulting in the death of six out of 18 infected individuals. Although drastic control measures and culling of the entire poultry population in Hong Kong contributed to the eradication of the disease, viruses of the HPAIV A(H5N1) subtype re-emerged in China and Vietnam in 2003. Since then, over 600 cases (as at 10 August 2012) have been confirmed in South-east Asia, the Middle East and Africa, of which approximately 54% were fatal. Most cases have been in children or young adults, and were epidemiologically linked to close

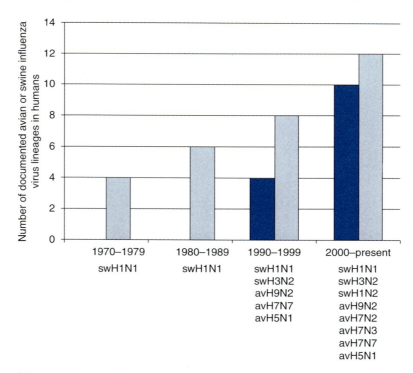

Fig. 4.2. Number of documented avian (dark blue bars) and swine influenza virus subtypes and lineages (light blue bars) in humans since 1970. Subtypes are indicated for each decade; sw: swine influenza virus; av: avian influenza virus.

L.A. Reperant and A.D.M.E. Osterhaus

contact with infected poultry or poultry products. Serological surveys revealed low levels of antibodies against HPAIV A(H5N1) in the healthy population. Like other avian influenza viruses, HPAIV A(H5N1) are not efficiently transmitted among humans. HPAIV A(H5N1) typically causes severe and fatal respiratory tract disease, characterized by pneumonia and acute respiratory distress syndrome. Other unconventional symptoms may also occur, such as gastrointestinal and neurological symptoms, in association with the presence of the virus in organs beyond the respiratory tract.

Several determinants of virulence have been identified in avian influenza viruses that have caused severe and fatal infection in humans, i.e. HPAIV A(H7N7) and HPAIV A(H5N1). They abundantly attach to and infect cells located in the deeper regions of the respiratory tract, mainly in the bronchioles and alveoli. Infection of these cells results in severe damage and strong immune responses at the origin of pneumonia. Several genetic and phenotypic characteristics of these viruses also account for their increased pathogenicity. In particular, their polymerase proteins, which control virus replication, are efficient in mammalian cells, allowing for high levels of viral production. HPAIV A(H5N1) also are resistant to certain components of the innate immune responses. They can evade these host defences, possibly resulting in massive production of cytokines in the deep lungs, which contributes to the severity of the disease.

Swine influenza in humans

Swine influenza viruses of the A(H1N1), A(H1N2) and A(H3N2) subtypes have caused human infection. Reports of swine influenza virus infection in humans have increased in the past decade. Most cases were found in children and young adults, and epidemiologically linked to close contacts with infected pigs or swine products. They typically caused influenza-like illness, with fever, nasal discharge, coughing and laboured breathing, sometimes requiring hospitalization. Six out of 48 reported cases died of severe pneumonia following infection with swine influenza viruses of the A(H1N1) subtype. Swine influenza viruses typically have a tropism for cells all along the respiratory tract, and can infect cells deep in the lungs, which may result in severe disease.

Most cases of swine influenza virus infection in humans have resulted from sporadic cross-species transmission; these viruses typically are not efficiently transmitted among humans. However, in 1976, a strain of swine influenza virus of the classical A(H1N1) lineage efficiently spread and infected 230 military personnel in a basic combat training camp at Fort Dix in New Jersey (USA). It was a transmissible virus, yet, for unknown reasons, did not further spread in the human population. In April 2009, another strain of swine influenza virus of the A(H1N1) subtype spread and infected humans in Mexico and subsequently worldwide, resulting in the first influenza pandemic of this century.

4.5 Origins of Pandemic Influenza

Pandemic influenza is caused by novel influenza A viruses introduced from animal reservoirs into the human population with no or little pre-existing immunity. All recorded influenza pandemics were caused by influenza viruses of avian or swine origin. The 1918 pandemic was caused by influenza virus of the A(H1N1) subtype. It resulted in an estimated 30 to 50 million deaths and infection of about one-third of the global population during the successive pandemic waves (Chapter 5). The animal origin of this virus is unclear, yet all gene sequences were found related to those of avian influenza viruses. Further analyses suggest that the different gene segments had circulated for several years in humans or swine before the onset of the pandemic, and that the pandemic virus likely resulted from reassortment events between avian and mammalian influenza viruses. Likewise, the 1957 pandemic was caused by influenza virus of the A(H2N2) subtype that was a reassortant between previously circulating A(H1N1) strains and an avian influenza A(H2N2) virus. The 1968 pandemic was caused by influenza virus of the A(H3N2) subtype that was a reassortant between previously circulating A(H2N2) strains and an avian influenza A(H3N2) virus. The host species in which these reassortment events occurred is not known.

The 2009 pandemic was caused by an influenza virus of swine origin, now termed A(H1N1)pdm09, resulting from reassortment events between swine, avian and human influenza virus strains. A set of genes originated from a triple-reassortant swine influenza virus circulating in North American pig populations. The source triple-reassortant itself comprised genes derived from avian, human A(H3N2) and classical swine A(H1N1) lineages. Another set of genes originated from the Eurasian avian-like swine influenza virus A(H1N1) lineage. Although the first human cases were detected in Mexico, the geographical origin of this swine influenza virus, bearing genes of both North American and Eurasian lineages of swine influenza viruses, is unknown.

Pandemic influenza viruses productively infect humans and are efficiently transmitted between individuals. The genetic and phenotypic changes that zoonotic influenza viruses must undergo to become efficiently transmitted in human populations are not fully understood. Productive infection of the upper regions of the respiratory tract is thought to be required for efficient transmission to occur. Any zoonotic influenza virus may pose a pandemic threat for humans. LPAIV A(H9N2) and some strains of avian influenza viruses of the A(H7) subtype can bind receptors typically used by human influenza viruses, and infect cells in the upper regions of the respiratory tract. As a result, the risk that these avian influenza viruses could initiate a pandemic is high. Similarly, swine influenza viruses can bind receptors used by both avian and human influenza viruses, and may readily reassort, making them strong candidates for triggering a future pandemic. HPAIV A(H5N1) typically do not productively infect the upper regions of the respiratory tract in humans, but their high pathogenicity in humans is unprecedented. The acquisition of human-to-human transmissibility by these viruses would have the most dreadful consequences.

4.6 Managing the Human and Public Health Consequences of Zoonotic Influenza

Surveillance of avian and swine influenza viruses in animal populations

The diversity of influenza viruses in bird and other animal populations represents a large pool of source viruses for future influenza pandemics in humans. The number of influenza outbreaks in domestic birds and the number of influenza virus subtypes and lineages in domestic pigs appear to be on the rise, and call for improved and extended influenza surveillance in animals. Phylogenetic studies of the reassortant virus at the origin of the 2009 influenza pandemic revealed a period gap in swine influenza surveillance, during which ancestral viruses had not been sampled. The circulation and evolution of precursor viruses with pandemic potential went undetected in pig populations for about a decade. Systemic surveillance of animal influenza viruses that may develop a transmissible phenotype in mammals is urgently needed to

improve our grasp of their epidemiological and evolutionary dynamics and assess relative risks of pandemic threats. In addition the improved surveillance of animal influenza viruses may further lead to the generation of a comprehensive bank of virus seeds for the development of future vaccines.

Management of outbreaks caused by avian influenza viruses of the A(H5) and A(H7) subtypes in poultry

Because of the significant impact of avian influenza on the poultry production sector, it is recommended to apply management and control measures to reduce the risk of transmission of LPAIV from wild bird to poultry populations by improving biosecurity. HPAIV outbreaks have devastating economic consequences and pose public health risks, thus the management of outbreaks caused by avian influenza viruses of the A(H5) and A(H7) subtypes in poultry is required. Detection of LPAIV and HPAIV of the A(H5) and A(H7) subtypes in poultry must be reported to the OIE (Organisation Mondiale de la Santé Animal–World Animal Health Organization) and appropriate measures should be taken according to national and international regulations. Following detection of HPAIV in wild or domestic birds, control and monitoring areas, where restrictions on movements of live poultry and poultry products apply, and where hunting of wild birds is banned, must be established. Domestic poultry must be kept indoors to prevent contact with and transmission to wild birds. Stamping out measures with large-scale culling of infected or potentially infected birds in the affected area, the adequate disposal of carcasses and disinfection of premises and equipment are necessary measures for the control and elimination of HPAIV in farms. Where culling is impractical or ineffective, e.g. in zoos with endangered or precious bird species or collections, or in backyards with small poultry flocks, alternative strategies like vaccination may be considered. However, this should only be implemented in compliance with national and international legislation. While vaccination may reduce the spread of influenza virus in bird populations, vaccinated birds may not be completely protected against infection, and may shed virus for prolonged periods without showing clinical signs if infected. Furthermore, vaccination has been claimed to lead to increased antigenic drift of avian influenza viruses in poultry populations, and therefore should be combined with regular updating of the vaccine composition to ensure its antigenic match with circulating strains. Upon an HPAIV outbreak in poultry, prevention and diagnosis of human infection are considered among the highest priorities today, which should go hand in glove with management of the outbreak in the birds. Protective measures when handling infected birds include the wearing of protective clothing and respiratory protective equipment, as well as disinfection of tools, utensils and vehicles. The implementation of prophylactic anti-viral treatment should be considered for people at increased risk of infection (including sustained exposure during incident response), and specific monitoring of virological, serological and clinical parameters performed. A treatment protocol should be available for people who become infected in spite of all precautionary measures. For avian influenza viruses of the A(H5N1) subtype, human vaccines have recently become available.

- Wild birds are the natural reservoir for influenza A viruses; avian influenza viruses encompassing virtually all possible combinations of the 17 HA and nine NA described to date have been isolated in wild aquatic birds. The degree of virus reassortment constantly taking place is immense. Coupled with favourable conditions for virus persistence in the immediate aquatic environment, conditions for the emergence of novel influenza viruses are almost ideal.
- Domestic (farmed) pigs appear susceptible to both avian and human influenza A viruses. As such they provide a 'mixing vessel' for viruses and facilitate cross-species transmission of viruses from birds to pigs to humans, and vice versa.
- Highly pathogenic avian influenza A(H5N1) viruses have become endemic in domestic poultry in parts of South-east Asia, the Middle East and West Africa. Because of their known ability to cause severe disease in humans, they pose a sustained pandemic threat to humans. The occurrence of the last pandemic due to A(H1N1)pdm09 has neither reduced nor increased the threat posed by A(H5N1) and other avian influenza viruses, notably those of the A(H7) and A(H9) subtypes.
- Major risk factors for zoonotic transmission of influenza to humans include: slaughtering, de-feathering, butchering and preparation of meat for consumption. There is serological evidence that occupational groups involved in close contact with poultry, swine and their raw products are at increased risk from cross-species transmission.

Further Reading

Belser, J.A., Bridges, C.B., Katz, J.M. and Tumpey, T.M. (2009) Past, present, and possible future human infection with influenza virus A subtype H7. *Emerging Infectious Diseases* 15, 859–865.

de Jong, J.C., Claas, E.C., Osterhaus, A.D., Webster, R.G. and Lim, W.L. (1997) A pandemic warning? *Nature* 389, 554.

Kreijtz, J.H., Osterhaus, A.D. and Rimmelzwaan, G.F. (2009) Vaccination strategies and vaccine formulations for epidemic and pandemic influenza control. *Human Vaccines* 5, 126–135.

Kuiken, T., Leighton, F.A., Fouchier, R.A., LeDuc, J.W., Peiris, J.S., Schudel, A., Stöhr, K. and Osterhaus, A.D. (2005) Public health. Pathogen surveillance in animals. *Science* 309, 1680–1681.

Myers, K.P., Olsen, C.W. and Gray, G.C. (2007) Cases of swine influenza in humans: a review of the literature. *Clinical Infectious Diseases* 44, 1084–1088.

Olsen, B., Munster, V.J., Wallensten, A., Waldenstrom, J., Osterhaus, A.D. and Fouchier, R.A. (2006) Global patterns of influenza a virus in wild birds. *Science* 312, 384–388.

Peiris, J.S., de Jong, M.D. and Guan, Y. (2007) Avian influenza virus (H5N1): a threat to human health. *Clinical Microbiology Reviews* 20, 243–267.

Peiris, M. (2009) Avian influenza viruses in humans. *Revue Scientifique et Technique de l'Office International des Epizooties* 28, 161–174.

Reperant, L.A., Rimmelzwaan, G.F. and Kuiken, T. (2009) Avian influenza viruses in mammals. *Revue Scientifique et Technique de l'Office International des Epizooties* 28, 137–159.

Shinde, V., Bridges, C.B., Uyeki, T.M., Shu, B., Balish, A., Xu, X., Lindstrom, S., Gubareva, L.V., Deyde, V., Garten, R.J., Harris, M., Gerber, S., Vagasky, S., Smith, F., Pascoe, N., Martin, K., Duffcy, D., Ritger, K., Conover, C., Quinlisk, P., Klimov, A., Bresee, J.S. and Finelli, L. (2009) Triple-reassortant swine influenza A (H1) in humans in the United States, 2005–2009. *New England Journal of Medicine* 360, 2616–2625.

5 History and Epidemiological Features of Pandemic Influenza

ARNOLD S. MONTO[1] AND CHLOE SELLWOOD[2]

[1]University of Michigan, Ann Arbor, Michigan, USA;
[2]NHS London, London, UK

- Which influenza A subtypes caused the most recent pandemics?
- When was the worst pandemic?
- Have pandemics occurred in earlier history?
- What can we predict about the epidemiology of the next pandemic?

5.1 Introduction

Influenza pandemics are rare but recurrent events that occur when a new type A influenza virus emerges that is able to spread easily from person to person and against which most or all of the population has little or no immunity. The result is an outbreak of influenza encompassing the whole world, lasting 12–18 months, with distinct waves of infection. In order for a pandemic to occur, four key criteria must be met:

1. A new influenza A virus substantially different (antigenically) from the circulating pre-pandemic strains must emerge or evolve and circulate in humans.
2. There must be little or no pre-existing immunity to the new subtype in major segments of the global population.
3. The new virus must cause significant clinical illness.
4. The virus must be able to spread efficiently from person to person and as a result spread globally.

This chapter discusses the pandemics prior to 2009; the 2009 pandemic is dealt with in Chapters 6 and 7.

5.2 Pandemics before the 20th Century

Influenza pandemics have probably occurred periodically throughout human history. Some are better documented than others, and there is considerable virological uncertainty prior to 1889; some so-called pandemics before this date may or may not have been due to other respiratory pathogens, but we have no way of telling. The three influenza pandemics of the 20th century (in 1918, 1957 and 1968, see later) are well reported and it is from studying these that much of our pandemic preparedness was based. However our thinking about future pandemics has been modified by experience from the 2009 pandemic.

Pandemics prior to 1918 are less well documented, but still help to inform thinking and are of interest. The first influenza pandemic may have been identified in 412 BC by Hippocrates, and accounts of 'epidemic fever' – rapidly spreading outbreaks of febrile respiratory illness which caused a high excess mortality – appear in texts dating back to the 1500s. As indicated in Table 5.1, they seem to have originated in Russia or Asia, and generally had high attack rates with variable mortality impact.

From 1889 until the 20th century

1889–1892: A(H2)? Asiatic or Russian flu

This is the first documented truly global pandemic, due to the availability of records from across the world and the development of health statistics. The pandemic started in Russia in May 1889. Two further waves of infection occurred in 1891 and 1892. Population attack rates ranged between 25% and 50%, and the number of deaths worldwide was estimated at 300,000. The majority of deaths were in the elderly, and in the later waves.

This is the earliest pandemic for which there is serological evidence about the origin of the virus. Studies on serum samples collected before 1957 from people who were alive in 1889 showed A(H2) antibodies, indicating exposure to an A(H2) virus prior to the 1957 A(H2N2) pandemic. When A(H2N2) caused the Asian flu pandemic in 1957, the majority of the population had not had previous contact with the virus and so were susceptible; but such prior exposure to an A(H2) virus at the end of the 1800s may explain the relatively lower attack rate seen in older people.

1898–1901: A(H3)?

The origin of this pandemic is unknown, and even its status as a pandemic has been questioned. There were large influenza epidemics in Europe, Australia, North America, Alaska, the Pacific Islands and Japan throughout 1898–1900. These outbreaks were mainly mild, and the main interest is based on serological studies trying to document the emergence of influenza A subtypes. As in the previous example, sera collected before 1968 from people alive in 1898 indicate the presence of antibodies to influenza A(H3) and there was lower mortality during the 1968 pandemic in people aged over 75 years, compared to those aged 65 to 74 years.

These two events indicate possible previous circulation of virus subtypes responsible for later pandemics, however exact details of the circulation of A(H2) and A(H3) have been debated.

5.3 Influenza Pandemics of the 20th Century

The three 20th century pandemics (Fig. 5.1) provide much of our knowledge upon which recent

Table 5.1. Influenza pandemics since 1580.

Year	Areas reported affected	Origin	Subtype
1580	Europe, N. America, Africa	Asia	Unknown
1729–1733	Europe, Americas, Russia	Russia	Unknown
1781/82	Europe, N. America, Russia, China, India	Russia/China	Unknown
1830–1833	Europe, N. America, Russia, China, India	China	Unknown
1889–1892	Global	Russia	A(H2)?
1898–1900	Europe, Americas, Australia	Unknown	A(H3)?
1918–1920	Global	USA/China	A(H1N1)
1957/58	Global	China	A(H2N2)
1968/69	Global	China	A(H3N2)
2009/10	Global	Mexico	A(H1N1)

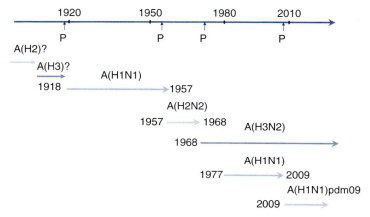

Fig. 5.1. Major influenza A subtypes.

influenza pandemic preparedness is based. Despite some similarities in these events, they differed with respect to the causative virus, epidemiology and disease severity, and number of separate waves, highlighting the need for flexible planning.

1918: A(H1N1) Spanish influenza

The 1918 pandemic coincided with the end of World War I and in a few months was responsible for more deaths than occurred during the preceding 4 years of war. It was caused by an unusually severe strain of influenza A(H1N1). Genetic sequencing of the virus now suggests this was of avian origin, and that it subsequently adapted to the human host over a period of time prior to the pandemic starting. It is difficult to reconstruct the early phases of the pandemic in the absence of virologic confirmation, and the true origin of the virus remains unclear (it is commonly referred to as 'Spanish flu' due to the amount of media reporting and attention the pandemic received in Spain). However, it appeared to spread across Europe in the spring of 1918 and rapidly reached epidemic proportions in France and other countries. The close confines of military accommodation and the mass deployment and movement of troops involved in World War I may have accelerated initial spread through Europe in early 1918 (Fig. 5.2). Many countries experienced a second (1918/19) severe wave and a third wave (1919/20) of infection.

In the UK, the 'Spanish flu' pandemic occurred in three distinct waves. The first was in spring 1918 and was relatively small. The number of cases reduced over the summer, before a resurgence and second peak in autumn/early winter 1918, although this time the pattern of infection was very different and the disease much more severe. There was a noticeable increase in both clinical attack rate and mortality among adults aged 20–40 years compared to the usual age groups affected by influenza. This became a defining characteristic of the 1918 pandemic. The third wave occurred in early 1919 and was of moderate intensity. Fear of a future 1918-like situation affecting young adults of working age is one particular concern in relation to a future pandemic, although a repeat of such a dramatic shift in age-specific mortality cannot be ruled in or out.

In the majority of cases, the 1918 virus caused the typical clinical symptoms of influenza: acute onset, chills, fever and muscle aches. However, bacterial pneumonia appears to have occurred as a complication in 15–20% of cases, and in a much smaller proportion of cases (around 1–2%) the disease was associated with rapid progression. An intense, haemorrhagic, rapidly fatal, viral pneumonitis was the unique feature of this pandemic, considered by contemporary observers not to have been seen before. Most data sources point to an average case fatality rate of 2.0–2.5%, but in young adults this was around 4%.

The reason for the enhanced severity in the second wave which disproportionately affected young adults is unknown. It is possible that the virus adapted to its new human host between waves and that the response to infection in young adults involved an intense cytokine response as described with human A(H5N1) infections (Chapter 4). The reconstitution of the 1918 virus from archived specimens has allowed study of its virulence in laboratory animals; there are as yet no definitive answers although suggestions are emerging.

While accurate figures are unavailable for many parts of the world, the pandemic is estimated to have infected 50% of the world's population; half of whom may have suffered a clinically apparent infection. Total excess mortality due to the pandemic is estimated to be at least 40 million although this figure may be quite inaccurate. In the USA more than 600,000 excess deaths occurred and in England and Wales civilian excess deaths numbered about 200,000.

The literature regarding deaths from many developing countries is unclear; however there is a general suggestion that case fatality rates were exceptionally high. In some populations, such as Alaska, southern Africa, India and Western Samoa extremely high deaths rates were recorded, and in some cases entire villages were reportedly wiped out. In Australia and New Zealand indigenous populations were generally more severely affected than non-native people. New Zealand Maoris were seven times more likely to die from influenza than New Zealanders of European origin, with a population death rate in excess of 4%, while indigenous Australians suffered a population mortality rate of almost 50% in some communities.

1957: A(H2N2) Asian influenza

The Asian flu pandemic was a global human outbreak of an adapted avian influenza A(H2N2) that started in Yunnan Province, China in February 1957. Virological evidence indicates that the pandemic virus was a reassorted human and avian influenza

A.S. Monto and C. Sellwood

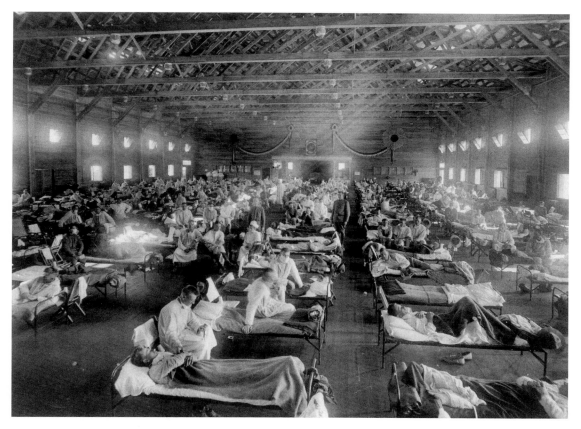

Fig. 5.2. Emergency hospital during the 1918 pandemic, Camp Funston, Kansas. (Courtesy of the National Museum of Health and Medicine, Armed Forces Institute of Pathology (NCP 1603).)

virus, a process that might have occurred in an intermediate mammalian host, such as the pig. A polymerase gene, the haemagglutinin and neuraminidase genes were most likely of avian origin, while the others were derived from the previously circulating A(H1N1) virus. Quarantine measures were largely ineffective (at best merely postponing transmission by a few weeks) and the pandemic spread across the world reaching most countries.

The majority of spread was along shipping lanes and infections were seen in ports before spreading to urban and rural areas. However there were two clear overland routes. The first was across Russia to Scandinavia and Eastern Europe as occurred in earlier events, while the second was less conventional. Almost 2000 people attended a large international conference in Iowa, USA. Many of the participants were from countries already experiencing epidemics of influenza, and consequently

200 cases occurred during the conference, while many people took the infection home when the event ended.

In Europe the infection was seeded from June 1957 and outbreaks started in September when the autumn school term started. Consequently the illness was first seen in schoolchildren, followed by preschool children and finally adults. Cases in the UK were concentrated in school-aged children and those crowded together, however the biggest impact on mortality was in the elderly. It was thought that the pandemic was over at the end of 1957; however a second wave of infection occurred early in 1958 and affected Europe, North America, Russia and Japan. The two waves were of similar severity in some countries, while in others the second wave caused higher rates of illness and increased fatalities.

The clinical presentation of A(H2N2) in humans was rather more typical than in 1918, although high mortality was noted in pregnant women and there was a preponderance of secondary bacterial pneumonia due to *Staphylococcus aureus*. The majority of deaths were in the very young or very old and were due to secondary bacterial pneumonia. The apparent attack rate in older people was lower than in other groups, and may have been due to previous exposure to an influenza A(H2) virus in earlier life (Focus Box 5.1). The case fatality rate was less than 0.5% and over 1 million people died globally. Although significant, such a level of mortality is several magnitudes lower than occurred in 1918.

1968: A(H3N2) Hong Kong influenza

The 1968 influenza pandemic also started in China through a process of antigenic reassortment where avian and human viruses recombined; the haemagglutinin and polymerase-coding gene came from the avian virus but the neuraminidase remained the same as in the 1957 pandemic virus. The outbreak spread to Hong Kong in July 1968 causing 500,000 cases in just 2 weeks (hence the name 'Hong Kong flu'), from where global spread was rapid. However, this was not as dramatic as in 1957, perhaps because of the timing of the arrival of the virus in many countries or the fact that the neuraminidase remained unchanged. For example, Japan experienced a spring wave of infections in 1968, but infections did not peak until January 1969.

The virus reached the USA in September 1968, reportedly via US Marines returning to California from Vietnam. By December 1968, the illness was widespread across the USA; morbidity was as high as in the 1957 pandemic, although mortality was lower. In Europe the disease was diagnosed from September 1968 onwards; symptoms were mild, excess deaths negligible and demands on medical services were not excessive. However, the number of fatalities due to influenza sharply increased in Europe one year later, during the 1969/70 winter season. The virus eventually reached South America and South Africa in mid-1969.

The majority of deaths in North America occurred during the first wave, while in Europe and Asia the majority occurred in the second wave. In many countries, local epidemics of the virus were small, causing mild symptoms, and the relative protection of the elderly suggests previous exposure to a similar virus. This theory is supported by serological evidence from samples collected prior

to the pandemic from older people who were alive during the 1898–1901 pandemic.

The virus was rapidly identified as influenza A(H3N2) and vaccine manufacture began within 2 months of the virus being isolated. However, only 20 million doses were ready by the time the epidemic peaked in the USA and, because of late deployment, this did not prove a useful control measure.

The 1968 pandemic is estimated to have caused between 1 and 3 million fatalities globally; an overall case fatality rate of less than 0.5%. In the UK there were over 30,000 excess deaths attributed to the pandemic, which was no larger than reported for subsequent severe seasonal epidemics in 1976 and 1989.

5.4 Seasonality

Whilst interpandemic influenza is recognized to be seasonal in the temperate zones, it was traditionally believed that pandemic influenza could start at any time of year. For example, the first wave of the 1918 pandemic in the northern hemisphere began in spring 1918. In the northern hemisphere, this wave was relatively small in size and mild in its clinical impact compared to the second wave in autumn 1918. It has since been suggested that the reason for the increased size and severity of the second wave might relate in part to seasonality. Likewise, the 'Hong Kong' pandemic virus of 1968 did not reach the UK until January 1969 and the main pandemic wave in the UK was observed in the following winter. In contrast the virus entered the USA in early autumn 1968 and produced a large pandemic wave in the 1968/69 winter. If this phenomenon is based on seasonality, then if a future pandemic were to begin in the spring, more time might be gained for preparation and vaccine production, compared with a novel virus appearing in early autumn or at the start of winter. Then again, much of what happens in a pandemic may be related to activities coinciding. For example, in 1957, the start of spread in August was linked to opening of schools.

5.5 1976: A(H1N1) Swine Flu – a False Alarm

In early 1976, an outbreak of swine influenza (A/H1N1/New Jersey/76) occurred at a USA military recruits base in Fort Dix, New Jersey. The outbreak lasted from 19 January until 9 February, and infected at least 230 military personnel, and caused

13 hospitalizations for acute respiratory disease and one death. Transmission was probably facilitated by the recruits' cramped living conditions on the military base.

There was great concern that this event could herald the start of the next pandemic, especially because of the recycling theory (Focus Box 5.1). A vaccine against the virus was rapidly developed and after a clinical trial of 3000 individuals, a mass vaccination programme of 43 million people was started in September 1976 in the USA, even though no transmission had been detected. However, the association of Guillain-Barré Syndrome (a rare neurological condition) with this vaccine led to the premature cessation of the programme. In retrospect, this episode represented the first of a number of subsequently documented episodes of unsustained human transmission of an influenza A virus of swine origin.

5.6 1977: Re-emergence of A(H1N1) – a Pseudo-pandemic

One year later, human influenza A(H1N1) re-emerged in humans. The virus did not displace A(H3N2), and instead co-circulated with A(H3N2) until 2009. Although the re-emergence of A(H1N1) was first reported in Russia in November 1977 (it was thus termed 'Russian flu'), it was later determined that is had been present in at least three Chinese provinces some months earlier. Throughout early 1978 it spread through the Americas, Europe, Middle East and Australia, reaching South America and New Zealand by June 1978. The outbreaks were all mild, and almost all those affected were under 25 years of age, who had not been exposed to the virus when it was circulating prior to the 1957 A(H2N2) pandemic. The highest weekly attack rates at the peak of the epidemic reached 13% in children aged 7 to 14 years.

This event is not generally described as a true pandemic, but some now argue that it could or should have been. The virus closely resembled strains which had circulated previously in human populations, and was molecularly identical to an isolate of A(H1N1) from 1950. It is unlikely that such a strain could have remained silently in a natural animal or human reservoir, either as a dormant infection or causing undetected cases, without significant antigenic drift. The resemblance was so great that many feel the re-emergence of this virus was due to an artificial introduction. In all previous pandemics for which there are virological data, the emergence of a new subtype has coincided with the disappearance of the older circulating subtype. This did not happen in 1977 and instead the previously unrecognized situation of two influenza A subtypes (A(H1N1) and A(H3N2)) co-circulating in human populations commenced.

5.7 1997 Onwards: Avian Influenza Viruses in Humans – a Pandemic Alert?

While it has been known that avian viruses were the original source of some genes in pandemic viruses, until recently it was not believed that these viruses could spread directly to humans causing a true infection and then transmit further. There are some notable exceptions, in particular A(H9N2) caused human cases in China and Hong Kong (in 1999, 2003 and 2008) and A(H7N7) spread to humans during major poultry outbreaks in 2003 (Chapter 4).

The situation with the avian influenza virus A(H5N1) is somewhat different. This virus is termed 'highly pathogenic' because of its near total lethality when poultry are infected. It first came to prominence in 1997, where an outbreak in Hong Kong poultry led to 18 clearly infected human cases, of whom six died. The outbreak was unprecedented, given the severity of the illnesses, and attracted global attention. Many thought this might be the start of the next pandemic, although there was little evidence of further person-to-person transmission. Because of the threat to humans, all poultry in Hong Kong were slaughtered in an attempt to contain the virus; an effort that appeared to be successful.

However, in 2003, when the world's attention was still directed to the outbreak of severe acute respiratory syndrome (SARS), major poultry outbreaks of A(H5N1) were recognized, principally in South-east Asia, with occasional transmission directly to humans. These cases reinforced the realization that the virus was lethal, with human case fatality initially of up to 80%. The basic features of the disease were well defined with primary viral pneumonia prominent, often characterized as acute respiratory distress syndrome (ARDS). Other features suggested that infections were possibly disseminated. As in 1918, many characteristics indicated a role of cytokine storm in producing the severity of the disease.

A(H5N1) was an avian virus which could occasionally transmit from poultry to humans and it was known that past pandemic viruses were of avian origin. Thus A(H5N1) posed (and still poses) the threat of a severe pandemic. This, as well as the spectre of the 2003 SARS outbreak, which virtually shut down some major cities in Asia, resulted in a global alert focusing on pandemic preparedness. While SARS transmission ended, A(H5N1) transmission continued, expanding into West Asia, Africa and Europe. Unexpectedly, when the next pandemic occurred in 2009, it turned out to be caused by the swine influenza derived A(H1N1)pdm09 virus.

5.8 2000 Onwards: Pandemic Planning – the Basis of the 2009/10 Response

During the first decade of the 21st century, planning for an influenza pandemic became a major focus of national and international organizations, especially from 2005 onwards. The call to action from the World Health Organization (WHO) was based in part on the continuing threat of an A(H5N1) pandemic. Indeed, in many respects, the thinking about pandemic response was based on the premise that it would be caused by that virus, that it would be severe and that it would emerge gradually from animal sources. Planning was largely based on learning from the three pandemics of the 20th century (Focus Box 5.2).

Focus Box 5.2. Assumptions used to plan for the 2009 pandemic.

A range of features of the influenza pandemics of the 20th century were used to inform pandemic preparedness in the early years of the 20th century:

- the data point to a clinical attack rate in the range of 25–40%;
- the distribution of deaths suggest that a pandemic wave may last about 4 months at national level;
- the number of distinct waves may vary from one to three;
- a pandemic is likely to be shorter and sharper at local level (and in closed communities such as prisons), with up to 50% of cases (and the associated deaths and demand for healthcare) occurring in a 2-week period around the local peak in incidence;

- more total deaths occurred in younger adults than in later years with the same virus; in 1918 high case fatality in this age group was the most prominent feature;
- pandemics can vary in severity – two of the 20th century pandemics could be classified as mild or moderate, and one as extremely severe;
- the interval between pandemics can vary between 10 and 40+ years;
- most pandemics seem to have originated in Asia*;
- the most likely pandemic threat was posed by A(H5N1)*; and
- viruses of animal origin could cause a severe pandemic.

Assumptions marked * were proved incorrect by the 2009 pandemic.

A.S. Monto and C. Sellwood

Strategies to respond to the next pandemic started to be discussed. These included how to contain the virus in the area where sustained human-to-human transmission began, expected to be South-east Asia, as well as specific pharmaceutical interventions. Vaccines against A(H5N1) were developed and tested, and, in order to make vaccines available as early as possible, mock-up dossiers were filed by manufacturers with the European Regulatory Authorities. These dossiers were deliberately flexible to allow rapid manufacture and licensure whatever pandemic virus emerged, and were valuable in the 2009 pandemic. Influenza antiviral drugs are the other key pharmaceutical intervention for pandemic control and in the first months of a pandemic would likely be the only intervention available for prophylaxis and treatment. Unlike vaccines, these antiviral drugs can be used against any pandemic influenza virus that emerges. However, since there is little surge capacity in the manufacturing process, they would have to be stockpiled – something many countries did in anticipation of an A(H5N1) pandemic.

It was recognized that if the next pandemic, particularly one caused by A(H5N1), was severe, the pharmaceutical interventions would be inadequate to handle its impact. This would be particularly true in low-resource regions. Therefore, various countries and the WHO developed elaborate plans to use a variety of societal measures such as voluntary isolation and quarantine as well as social distancing to mitigate the pandemic. Modelling studies were carried out to identify the probable impact of each intervention if used in a current response as well as to determine the contribution of various measures employed in the 1918 pandemic, with the conclusion that in certain circumstances and when used in combination, these measures could have an appreciable impact (Chapter 16).

Pandemic planning at the WHO was handled in the context of the International Health Regulations 2005 (IHR), which went into effect in 2007 (Chapter 17) and followed the broad phases set out in Table 5.2.

Table 5.2. WHO Pandemic Phases, April 2009 onwards.

Phase 1	No viruses circulating among animals have been reported to cause infection in humans	Predominantly animal infections; few human infections. Pandemic probability uncertain
Phase 2	An animal influenza virus circulating among domesticated or wild animals is known to have caused infection in humans and is therefore considered a specific potential pandemic threat	
Phase 3	An animal or human–animal influenza reassortant virus has caused sporadic cases or small clusters of disease in people (e.g. when there is close contact between an infected person and an unprotected caregiver), but has not resulted in human-to-human transmission sufficient to sustain community-level outbreaks	
Phase 4	Human-to-human transmission of an animal or human–animal influenza reassortant virus able to sustain community-level outbreaks has been verified	Sustained human-to-human transmission. Pandemic probability medium to high
Phase 5	The same identified virus has caused sustained community-level outbreaks in two or more countries in one WHO region	Widespread human infection. Pandemic probability high to certain (Phase 5)
Phase 6	In addition to the criteria defined in Phase 5, the same virus has caused sustained community-level outbreaks in at least one other country in another WHO region	
Post-peak period	Levels of pandemic influenza activity in most countries with adequate surveillance have declined below peak levels	Possibility of recurrent events
Post-pandemic period	Levels of influenza activity have returned to levels seen for seasonal influenza in most countries with adequate surveillance	Disease activity at seasonal levels

See: http://www.who.int/csr/disease/swineflu/phase/en/index.html

5.9 Preparedness for Future Pandemics

There is no way at present of predicting the severity of a future pandemic; it may be as globally devastating as the 1918 pandemic, or the same as the 2009 pandemic. The northern hemisphere has not experienced a severe winter epidemic since 1989/90, and while medical facilities continue to improve, many health-care workers have minimal experience of caring for influenza patients with severe disease. Furthermore, the interval between pandemics is irregular. Only 11 years passed between 1957 and 1968, but 41 years between 1968 and 2009. Therefore, complacency is misplaced, even though it is not long since the last pandemic was officially declared over in 2010.

Some have talked about the possible return of A(H2N2), given the recycling theory. Others, noting continual spread of A(H5N1) amongst poultry and to humans, remind us that the threat of this virus still exists.

- The pandemics of the 20th century were caused by three different subtypes of influenza: A(H1N1), A(H2N2) and A(H3N2). The first pandemic of the 21st century was caused by an A(H1N1) virus different from the one in 1918. All varied in the age groups affected and numbers of deaths.
- The 1918 A(H1N1) pandemic was the worst pandemic on record. Cases occurred over three waves, with the second wave being the most severe in most countries, and an estimated 40 million deaths occurring worldwide. Young adults aged 20–40 were severely affected by the virus.
- Pandemics appear to have occurred throughout history, the first being recognized in 1580; however we cannot be certain that pandemic events prior to 1889 were definitely attributable to influenza. There is evidence of antigenic recycling of subtypes A(H1), A(H2) and A(H3).
- Reviewing previous pandemics can give an indication of what might be expected, however nothing is certain. It is impossible to predict the next pandemic virus or its impact, as demonstrated by the 2009 A(H1N1) pandemic.

Further Reading

Ahmed, R., Oldstone, M.B. and Palese, P. (2007) Protective immunity and susceptibility to infectious diseases: lessons from the 1918 influenza pandemic *Nature Immunology* 8(11), 1188–1193.

Hsieh, Y.C., Wu, T.Z., Liu, D.P., Shao, P.L., Chang, L.Y., Lu, C.Y., Lee, C.Y., Huang, F.Y. and Huang, L.M. (2006) Influenza pandemics: past, present and future *Journal of the Formosan Medical Association* 105(1), 1–6.

Kilbourne, E.D. (2006) Influenza pandemics of the 20th century. *Emerging Infectious Diseases* 12(1), 9–14.

Morens, D.M. and Fauci, A.S. (2007) The 1918 influenza pandemic: insights for the 21st century *Journal of Infectious Diseases* 195(7), 1018–1028.

Monto, A.S., Black, S., Plotkin, S.A. and Orenstein, W.A. (2011) Reponse to the 2009 pandemic: effect on influenza control in wealthy and poor countries *Vaccine* 29, 6427–6431.

Potter, C.W. (2001) A history of influenza. *Journal of Applied Microbiology* 91(4), 572–579.

Viboud, C., Grais, R.F., Lafont, B.A., Miller, M.A. and Simonsen, L.; Multinational Influenza Seasonal Mortality Study Group (2005) Multinational impact of the 1968 Hong Kong influenza pandemic: evidence for a smouldering pandemic *Journal of Infectious Diseases* 192(2), 233–248.

A.S. Monto and C. Sellwood

6 Epidemiology of Pandemic Influenza A(H1N1)pdm09

Jim McMenamin[1] and Jonathan Van-Tam[2]

[1]Health Protection Scotland, Glasgow, UK; [2]University of Nottingham, UK and Health Protection Agency (East Midlands), Nottingham, UK

- What were the main timelines of the 2009 pandemic?
- What were the characteristic epidemiological features of A(H1N1)pdm09?
- What was the mortality impact of the 2009 pandemic?
- What will happen next regarding the A(H1N1)pdm09 virus?

6.1 Introduction

For many countries pre-pandemic preparedness work reached a crescendo in the period 2006–2009. However, rather than the more widely expected avian influenza challenge, it was a virus of swine origin which caused the first pandemic of the 21st century. The 2009 pandemic attributable to the influenza A(H1N1)pdm09 virus is the most intensively studied pandemic to date. Its epidemiology is captured by consideration of time, place and person characteristics as discussed below.

6.2 Time and Place

In early 2009, public health authorities in Mexico began to identify clusters of influenza and an increased number of non-typeable influenza samples. By mid-March, morbidity reports showed an increased number of acute respiratory disease, cases with high attack rates in some communities, and referral centres noted an abnormally high number of patients with severe influenza-like illness (ILI) and severe pneumonia, most of whom were young and previously healthy. Samples from non-typeable influenza A cases were sent to reference laboratories in Canada and the USA.

On 23 April 2009 the US Centers for Disease Control and Prevention (CDC) announced a small number of human influenza A infections in its southern states, mainly those bordering Mexico, that initially could not be subtyped. In the next few days, a novel influenza A(H1N1) virus containing six genes from a North American swine flu virus and two from a Eurasian swine virus was identified from respiratory samples taken from two unrelated children in San Diego, California. It was designated A/California/7/2009(H1N1) – 'swine flu', later designated A(H1N1)pdm09. The Mexican cases were subsequently identified as being due to the same virus, at which point it became clear that a novel influenza virus of swine origin was already spreading amongst humans in both Mexico and the USA. A Public Health Emergency of International Concern (PHEIC) was declared by Mexico on 25 April 2009 (Chapter 17). The World Health Organization (WHO) Pandemic Phase 4 was triggered on 27 April, followed by Pandemic Phase 5 on 29 April 2009 after the identification of cases in Europe (mainly the UK and Spain), Canada and New Zealand (see Chapter 5 for definition of phases). By late May 2009, driven initially by international travel and limited community spread, thousands of cases had been reported in North and South America, Europe, the Middle East, Asia and Australasia.

By 6 June 2009, the novel A(H1N1) virus had affected over 214 countries across all major continents of the world and significant community transmission was documented as occurring in more than one WHO world region (North America and Europe). With the fulfilment of the last of its predetermined conditions, WHO declared a pandemic on 11 June 2009.

In the southern hemisphere a single wave of infection was then documented in 2009 over the winter season; for example, in Australia, over a period of 18 weeks from mid-May to mid-September 2009 (Fig. 6.1). A second pandemic wave occurred in 2010, again over the same period that is 'usual' for seasonal influenza, just falling within the WHO defined pandemic period.

In many northern hemisphere countries, a single wave of infection was described (Fig. 6.2) with significant increases in cases following the pattern of schools re-opening after their summer vacation. However some countries (including England, Scotland and Ireland) described two waves of infection, where the number of new cases dropped over the early summer only to recrudesce following the return of pupils to school after the summer vacation. In this respect there was greater similarity between these countries and North America (USA and Canada) than with the majority of EU countries. The explanation for this is uncertain: one hypothesis is that the UK has substantially more air traffic from North America compared with many European countries and thus experienced multiple introductions/seeding events during spring 2009 onwards. Detailed UK molecular virological investigation appears to offer support for this premise.

In the UK the first wave peaked in mid/late-July 2009. The UK regions most affected initially were central Scotland, the West Midlands and London, the latter attributable to several early, large, school-based outbreaks. Overall England and Wales experienced higher clinical activity levels in the first wave compared to Scotland and Northern Ireland, which may have been due to the earlier closure of Scottish and Northern Irish schools for summer holidays. The second wave in each of the UK countries started with the return to school in the autumn, with a peak in mid-October 2009 (Fig. 6.3). Similar evidence supporting the importance of the timing of school vacation periods in slowing or accelerating spread has since been documented in Canada and South-east Asia.

Pandemic activity in Hong Kong peaked in a second wave in early September 2009 after an

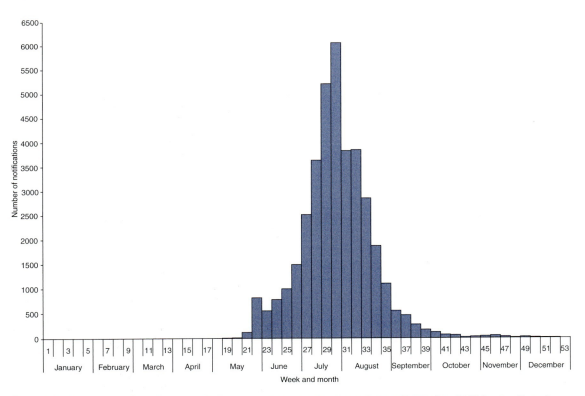

Fig. 6.1. Laboratory-confirmed cases of influenza A(H1N1)pdm09 in Australia, to December 2009 by month and week number.

J. McMenamin and J. Van-Tam

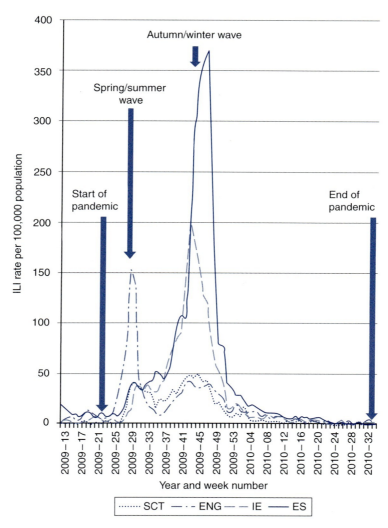

Fig. 6.2. Pandemic influenza 2009/10 – spring/summer and autumn/winter waves of infection seen in some EU countries (ILI cases per 100,000 population for Scotland (SCT), England (ENG), Eire (IE) and Spain (ES)). (Adapted from ILI data submitted to ECDC through TESSy. Denominator data inserted for Spain for the period to 2010 week 13.)

initial first wave. South Africa was unique in documenting an early A(H3N2) season followed by a wave of pandemic influenza. In contrast Argentina and Chile experienced a single wave of infection in mid-2009, similar to Australia and New Zealand. However, sub-Saharan Africa, particularly West Africa, experienced a single wave of infection in early to mid-2010.

The post-pandemic phase was formally declared by WHO on 10 August 2010. It is however important to remember that, as emphasized in Chapter 1,

the distinction between a pandemic virus and an immediately post-pandemic virus may be somewhat artificial. Although lying outside the officially defined pandemic period, the upsurge in A(H1N1)-pdm09 activity in the southern hemisphere in mid-2010 and the same in the northern hemisphere in late 2010, both classified as 'seasonal epidemics', were in epidemiological terms second and third waves respectively of the pandemic virus in these territories and arguably at least as severe in their impact.

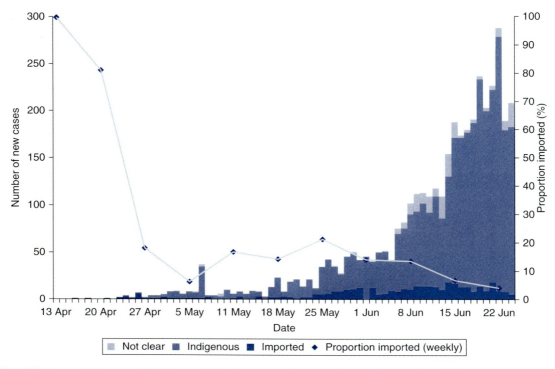

Fig. 6.3. Cases of influenza A(H1N1)pdm09 infection by onset date and route of acquisition of infection and weekly proportion imported, UK (to 1 July 2009). (Kindly provided by the Health Protection Agency, see http://www.hpa.org. uk/hpr/archives/2010/hpr4310_rsprtry_spplmnt.pdf.)

6.3   Person Characteristics

Whilst the virulence of the virus itself may change the impact of a pandemic (Chapters 3 and 5), epidemiologists must also consider the relative contribution of age, sex, and other demographic and host factors (e.g. pre-existing immunity; predisposition by: race/ethnicity, presence or absence of chronic or physiological conditions, nutritional status, obesity/body mass index; and relationship to behavioural or environmental factors).

Age and sex

It became quickly apparent during the first wave of infection that laboratory-confirmed cases of influenza A(H1N1)pdm09 showed a relative sparing of individuals born prior to the 1950s. Within this birth cohort this appeared consistent with cross-protection afforded by prior exposure to circulating variant strains of influenza A(H1N1) that followed the pandemic strain responsible for the 1918

pandemic, i.e. viruses that were seasonal influenza strains up until 1956. These influenza A strains were then replaced in human circulation, first by A(H2N2) and more recently by A(H3N2) and A(H1N1), the latter of which was only distantly related to the 1918 pandemic strain type (Chapters 1 and 5). There was then a significant majority of the population (all of those born after 1956 plus a minority born before) at risk of acquisition of the new influenza A(H1N1)pdm09 virus. Serological data (studies of antibody levels in the population), described later on in this chapter, show that the level of susceptibility varied between countries.

The maximal burden of illness resulting in presentation to a general practitioner/community physician or subsequent hospitalization in the UK was seen in the age groups 0–4 and 5–14 years in most countries. While fatal cases were reported in small numbers across all age groups, case fatality rates were maximal in the elderly and patients with underlying medical conditions – i.e. a similar pattern to that seen in seasonal influenza. The increased

J. McMenamin and J. Van-Tam

rates of hospitalization, complications and mortality in pregnancy, observed in some studies, mirrored the findings of prior pandemics.

In the UK during the 'containment phase', pandemic cases were identified aged from 0 to 90 years; the age structure for confirmed cases up to 1 July 2009 was much younger than in previous pandemics of the 20th century, with evidence of marked geographic variation by region and a median age of 14 years (inter-quartile range: 9–25 years). The 5–14 year age group had the highest cumulative population incidence rate (42 per 100,000) by 1 July 2009 (Fig. 6.4). Age groups over 45 years had the lowest cumulative population incidence rates. Median age varied by region; in London and the West Midlands, where there had been several large school outbreaks, it was 12 years whereas in other UK regions it was somewhat higher (Scotland – 17 years; North West England – 25 years). There was an approximately equal sex distribution (48% female).

In countries with two distinct waves of infection separated by the summer vacation period, there was an increase in the average age of those affected between waves as evidenced by data from general practitioner/physician consultations and hospital admissions. This is consistent with the reducing number of susceptible individuals in the younger age groups as the pandemic progressed.

Serology

It is well recognized that the number of individuals who are exposed to and develop an immune response to most infections (serological attack rate) is greatly in excess of the number who become ill with symptoms (clinical attack rate, CAR). Historically this was known to be case for influenza (Chapter 1) and was seen clearly with influenza A(H1N1)pdm09, when it was apparent from early on in the pandemic that many individuals who had a throat or nasal swab that was positive for the virus either had no symptoms or very few (insufficient to satisfy most national case definitions). It was therefore not surprising when the first of the serological studies published from the UK indicated that a much larger proportion of the population had been exposed to the virus (developing antibodies) than had become unwell with symptoms. What was not anticipated was the magnitude of the difference between the proportion of the population affected by the pandemic as indicated by symptoms and the much larger proportion who had clearly been exposed and developed antibodies.

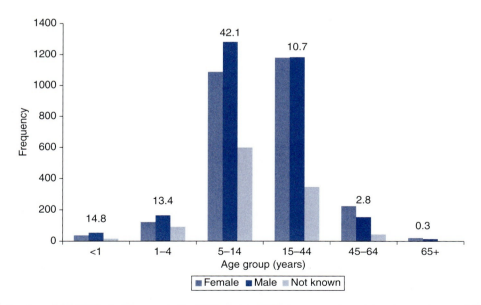

Fig. 6.4. Number of A(H1N1)pdm09 cases in the UK to 1 July 2009, by age and sex (showing crude cumulative rate per 100,000 population above each age group).

For example, in England serological data that became available in September 2009 revealed that the size of the first wave in May–July had been hugely underestimated. This was particularly the case in children in whom the ratio of undiagnosed influenza compared to clinical recognized illness may have been as high as 10 to 1. In contrast to the initial data in which the UK second wave dwarfed the first wave, the overall sizes of the first and second wave were probably approximately equivalent (Fig. 6.5). Globally by the end of the first (or only) pandemic wave, serology positivity rates had increased with maximum values found in school-aged children (up to 65%).

Socio-economic status and ethnicity

In the early stages of the pandemic, observational studies from laboratory-confirmed cases of A(H1N1)pdm09 demonstrated that the CAR in households from lowest socio-economic groups was higher than from households of the highest socio-economic groups.

Increased morbidity and mortality in previous pandemics is well described for indigenous peoples, and similarly there were initial reports in the first summer 2009 wave of higher than expected clinical attack, hospitalization and death rates in indigenous populations such as those in North America, Australia and New Zealand. However such reports are difficult to interpret due to multiple potential confounders factors such as:

- lower background seasonal influenza vaccination uptake (repeat annual vaccination with a seasonal vaccine used in the period prior to the pandemic could have conveyed some level of protection in recipients);
- increased rurality or social isolation resulting in an increased chance of the population being immunologically naïve to previously circulating influenza strains which could afford partial or full protection;
- increased prevalence of chronic medical conditions and obesity in these population groups;
- lower socio-economic status;
- different healthcare seeking behaviour;
- different access to acute medical services.

Similar trends were seen in UK Indian/Pakistani populations; however this population represents a well-established migrant community, and not an indigenous population group.

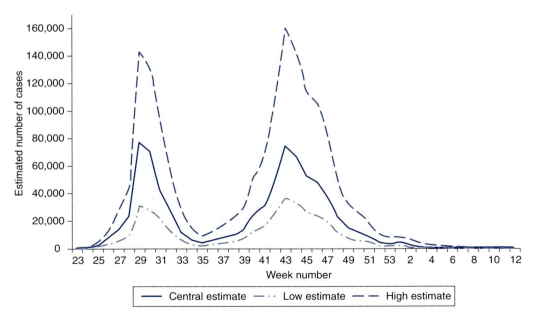

Fig. 6.5. Estimated number of clinical cases of influenza A(H1N1)pdm09 infection in England, June 2009–March 2010. (Kindly provided by the Health Protection Agency, see http://www.hpa.org.uk/hpr/archives/2010/hpr4310_rsprtry_spplmnt.pdf.)

J. McMenamin and J. Van-Tam

Clinical attack rates

High-quality data on a series of early cases were collected in the UK. The 'First Few Hundred' (FF100) approach (Chapter 2) demonstrated that the overall household secondary attack rate (SAR) (for virologically confirmed influenza A(H1N1)pdm09) was estimated as 8.2% (95% CI 6.4–10.3%) during the first wave of the pandemic. This was significantly affected by the use of antivirals to treat index cases and as prophylaxis for close household contacts (Chapter 14). There was also evidence of a differing SAR by age group; with the rates in children and young adults significantly higher than the rate in adults aged over 50 years.

In one early school outbreak in England, 91 symptomatic cases were identified between 15 April and 15 May 2009 of which 33 were confirmed to be positive for influenza A(H1N1)pdm09. In this outbreak an overall virologically confirmed attack rate in the school pupils of 2% was observed, though in the most affected age group this increased to 15%. Transmission was documented in several households of the pupils, with a 17% virologically confirmed SAR in household contacts. A large, late-recognized, outbreak of influenza A(H1N1)pdm09 infection in an English primary school had a CAR of 30% in the pupils, with a virologically confirmed attack rate of 13% overall (ranging from 5% to 23% in different age groups). These data illustrate the considerable variability according to individual setting.

A later overview of the initial CAR and clinical spectrum of illness was provided by WHO. The highest attack rates were reported among children and young adults; 60% of laboratory-confirmed infections and 32–45% of hospitalized cases in the first wave in the USA occurred in persons under 18 years of age, and cases younger than 65 years accounted for approximately 90% of deaths. Thus in epidemiological terms, disease burden was far greater among children and young adults than in the elderly, a pattern also seen very clearly in 1918.

Basic reproduction number – R_0

One key epidemiological parameter required for epidemic or pandemic analysis is the basic reproduction number, R-nought, or R-zero (R_0); defined as the number of additional cases one infected person generates on average over the course of their infectious period (Chapter 13). The WHO estimated that R_0 during the 2009 pandemic ranged from 1.3 to 1.7 in most populations, but individual studies around the world reported values from 1.4 to 2.3. Initially the R_0 was estimated to be between 1.4 and 1.6 in Mexico, higher in children than adults, similar to or slightly higher than estimates for seasonal influenza.

There are pitfalls for the unwary in interpreting such values and multiple methods for generation of R_0. In the UK much lower R_0 values were seen during the first summer wave; R_0 was estimated to be close to 1 but with considerable uncertainty from early May until mid-June 2009, after which it rose consistently above 1.0 (Fig. 6.6). This fluctuation in the estimate is to be expected due to stochastic effects (randomness) when numbers of infected individuals are low.

6.4 Hospitalization and Death

Case fatality rates

Internationally there has been much variation in the estimated case fatality rate (CFR) and consequent estimates of the overall number of deaths within and between countries, attributable to A(H1N1)-pdm09 over the course of the pandemic. Such a wide range of estimates presented policy makers with significant challenges particularly in the early days of the pandemic; for example, contrast the first estimated CFR for Mexico of 1.9% versus 0.14% in the USA early in the pandemic. The upper value would have placed the 2009 pandemic in a similar severity range to 1918, whereas the lower value would indicate something less severe than in 1968.

A closer examination of the UK data reveals important details underpinning the quantification and description of deaths attributable to pandemic influenza. The first UK death due to A(H1N1)-pdm09 occurred on 14 June 2009. A total of 474 deaths certified due to A(H1N1)pdm09 were reported in the UK up to 15 April 2010. Whilst a number of deaths occurred in the spring/summer wave, the vast majority (83%) occurred over the autumn/winter. Seventy-two per cent of fatal cases were reported to have an underlying risk factor for severe disease. In the UK the finally calculated CFR was 0.026% overall – this was lower than most estimates made in the pandemic prior to this date. Most other estimates available to this date used laboratory-confirmed cases in their denominator, resulting in rates of 0.1–0.9%.

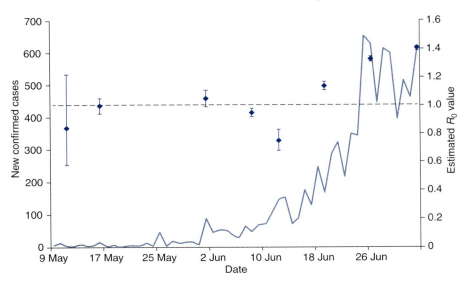

Fig. 6.6. Estimated R_0 by date of estimation with the number of new confirmed cases of pandemic influenza A(H1N1)pdm09, UK, April–June 2009. (Kindly provided by the Health Protection Agency, see http://www.hpa.org.uk/hpr/archives/2010/hpr4310_rsprtry_spplmnt.pdf.)

However, by confining the denominator to laboratory-confirmed cases these previous studies provided a gross underestimate of the incidence of true symptomatic cases and therefore a substantial overestimate of the fatality rate for symptomatic cases. Subsequent international review of studies reported gives an overall estimated infected CFR of 0.02%.

Excess mortality

In England and Wales, no excess of weekly all-cause death registrations above the threshold was observed over the summer of 2009. In the 2009/10 winter season 3261 excess deaths were estimated to have occurred in weeks 52 and 53; however this is somewhat unlikely to be due to influenza, as all other influenza indicators were showing low activity at that time. The deaths were concentrated in the elderly, and coincided with a period of very cold weather.

Estimated number of deaths and years of life lost

There were an estimated 7500 to 44,100 deaths in the USA attributable to the A(H1N1)pdm09 virus

for the period May to December 2009; compared with the estimated 500,000 excess deaths in the same country in 1918 this seems very small, taking into account population growth, and instead is rather more typical of a 'normal' winter seasonal epidemic. Indeed, one of the criticisms levelled at the WHO and individual governments after the 2009 pandemic related to whether the response mounted was proportional to the mildness of the pandemic. However this assessment fails to take into account that deaths that occurred in the 2009 pandemic were from younger age groups than for seasonal influenza and both pandemics in 1957 and 1968. The resulting effect on years of life lost suggests a much more severe picture (Table 6.1).

Putting this into context, in terms of years of life lost, the 2009 pandemic would appear to be rather similar to the 1968 pandemic. Early global estimates for the 2009 pandemic are that 9.9 million life years were lost. It is of note however that the unexpectedly severe impact of seasonal influenza observed in the northern hemisphere 2010/11 winter due to the same A(H1N1)pdm09 virus means that the final burden attributable to the virus may yet greatly exceed these initial estimates.

Table 6.1. Estimated number of deaths,[a] mean age and years of life lost[a] in US citizens by pandemic year and compared with seasonal influenza.

Year	Number of deaths	Mean age	Years of life lost
2009	44,100	37.4	1,973,000
1968	86,000	62.2	1,693,000
1957	150,600	64.6	2,698,000
1918	1,272,300	27.2	63,718,000
Average A(H3N2) interpandemic season, 1979–2001	47,800	75.7	594,000

[a]Estimates based on all-cause mortality and adjusted to 2000 population. (Adapted with permission from Viboud, C. *et al.* (2010) *PloS Currents* doi:10.1371/currents.RRN1153.)

6.5 Hospital Admissions, Critical Care Needs and Risk Groups

Whilst the overall burden of infection demonstrated a rough equivalence between the total number of estimated cases in the community in both waves in the UK, the pattern of hospital admissions shows that the number of hospitalizations with confirmed A(H1N1)pdm09 infection was substantially higher in the second wave. Across the UK, as in most countries, the hospitalization rate decreased with age, with children aged 5 years and under having the highest population hospitalization rate (about 28 per 100,000 compared with 3 per 100,000 in those aged 65 years and over).

The UK FLU-CIN study collected information on 1520 patients admitted to 75 UK hospitals with confirmed A(H1N1)pdm09 infection during both pandemic waves. This in-depth study found that non-white and pregnant patients were over-represented and 55% of patients did not have an underlying medical condition. Of the 80 patients who died (5%), 41% were previously healthy and had no recorded co-morbidities; although this is not a pattern usually associated with seasonal influenza, similar observations were again made in winter 2010/11 in the UK associated with A(H1N1)pdm09.

Risk groups

Data from the UK FF100 surveillance project showed that people between 6 months and 65 years of age with underlying medical conditions, such as chronic respiratory, neurological or heart disease, were not at significantly greater risk of clinical infection in the early stages of the pandemic. However, these people were ten times more likely to be hospitalized with confirmed A(H1N1)-pdm09 infection compared to those of the same age without an underlying condition, and 18 times more likely to die from the infection. The underlying conditions with the highest risk of hospitalization with pandemic A(H1N1)pdm09 infection were immunosuppression, chronic renal disease and chronic neurological disease (including stroke). For death, the risks were highest for chronic neurological disease (excluding stroke), chronic liver disease and immunosuppression. The pandemic risk groups closely map those seen for seasonal influenza.

Obesity

One new observation in 2009 was that obesity appeared to be a risk factor for hospitalization, intensive care admission and death; this new phenomenon was especially well described in North America. Whilst this observation was difficult to disentangle from other obesity-associated risk factors found in the same patients (e.g. cardio-respiratory disease and diabetes), it has since been shown to be an independent risk factor by many researchers. Among patients with severe or fatal cases of A(H1N1)pdm09 virus infection, severe obesity (body mass index (weight in kilograms divided by the square of the height in metres) ≥35) and morbid obesity (body mass index ≥40) were reported at rates higher by a factor of five to 15 than those seen in the general population. Possible adverse immunologic effects, respiratory compromise related to physical size and management problems related to obesity may also explain this association.

Pregnancy

Pregnant women became a focus of many national pandemic influenza vaccination campaigns. This was on the basis of the preliminary information from the first wave of increased severity of illness and mortality in pregnant mothers and increased fetal loss. Pregnant women were not at an elevated risk of becoming cases, but were five times more likely to be hospitalized and seven times more likely to die, once infected, compared to females of child-bearing age (15–44 years) with no underlying condition, although not all studies have found such effects. Newer data suggest that the threshold for hospital admission may have been lower for pregnant women in some healthcare settings.

6.6 Outbreaks in Closed Settings and Nosocomial Disease

Immunocomprised patients often serve as the indicators of the success or failure of infection control in hospital environments. Nosocomial influenza is well documented during interpandemic periods as was also the case during the 2009 pandemic. Of 1520 patients in the FLU-CIN study, 30 (2%) met the criteria for nosocomial influenza due to A(H1N1)pdm09; 26 of these also had serious underlying illnesses such as haematologic malignancy in adults, and congenital abnormalities, prematurity or malignancy in children. Almost one third died due to influenza.

Three sources were postulated:

- infection could have been acquired from other patients;
- transmission may have occurred from visitors of patients;
- transmission may have occurred from an infectious healthcare worker (because it is known that some staff continue to work when infected with influenza, usually because the illness goes unrecognized).

These findings highlight the need for adherence to infection control guidelines for staff and visitors (Chapter 8)

6.7 Persistence of A(H1N1)pdm09 as a Seasonal Virus in 2010/11 and Beyond

In previous pandemics it has been well documented that pandemic viruses continue to circulate as a cause of illness in subsequent non-pandemic seasons (Chapter 1). Indeed this rationale, along with detailed virological evidence, explains the inclusion of A(H1N1)pdm09 as one of the three antigens in the trivalent seasonal influenza vaccine for both northern and southern hemispheres for 2010/11 through at least 2012/13.

Following the 2009 pandemic, serological data across age groups were available in some countries to predict whether it was likely that significant outbreaks of influenza A(H1N1)pdm09 would be likely in the influenza seasons that followed the pandemic. The 2010/11 season in the northern hemisphere was followed with much interest to observe the accuracy of these predictions. In the UK one such serological study concluded, based on the available evidence, that it was unlikely there would be a significant 'third wave' of activity in the UK in the 2010/11 season; nevertheless significant activity did occur and severe cases put pressure on intensive care facilities and, overall, mortality was possibly higher than in 2009/10. This unexpectedly high activity is worthy of further consideration. Statistical modelling of the UK data is consistent with a modest increase in transmissibility of the A(H1N1)pdm09 virus among those in the population who remained susceptible within the population (those slightly older than in the pandemic period); this then generated increased rates of clinical presentation among adults and increased rates of admission to intensive care. Although this pattern was replicated in most parts of Europe, North America witnessed a 2010/11 season dominated by A(H3N2) activity.

Whilst a range of influenza A types were described in the first post-pandemic year, it remains to be seen whether subsequent antigenic drift within the A(H1N1)pdm09 will allow it to become established as the principal cause of influenza A infections in the next decade.

6.8 Summary

The first pandemic of the 21st century originated from a virus of swine not avian origin. It produced an atypical summer first (and for some second) wave in some northern hemisphere countries and rapidly spread across the globe, with southern hemisphere peaks in mid-2009 and widespread northern hemisphere peaks towards the end of 2009. R_0 was estimated to lie between 1.3 and 1.7. The elderly appeared comparatively spared, most likely as a consequence of cross-protection from historical exposure to a similar virus before 1957. The pandemic virus produced a range of symptoms which in the main were mild to moderate in severity. Clinical attack rates were maximal in school-aged children. Serological investigation following the first wave demonstrated that, in children, unrecognized or mild infection far exceeded the number of symptomatic cases presenting for medical care. Clinical attack rates were increased in the most deprived and in some ethnic groups. A significant minority of cases developed complications prompting their admission to hospital, which for some resulted in intensive care admission and/or death. Like seasonal influenza a similar profile of patients with specific clinical illness were most at risk of complications, but pregnancy and morbid obesity were identified as independent risk factors, the latter for the first time. However the majority of hospital admissions and deaths were in patients without recognized clinical risk factors. Overall, whilst the estimated number of deaths attributable to the pandemic was far smaller than in the pandemics of the 20th century, in terms of estimated life years lost, the 2009 pandemic was comparable to the 1968 pandemic.

- The 2009 pandemic was officially declared on 11 June 2009. In reality, the first cases of A(H1N1)pdm09 occurred in Mexico between January and March 2009, followed shortly by early first waves in North America, the UK and across the southern hemisphere countries in spring 2009; and a second more widespread northern hemisphere wave in autumn/winter of the same year. Of note, many central and sub-Saharan parts of Africa did not experience appreciable pandemic activity until the early months of 2010. After the pandemic was declared over on 10 August 2010 there were effective 'third waves' of A(H1N1)pdm09 disease in both the southern and then the northern hemisphere in the following winter seasons.
- Epidemiologically, the 2009 pandemic was characterized by highest attack rates in children (of whom at least one half had asymptomatic illness) and very substantial sparing of people born before 1956. Known risk factors for severe disease (underlying chronic illnesses and pregnancy) were confirmed along with new ones such as obesity. As in previous pandemics, a high burden of disease was noted in some indigenous populations.
- Although generally mild with an estimated case fatality rate of 0.02%, and low impact on excess mortality, the age distribution of deaths due to A(H1N1)pdm09 implies that, in terms of years of life lost, the impact of the 2009 pandemic was not dissimilar to the 1968 A(H3N2) pandemic.
- The influenza A(H1N1)pdm09 virus seems to have entirely replaced the old 'seasonal' A(H1N1) virus that circulated previously. However, in the immediate post-pandemic period it has not exerted clear dominance over A(H3N2) and influenza B, both of which continue to circulate alongside the new virus. What happens next is unknown, and simply cannot be guessed at.

Further Reading

Centers for Disease Control and Prevention (2009) Swine influenza A (H1N1) infection in two children – Southern California, March–April 2009. *Morbidity and Mortality Weekly Report* 58, 400–402. Available at http://www.cdc.gov/mmwr/preview/mmwrhtml/mm58d0421a1.htm (accessed 9 April 2012).

Donaldson, L.J., Rutter, P.D., Ellis, B.M., Greaves, F.E., Mytton, O.T., Pebody, R.G. and Yardley, I.E. (2009) Mortality from pandemic A/H1N1 2009 influenza in England: public health surveillance study. *British Medical Journal* 339, b5213.

Fraser, C., Donnelly, C.A., Cauchemez, S., Hanage, W.P., Van Kerkhove, M.D., Hollingsworth, T.D., Griffin, J., Baggaley, R.F., Jenkins, H.E., Lyons, E.J., Jombart, T., Hinsley, W.R., Grassly, N.C., Balloux, F., Ghani, A.C., Ferguson, N.M., Rambaut, A., Pybus, O.G., Lopez-Gatell, H., Alpuche-Aranda, C.M., Chapela, I.B., Zavala, E.P., Guevara, D.M., Checchi, F., Garcia, E., Hugonnet, S. and Roth, C.; WHO Rapid Pandemic Assessment Collaboration (2009) Pandemic potential of a strain of influenza A (H1N1): early findings. *Science* 324(5934), 1557–1561.

Ghani, A., Baguelin, M., Griffin, J., Flasche, S., van Hoek, A.J., Cauchemez, S., Donnelly, C., Robertson, C., White, M., Truscott, J., Fraser, C., Garske, T., White, P., Leach, S., Hall, I., Jenkins, H., Ferguson, N. and Cooper, B. (2009) The early transmission dynamics of H1N1pdm influenza in the United Kingdom. *PLoS Currents* 1, RRN1130. Available at http://www.ncbi.nlm.nih.gov/pmc/articles/PMC2780827/?tool=pubmed (accessed 9 April 2012).

Health Protection Agency (2010) Epidemiological report of pandemic (H1N1) 2009 in the UK; April 2009–May 2010. Available at http://www.hpa.org.uk/webc/HPAwebFile/HPAweb_C/1284475321350 (accessed 9 April 2012).

Kwong, J.C., Campitelli, M.A. and Rosella, L.C. (2011) Obesity and respiratory hospitalizations during influenza seasons in Ontario, Canada: a cohort study. *Clinical Infectious Diseases* 53(5), 413–421.

McLean, E., Pebody, R.G., Campbell, C., Chamberland, M., Hawkins, C., Nguyen-Van-Tam, J.S., Oliver, I., Smith, G.E., Ihekweazu, C., Bracebridge, S., Maguire, H., Harris, R., Kafatos, G., White, P.J., Wynne-Evans, E., Green, J., Myers, R., Underwood, A., Dallman, T., Wreghitt, T., Zambon, M., Ellis, J., Phin, N., Smyth, B., McMenamin, J. and Watson, J.M. (2010) Pandemic (H1N1) 2009 influenza in the UK: clinical and epidemiological findings from the first few hundred (FF100) cases. *Epidemiology and Infection* 138(11), 1531–1541.

Myles, P.R., Semple, M.G., Lim, W.S., Openshaw, P.J., Gadd, E.M., Read, R.C., Taylor, B.L., Brett, S.J., McMenamin, J., Enstone, J.E., Armstrong, C., Bannister, B., Nicholson, K.G. and Nguyen-Van-Tam, J.S.; on behalf of the Influenza Clinical Information Network (FLU-CIN) (2012) Predictors of clinical outcome in a national hospitalised cohort across both waves of the influenza A/H1N1 pandemic 2009–2010 in the UK. *Thorax* 67(8), 709–717.

Presanis, A.M., De Angelis, D., New York City Swine Flu Investigation Team, Hagy, A., Reed, C., Riley, S., Cooper, B.S., Finelli, L., Biedrzycki, P. and Lipsitch, M. (2009) The severity of pandemic H1N1 influenza in the United States, from April to July 2009: a Bayesian analysis. *PLoS Medicine* 6(12), e1000207.

Riley, S., Kwok, K.O., Wu, K.M., Ning, D.Y., Cowling, B.J., Wu, J.T., Ho, L.M., Tsang, T., Lo, S.V., Chu, D.K., Ma, E.S. and Peiris, J.S. (2011) Epidemiological characteristics of 2009 (H1N1) pandemic influenza based on paired sera from a longitudinal community cohort study. *PLoS Medicine* 8(6), e1000442.

Yin, J.K., Chow, M.Y., Khandaker, G., King, C., Richmond, P., Heron, L. and Booy, R. (2012) Impacts on influenza A(H1N1)pdm09 infection from cross-protection of seasonal trivalent influenza vaccines and A(H1N1)pdm09 vaccines: systematic review and meta-analyses. *Vaccine* 30(21), 3209–3222.

7 Clinical Features and Treatment of Pandemic Influenza A(H1N1)pdm09

SEEMA JAIN

Centers for Disease Control and Prevention, Atlanta, Georgia, USA

- What were the main presenting symptoms of A(H1N1)pdm09 infection?
- Once infected what was the likely prognosis?
- What are the cornerstones of modern medical care for severe influenza?
- Were there any special features of A(H1N1)pdm09 infection?

7.1 Introduction

In April 2009, the US Centers for Disease Control and Prevention (CDC) confirmed the first two cases of human infection with the A(H1N1)pdm09 virus in the USA. This virus contained a unique combination of gene segments that had not previously been recognized among human or animal influenza viruses. Since spring of 2009, the virus has spread throughout the world and continues to circulate globally. Detailed information on the epidemiology of A(H1N1)pdm09 infection is available in Chapter 6.

7.2 Presenting Symptoms

The clinical features of people with A(H1N1)-pdm09 infection are generally similar to those reported during seasonal influenza epidemic periods with an acute onset of respiratory illness. The most common symptoms include fever or feverishness and/or chills, cough and sore throat, which are reported in >50% of confirmed cases. It is important to note that not everyone with symptomatic A(H1N1)pdm09 infection will develop a fever. Fatigue or weakness, rhinorrhoea, myalgia and headache are also commonly reported. Patients can also present with shortness of breath, particularly among those hospitalized with pneumonia, and this has been reported in >50% of hospitalized confirmed cases. In addition, among outpatients and hospitalized patients, vomiting or diarrhoea was commonly reported during the 2009 pandemic,

occurring in 20–40% of confirmed cases, which is higher than the proportion reported among confirmed cases during seasonal influenza epidemic periods (5–10%).

7.3 Disease Severity and Prognosis

Similar to seasonal influenza, illness due to A(H1N1)pdm09 infection usually lasts a few days and in most individuals is self-limiting. However, hospitalization occurs in less than 1% of people with A(H1N1)pdm09 infection; risk of death is even lower. The most common complications due to A(H1N1)pdm09 infection are pneumonia, bronchitis, sinus and ear infections, bacterial or viral co-infections, dehydration, and exacerbations of underlying conditions such as asthma or congestive heart failure. Febrile seizures can occur in young children. More rarely, the virus can cause inflammation of various organ systems, which can lead to encephalitis, myelitis, myositis, myocarditis and pericarditis.

As for seasonal influenza virus infections, people at higher risk of complications due to A(H1N1)-pdm09 infection include: children aged under 5 years (especially those aged under 2 years); adults >65 years; people with chronic pulmonary, cardiovascular, renal, hepatic, haematologic (including sickle cell disease), metabolic (including diabetes), neurological or immunosuppressive (either due to HIV or medication) conditions; pregnant women; people aged ≤18 years old receiving long-term aspirin therapy; members of indigenous/aboriginal communities; people who are morbidly obese (body mass index ≥40); and nursing home or chronic care facility residents.

It is important to note several important features of A(H1N1)pdm09 infection. First, despite a low attack rate in the elderly probably attributable to cross-reactive immunity, once infected, the elderly and young children had the highest risk for complications. Second, while many infected people who developed complications had an underlying medical condition, this varied from country to country and 20–40% of people, especially children, had no known underlying medical condition. Third, pregnancy was known from seasonal epidemics and past pandemics to be a risk factor for influenza complications; the risk of complications for pregnant (especially those in the third trimester) and postpartum women was again seen during the 2009 pandemic. Fourth, for the first time during the 2009 pandemic, morbid obesity emerged as a risk factor for complications and has now, in many countries, become a prioritized group for interventions including influenza vaccination and antiviral treatment. Lastly, in certain parts of the world, indigenous or minority populations, including American Indians, Alaskan Natives and Aborigines in the Australia–Pacific region, were at higher risk for influenza-associated complications, including hospitalization and death; this observation may also hold true for interpandemic influenza.

7.4 Management of Community Cases

Most people infected with the A(H1N1)pdm09 virus have mild illness and do not need immediate medical care. These people should stay home and avoid contact with others so they do not spread the virus. However, people who are at higher risk of complications (as described above) should talk to a healthcare provider and may need to be examined. People should seek immediate care if they have trouble breathing, chest pain, signs of dehydration, prolonged or persistent illness, confusion, dizziness, persistent vomiting or inability to eat, and among children, extreme lethargy with lack of interaction and trouble waking. In addition, if fever and cough develop after resolution of initial symptoms of A(H1N1)pdm09 infection, this may indicate a bacterial co-infection and the need for medical evaluation.

7.5 Management of Hospitalized Cases

Reasons for admission

People with A(H1N1)pdm09 infection are admitted to hospital for a variety of reasons and this may differ depending on clinical practice and resources in many parts of the world. One of the most common complications of influenza is pneumonia, which was reported in 40% or more of patients admitted to hospital through various case series conducted during the 2009 pandemic in different countries including Canada, Mexico and the USA. In addition, similar to infection during peak periods of seasonal influenza, people were also hospitalized due to exacerbations of underlying conditions such as asthma or because they were at higher risk for complications due to an underlying condition. It is difficult to know how many people with underlying conditions were hospitalized due to precautionary medical practice and lowered threshold for admission due to the potential for complications. However, the majority of patients admitted presented with acute respiratory illness and severe infection was observed among those hospitalized.

Inpatient management and reasons for escalation of care

Management of people with A(H1N1)pdm09 infection is not only similar to those with seasonal influenza but also to those with other acute respiratory infections. A(H1N1)pdm09 infection can present like other respiratory illnesses and if there is a delay in confirming a diagnosis, many entities may be considered, both infectious and non-infectious. As such, patients should be stabilized and if presenting with acute respiratory signs, may require oxygen or more invasive procedures such as mechanical ventilation. Patients with dehydration should be re-hydrated with oral or intravenous fluids. Those with underlying medical conditions should be treated for exacerbations of their underlying medical conditions. For instance, a patient with asthma and A(H1N1)-pdm09 influenza may require inhaled beta-agonists and steroids to treat the asthma exacerbation. If patients do not respond to primary treatments meant to stabilize their condition, including oxygen, antimicrobials (both influenza antiviral drugs and antibiotics), fluids and treatments for underlying conditions, they may require escalating care. Therefore, timely interventions are paramount to help prevent severe disease.

Intensive care management including use of radical interventions

In almost all reports of A(H1N1)pdm09 infection, a proportion of patients require management in an intensive care unit (ICU) – typically 15–20% of those hospitalized. For patients who do require ICU management, it is frequently due to more severe disease that often requires mechanical ventilation, and can also result in worse outcomes, such as acute respiratory distress syndrome (ARDS) and death. The use of ICU management for A(H1N1)-pdm09 infection varies greatly from country to country depending on availability of critical care beds, clinical practice patterns, and how severe infection and the need for critical care are defined. In the USA, approximately 23–34% of patients hospitalized with A(H1N1)pdm09 infection during the 2009 pandemic were admitted to the ICU. Non-invasive methods of ventilation such as bi-level positive airway pressure can be used initially and may make intubation and invasive mechanical ventilation unnecessary.

Patients who are at greater risk for requiring ICU management include those with underlying medical conditions and those who present with respiratory distress or pneumonia. However, it is important to note that patients without underlying conditions can require ICU admission. In some cases, patients can deteriorate rapidly and may not have time to develop signs of pneumonia or other complications that are recognized before they are in respiratory distress or have another life-threatening complication requiring ICU admission. In one study conducted in Canada, during the 2009 pandemic, the main presenting conditions for patients with A(H1N1)pdm09 infection treated in the ICU were bacterial pneumonia, severe low blood pressure requiring intravenous medications to maintain adequate blood pressure, asthma or chronic obstructive pulmonary disease exacerbation, altered mental status, acute kidney injury and chest pain.

In very severe A(H1N1)pdm09 infections, radical interventions might be necessary, including extracorporeal membrane oxygenation (ECMO). ECMO provides both cardiac and pulmonary support that allows for adequate oxygenation in patients whose heart and lungs are severely damaged and are functioning at very low capacity or have failed. ECMO is usually a last resort in most countries where it is available, and is not available at all in most resource-poor settings. It is unclear whether ECMO has substantial benefits as observational studies include few patients and there are no randomized controlled trials that examine the utility of ECMO for severe A(H1N1)-pdm09 infection.

Prognostic indicators

Patients hospitalized with A(H1N1)pdm09 infection are similar to patients with seasonal influenza and also other respiratory infections in that they should be monitored for resolution of symptoms and clinical findings, return of their laboratory measures to baseline levels, and decreased need for life-saving interventions such as mechanical ventilation. These factors are reviewed to determine stability for discharge from the hospital. Several severity scores, including the Acute Physiology and Chronic Health Evaluation (APACHE), Sequential Organ Failure Assessment (SOFA), Pandemic Medical Early Warning Score (PMEWS) and CURB-65 (severity score for community-acquired pneumonia), most of which have been validated in other patient groups prior to the 2009 pandemic, have been reported to be useful in helping to identify which patients are at higher risk for death. These severity scores incorporate clinical and laboratory findings that focus on respiratory, cardiac and systemic organ function to help determine possibility of death. These scores could be useful to help triage patients with A(H1N1)pdm09 infection and optimize aggressive treatments for the sickest patients, especially if resources are limited. However, there are at present no severity or triage scoring systems that perform particularly well when applied to pandemic influenza.

7.6 Influenza-associated Pneumonia, Community-acquired Pneumonia and Bacteriological Findings

Bacteria, viruses, fungi and other infectious agents can cause pneumonia. While useful in the diagnosis of pneumonia, clinical and radiographic findings do not help distinguish among possible aetiologies. Most studies reporting pneumonia cases during the 2009 pandemic were done among laboratory-confirmed or suspected A(H1N1)pdm09 infection, but few of these studies comprehensively explored all possible aetiologies of pneumonia. Therefore, a true understanding of the contribution of different aetiologies to pneumonia during the 2009 pandemic is lacking.

Influenza-associated pneumonia, including that due to A(H1N1)pdm09 virus, can manifest with viral pneumonia, secondary bacterial infection and also concomitant viral–bacterial pneumonia. Pneumonia and bacterial co-infections are known complications of seasonal influenza and are also well documented during the 2009 pandemic. Pneumonia was the most commonly reported complication among patients hospitalized with A(H1N1)pdm09 infection in many parts of the world. In addition, results from animal studies and human autopsy reports indicated that A(H1N1)-pdm09 infection caused severe diffuse alveolar damage that may have led to more severe lower-tract respiratory disease and respiratory failure than reported during previous seasonal influenza periods. In many reports, radiographic findings of A(H1N1)pdm09 pneumonia included bilateral infiltrates or multilobar infiltrates that are classically associated with viral pneumonia.

Reports on bacteriological findings in relation to A(H1N1)pdm09 infection are highly variable so the true prevalence of secondary infection is difficult to discern. One additional challenge is that patients with A(H1N1)pdm09 infection can have resolution of their flu-like symptoms and then, shortly afterwards, develop new fever and cough that could represent a secondary bacterial infection; these might be difficult to ascertain unless the patient is ill enough to present for medical care during the second course of illness. In addition, diagnostics for both influenza viruses and bacteria are not always available in some settings and have limitations to their detection. For influenza, in many settings, polymerase chain reaction (PCR) or viral culture is not available and only rapid diagnostic tests are available, which have low sensitivity; even rapid tests are often unaffordable in resource-poor settings. Additionally, there are no rapid diagnostics routinely available to diagnose bacterial pneumonia, the yield of gold standard techniques such as blood culture is low for *Streptococcus pneumoniae*, and the sensitivity of cultures is often further reduced by use of antibiotics. Despite these limitations, among patients hospitalized or who died with A(H1N1)pdm09 infection, bacterial co-infections with *S. pneumonia, Staphylococcus aureus* and *Streptococcus pyogenes* were commonly reported.

7.7 Antiviral Treatment

The Advisory Committee on Immunization Practices (ACIP) recommends neuraminidase inhibitors (oral oseltamivir or inhaled zanamivir) for the treatment of suspected or confirmed influenza in hospitalized patients, outpatients who are at higher risk for complications, and people with clinical deterioration or severe illness such as lower respiratory tract infection. While evidence of benefit from the use of influenza antiviral agents is strongest when treatment is initiated <48 h of symptom onset, three observational studies of hospitalized patients with laboratory-confirmed seasonal influenza indicated a reduction in mortality and shorter duration of hospitalization with oseltamivir treatment, even when antiviral drugs were initiated >48 h after symptom onset. Observational data from the 2009 pandemic also suggested that early antiviral treatment was associated with increased survival, including in pregnant women, children and severely ill patients. Despite the absence of definitive clinical effectiveness data, antiviral agents should be initiated in patients with suspected A(H1N1)pdm09 infection who are hospitalized or outpatients with underlying medical conditions, even if >48 h after illness onset, regardless of vaccination status. Detailed information on the influenza antiviral treatment is available in Chapter 14.

7.8 Summary

The A(H1N1)pdm09 virus emerged in April 2009 and caused a generally mild pandemic, albeit with a small proportion of severe hospitalized cases; it continues to circulate throughout the world as a seasonal influenza virus. The clinical findings among patients with seasonal influenza and A(H1N1)pdm09 infection are similar with few discerning features. While hospitalizations and deaths occur in <1% of people infected with A(H1N1)pm09 virus, there is a substantial burden on healthcare systems, especially in resource-limited settings. People at highest risk for complications due to A(H1N1)pdm09 infection include young children, the elderly and people with underlying medical conditions, including pregnant women and those who are morbidly obese. While most people infected with A(H1N1)pdm09 infection will have mild illness, people should seek immediate care if they have trouble breathing, chest pain, signs of dehydration, prolonged or persistent illness, confusion, dizziness, persistent vomiting or inability to eat, and among children, extreme lethargy with lack of interaction and trouble waking. Pneumonia is the most commonly reported complication with A(H1N1)pdm09 infection and can be due to a primary viral pneumonia, secondary bacterial infection or concomitant viral–bacterial co-infection. Influenza vaccination is recommended for prevention of A(H1N1)pdm09 infection and antiviral agents for treatment of selected patients who become infected with this virus.

- Patients with A(H1N1)pdm09 presented with a wide variety of symptoms that were not readily distinguishable from those encountered with interpandemic or seasonal influenza, although vomiting and diarrhoea were both considerably more common.
- Most patients experienced mild or asymptomatic disease, and only around 1% required hospitalization. Once infected the elderly and the very young carried the highest risk of complications and although rarely infected, case fatality rate was highest in the elderly. The prognosis was observed to be worse in patients with underlying conditions, pregnant women and the morbidly obese.
- The cornerstones of medical treatment for patients with severe disease are (according to need): supplemental oxygen, restoration of fluid balance, influenza antiviral agents and antibiotics (for bacterial complications).
- In hospitalized patients, a notable and somewhat unexpected feature of A(H1N1)pdm09 was the very high proportion (15–20%) of patients who required management on an intensive care unit. For the first time, extracorporeal membrane oxygenation (ECMO) was deployed in well-resourced settings to manage the most gravely ill patients.

Further Reading

The Australia and New Zealand Extracorporeal Membrane Oxygenation (ANZ ECMO) Influenza Investigators; Davies, A., Jones, D., Bailey, M., Beca, J., Bellomo, R., Blackwell, N., Forrest, P., Gattas, D., Granger, E., Herkes, R., Jackson, A., McGuinness, S., Nair, P., Pellegrino, V., Pettilä, V., Plunkett, B., Pye, R., Torzillo, P., Webb, S., Wilson, M. and Ziegenfuss, M. (2009) Extracorporeal membrane oxygenation for 2009 influenza A (H1N1) acute respiratory distress syndrome. *Journal of the American Medical Association* 302(17), 1888–1895.

Dominguez-Cherit, G., Lapinsky, S.E., Macias, A.E., Pinto, R., Espinosa-Perez, L., de la Torre, A., Poblano-Morales, M., Baltazar-Torres, J.A., Bautista, E., Martinez, A., Martinez, M.A., Rivero, E., Valdez, R., Ruiz-Palacios, G., Hernández, M., Stewart, T.E. and Fowler, R.A. (2009) Critically ill patients with 2009 influenza A (H1N1) in Mexico. *Journal of the American Medical Association* 302(17), 1880–1887.

Jain, S., Kamimoto, L., Bramley, A.M., Schmitz, A.M., Benoit, S.R., Louie, J., Sugerman, D.E., Druckenmiller, J.K., Ritger, K.A., Chugh, R., Jasuja, S., Deutscher, M., Chen, S., Walker, J.D., Duchin, J.S., Lett, S., Soliva, S., Wells, E.V., Swerdlow, D., Uyeki, T.M., Fiore, A.E., Olsen, S.J., Fry, A.M., Bridges, C.B. and Finelli, L.; 2009 Pandemic Influenza A (H1N1) Virus Hospitalizations Investigation Team (2009) Hospitalized patients with 2009 H1N1 influenza in the United States, April–June 2009. *New England Journal of Medicine* 361(20), 1935–1944.

Kumar, A., Zarychanski, R., Pinto, R., Cook, D.J., Marshall, J., Lacroix, J., Stelfox, T., Bagshaw, S., Choong, K., Lamontagne, F., Turgeon, A.F., Lapinsky, S., Ahern, S.P., Smith, O., Siddiqui, F., Jouvet, P., Khwaja, K., McIntyre, L., Menon, K., Hutchinson, J., Hornstein, D., Joffe, A., Lauzier, F., Singh, J., Karachi, T., Wiebe, K., Olafson, K., Ramsey, C., Sharma, S., Dodek, P., Meade, M., Hall, R. and Fowler, R.A.; Canadian Critical Care Trials Group H1N1 Collaborative (2009) Critically ill patients with 2009 influenza A (H1N1) infection in Canada. *Journal of the American Medical Association* 302(17), 1872–1879.

Novel Swine-Origin Influenza A (H1N1) Virus Investigation Team; Dawood, F.S., Jain, S., Finelli, L., Shaw, M.W., Lindstrom, S., Garten, R.J., Gubareva, L.V., Xu, X., Bridges, C.B. and Uyeki, T.M. (2009) Emergence of a novel swine-origin influenza A (H1N1) virus in humans. *New England Journal of Medicine* 360(25), 2605–2615.

Shrestha, S.S., Swerdlow, D.L., Borse, R.H., Prabhu, V.S., Finelli, L., Atkins, C.Y., Owusu-Edusei, K., Bell, B., Mead, P.S., Biggerstaff, M., Brammer, L., Davidson, H., Jernigan, D., Jhung, M.A., Kamimoto, L.K.,

Merlin, T.L., Nowell, M., Redd, S.C., Reed, C., Schuchat, A. and Meltzer, M.I. (2011) Estimating the burden of 2009 pandemic influenza A (H1N1) in the United States (April 2009–April 2010). *Clinical Infectious Diseases* 52(Suppl 1), S75–S82.

Siston, A.M., Rasmussen, S.A., Honein, M.A., Fry, A.M., Seib, K., Callaghan, W.M., Louie, J., Doyle, T.J., Crockett, M., Lynfield, R., Moore, Z., Wiedeman, C., Anand, M., Tabony, L., Nielsen, C.F., Waller, K., Page, S., Thompson, J.M., Avery, C., Springs, C.B., Jones, T., Williams, J.L., Newsome, K., Finelli, L. and Jamieson, D.J.; Pandemic H1N1 Influenza in Pregnancy Working Group (2010) Pandemic 2009 influenza A (H1N1) virus illness among pregnant women in the United States. *Journal of the American Medical Association* 303 (15), 1517–1525.

Van Kerkhove, M.D., Vandemaele, K.A., Shinde, V., Jaramillo-Gutierrez, G., Koukounari, A., Donnelly, C.A., Carlino, L.O., Owen, R., Paterson, B., Pelletier, L., Vachon, J., Gonzalez, C., Hongjie, Y., Zijian, F., Chuang, S.K., Au, A., Buda, S., Krause, G., Haas, W., Bonmarin, I., Taniguichi, K., Nakajima, K., Shobayashi, T., Takayama, Y., Sunagawa, T., Heraud, J.M., Orelle, A., Palacios, E., van der Sande, M.A., Wielders, C.C., Hunt, D., Cutter, J., Lee, V.J., Thomas, J., Santa-Olalla, P., Sierra-Moros, M.J., Hanshaoworakul, W., Ungchusak, K., Pebody, R., Jain, S. and Mounts, A.W.; WHO Working Group for Risk Factors for Severe H1N1pdm Infection (2011) Risk factors for severe outcomes following 2009 influenza A (H1N1) infection: a global pooled analysis. *PLoS Medicine* 8(7), e100105.

8 Influenza Transmission and Infection Control Issues

JOANNE ENSTONE AND BEN KILLINGLEY

University of Nottingham, Nottingham, UK

- What factors influence influenza transmission?
- Based on the available evidence, what can be said definitively about routes of transmission?
- What practical measures can be used to reduce influenza transmission in healthcare settings?
- Do face masks and respirators work in preventing influenza?

8.1 Introduction

Reducing the impact and spread of influenza epidemics and pandemics is central to national and international preparedness plans. Mitigation strategies include vaccination, antiviral use and non-pharmaceutical interventions (e.g. social distancing, respiratory etiquette, face masks and hand hygiene). However, the effectiveness of the latter depends on the dynamics and determinants of influenza transmission. During a pandemic such non-pharmaceutical interventions have a crucial part to play in limiting transmission, as vaccines and antivirals, whilst having a major role, may not be available in time, or at all, in resource-poor settings.

8.2 Transmission

Transmission of an infectious disease is the process by which an infectious organism moves from one host to another. There are many factors that contribute to and influence this process. Influenza replicates in epithelial cells throughout the respiratory tree (both upper and lower tracts). As a result both virus entry and exit in humans occurs through the respiratory tract, i.e. mouth and nose. Virus is released from a host during events such as coughing and sneezing, which produce a 'respiratory spray' of different sized particles in which virus travels. Virus gains entry to a new host via respiration (droplet nuclei) and/or inhalation (droplets) and/or direct contact (droplets) or indirect contact

(settled droplets and droplet nuclei) (see Section 8.3 for definitions). The potential of the conjunctivae to mediate transmission of human influenza viruses remains uncertain and there is very little evidence to suggest that the faecal–oral or waterborne route of transmission occurs in humans, which contrasts with transmission in birds (Chapter 4). A number of factors can influence transmission pathways (Fig. 8.1).

The concept of super-spreading, transmission to an unusually large number of secondary cases from a source case, has been proposed for influenza but not definitively proved. However, evidence suggests that there exists significant variation between individuals in the numbers of virus-containing particles produced during breathing, coughing, sneezing and talking. If influenza 'super-spreaders' exist, this may have important implications for our understanding of influenza transmission and for control strategies.

Some individuals shed virus but do not experience symptoms. This may happen early in the course of infection (pre-symptomatic) or be present throughout the course of an infection (asymptomatic). Such individuals may not seek treatment or self-isolate and therefore may be an important group for transmission. Data obtained during the 2009 pandemic showed asymptomatic infection rates of approximately 10% among cases diagnosed by PCR, although estimates based on serology suggest that at least 50% of infections were asymptomatic; and it has been estimated that

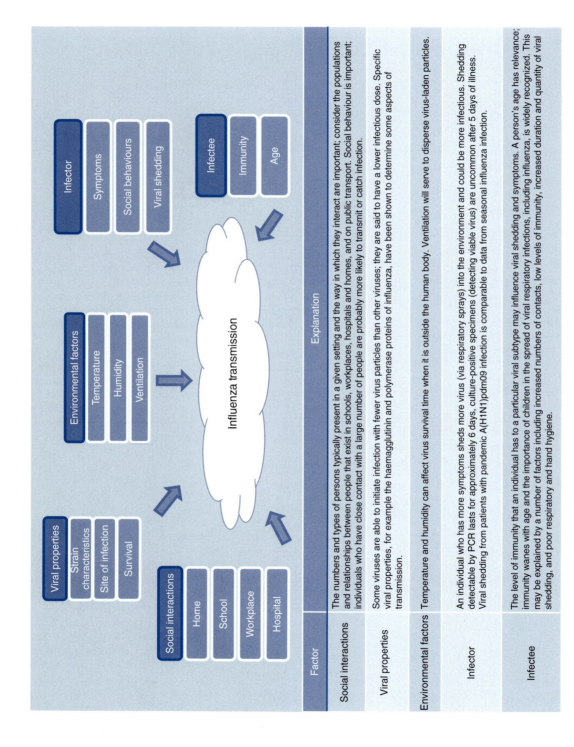

Factor	Explanation
Social interactions	The numbers and types of persons typically present in a given setting and the way in which they interact are important; consider the populations and relationships between people that exist in schools, workplaces, hospitals and homes, and on public transport. Social behaviour is important; individuals who have close contact with a large number of people are probably more likely to transmit or catch infection.
Viral properties	Some viruses are able to initiate infection with fewer virus particles than other viruses; they are said to have a lower infectious dose. Specific viral properties, for example the haemagglutinin and polymerase proteins of influenza, have been shown to determine some aspects of transmission.
Environmental factors	Temperature and humidity can affect virus survival time when it is outside the human body. Ventilation will serve to disperse virus-laden particles.
Infector	An individual who has more symptoms sheds more virus (via respiratory sprays) into the environment and could be more infectious. Shedding detectable by PCR lasts for approximately 6 days, culture-positive specimens (detecting viable virus) are uncommon after 5 days of illness. Viral shedding from patients with pandemic A(H1N1)pdm09 infection is comparable to data from seasonal influenza infection.
Infectee	The level of immunity that an individual has to a particular viral subtype may influence viral shedding and symptoms. A person's age has relevance; immunity wanes with age and the importance of children in the spread of viral respiratory infections, including influenza, is widely recognized. This may be explained by a number of factors including increased numbers of contacts, low levels of immunity, increased duration and quantity of viral shedding, and poor respiratory and hand hygiene.

Fig. 8.1. Factors influencing influenza transmission.

J. Enstone and B. Killingley

1–8% of infections are transmitted from asymptomatic or pre-symptomatic individuals. However, the amount and duration of viral shedding from asymptomatic patients is usually low and it remains to be proven that asymptomatic individuals effectively transmit influenza.

To formulate and implement effective preventative measures such as respiratory and hand hygiene, social distancing and infection control, it is critical to understand the above factors. Each of these in turn can have a bearing on the route(s) of transmission that is dominant in a given situation.

8.3   Routes of Transmission

Despite the fact that influenza has impacted on human health for many centuries and that the virus was first identified in humans in 1933, remarkably little is known definitively about its modes of transmission. A sound understanding of influenza transmission is key to developing evidence-based policies for infection prevention and control.

One of the difficulties in understanding routes of transmission is the inconsistency and variety of terms that are used. Airborne transmission has generally been used to refer to infections that spread over long distances via particles in the air, for example tuberculosis. Only droplet nuclei remain suspended in the air and can travel over long distances; however some confusion can arise because droplet nuclei can transmit infection over short distances as well as long; in fact, because droplet nuclei are more concentrated nearer their source, they are more likely to transmit over short distances than long.

The following terms will be used in this chapter:

- **Contact transmission:**
  - direct contact – transmission via direct physical contact, e.g. kissing;
  - indirect contact – transmission via an intermediate contaminated object, e.g. a door handle.
- **Droplet transmission:** transmission of influenza by droplet particles (>5 μm) emitted by an infected host (e.g. by coughing) which deposit on mucous membranes in the upper respiratory tract either directly or by inhalation.
- **Aerosol transmission:** transmission of influenza through the air by droplet nuclei (≤5μm). Such particles are small enough to remain suspended in air for prolonged periods of time. As well as depositing in the upper respiratory tract following inhalation, they can be respired and penetrate the lower respiratory tract. Infection could theoretically be initiated at either site.

The evidence base for influenza transmission is largely derived from studies that have assessed a range of factors including: virus deposition and survival in the environment; the epidemiology of disease in hospitals, nursing homes and other semi-closed settings; prospective pharmaceutical and non-pharmaceutical interventions in the setting of natural infection; human influenza challenge studies; animal models; and mathematical modelling of transmission. A particular weakness of the evidence is that investigating routes of transmission has seldom been the primary aim of such studies. Whilst most contribute in some way to the evidence base, very few are conclusive; some (especially retrospective observations) are weakened by confounding factors and others (animal and laboratory studies) can be difficult to interpret in the context of 'normal' human interactions.

Transmission almost certainly occurs through multiple routes but a clear hierarchy has not been established. The relative significance of each route will depend on a set of circumstances acting at a certain time. Table 8.1 provides a summary of what is currently known and unknown about influenza transmission.

Contact transmission

There is sound evidence supporting influenza virus survival on fomites; the virus survives for up to 48 h on hard surfaces (e.g. stainless steel and plastic) and for up to 12 h on soft items (e.g. clothing and paper). Similarly virus has been shown to survive on hands for several minutes, long enough to allow transmission. However, few studies have demonstrated the recovery of viable virus from hands or surfaces contaminated by patients with influenza in natural settings.

In a trial in Thailand to investigate hand hygiene and surface contamination during the 2009 pandemic, the hands of index cases (infected children) and secondary cases within the household were swabbed. The hands of 15/90 (17%) index cases were positive by PCR, one (1%) was culture positive, whilst 1/59 (2%) secondary cases were PCR positive and none were culture positive. Fomites in households were also swabbed: 540 swabs were collected, 3% were

Table 8.1. Summary of 'knowns' and 'unknowns' regarding influenza transmission.

What is known about influenza transmission?	What is unknown or uncertain about influenza transmission?
• Influenza is transmitted via respiratory sprays released by infected persons • The amount of viral shedding correlates with the severity of symptoms and the presence of fever; this peaks early in the course of the illness • Pre-symptomatic and asymptomatic viral shedding occurs • Long-range transmission of influenza is not supported by the available evidence • Influenza can survive on surfaces for several hours • Influenza can be detected in air and is associated with both respirable and inhalable sized particles	• The relative importance of droplet, contact and aerosol transmission and how this might change depending on circumstance • The infectious doses needed to initiate infection via each route • Why some individuals with influenza appear to be more infectious than others • Whether contact with contaminated surfaces commonly results in infection • The distances involved in respiratory droplet transmission • The relationship between pre-symptomatic and asymptomatic viral shedding with infectivity • Whether transmission of influenza via the conjunctiva of the eye causes respiratory infection

positive by PCR, none was culture positive. In another study, 648 fomite swabs were collected from the homes and hospital rooms of confirmed influenza cases. Virus was detected by PCR on 36 occasions (from 6% of samples taken, and from 38% of individuals) and live virus was recovered from one surface. These data suggest that virus deposited by infected patients does not contaminate the vast majority of fomites in high titre. However, it is important to appreciate the limitations that exist with regard to virus sampling and detection methods.

Droplet transmission

Droplet transmission is frequently assumed to be significant as epidemiological investigations often note that close proximity to a source patient is necessary for transmission to occur. However, data generated from clinical studies to back this up are lacking and it should be recognized that close proximity spread does not adequately differentiate droplet from aerosol transmission.

Droplets behave ballistically and fall from the air within a few feet of their source; they can be inhaled but not respired (due to their size). Aerobiological studies reveal that the vast majority of pathogens excreted in respiratory sprays are contained within droplet-sized particles; this is because droplets constitute 99% of the volume of a respiratory spray. This does not necessarily imply that droplet transmission produces the greatest number of secondary infections; in order to transmit effectively droplets in coughs and sneezes must

be precisely targeted towards fomites or a susceptible contact and be able to reach them.

Aerosol transmission (airborne/droplet nuclei transmission)

Aerosols can be generated by coughing, sneezing, talking and breathing and may transmit infection upon being respired into the respiratory tract. Influenza can survive in the air for periods long enough to allow transmission. Survival is prolonged (up to 24 h) at low relative humidity.

There are few data to support long-range influenza transmission but this does not preclude a significant role for short-range spread via droplet nuclei in some circumstances, at ranges normally or traditionally attributed to droplets. A number of influenza outbreak investigations have reported circumstances that seem to have facilitated aerosol transmission. Furthermore, advances in microbiological techniques and technology have recently led to the detection of influenza in aerosols released into the environment through respiration, coughing and sneezing by infected patients. Detection is usually achieved by PCR; only rarely has viable virus been detected though this probably reflects methodological limitations.

In animal studies both droplet and aerosol routes appear to play significant roles though it is often not possible to discriminate between them. However, extrapolating animal findings to humans may not always be appropriate as physical and social behaviours will differ.

8.4 Generic Infection Control Precautions for Use in Healthcare Settings

Infection control precautions can be usefully classified into two main categories: standard infection control precautions and transmission-based precautions.

Standard infection control precautions (or principles) were developed from the concept of 'universal precautions', introduced during the 1980s by the Centers for Disease Control and Prevention (CDC) in the USA, to reduce the transmission of blood-borne and other pathogens. They should be used for every patient irrespective of infection status (on the principle that some infections may not be immediately evident) and include hand hygiene, environmental hygiene, the use of PPE (personal protective equipment) and the safe use and disposal of sharps. Following the SARS (severe acute respiratory syndrome) epidemic in 2003, standard precautions were extended to include respiratory hygiene.

Transmission-based precautions, again initially devised by CDC, are used in addition to standard precautions whenever it seems likely that transmission would not be interrupted by standard precautions alone. The three key categories of transmission-based precautions mirror the three main categories of transmission, namely *droplet precautions*, *contact precautions* and *airborne (aerosol) precautions*.

8.5 Counteracting Transmission

There are a variety of ways of counteracting transmission, using barriers, hygiene and distance, depending on which method of transmission is being considered.

Counteracting droplet and contact transmission

Distancing

There is international debate about the maximum distance over which droplet transmission might occur. Following SARS in 2003, questions were raised about whether the distance that droplets travel may be closer to 6–10 ft rather than 3 ft as traditionally described. In the USA, current advice is to treat the '3 ft rule' as an example of a short distance from a patient, not a precise cut-off point. With no consensus on this, definitive studies could usefully be performed to give a robust answer. Around 3 ft from the source is the distance currently advised for donning a surgical face mask (SFM) to prevent infections transmitted by the droplet route, and the minimum distance historically between beds on a ward, although modern facilities' regulations demand a greater distance (6–10 ft from the centre of one bed to the centre of the next is now more the norm).

Personal protective equipment (PPE)

PPE includes disposable gloves, aprons, gowns and eye protection. Gloves help prevent contact transmission between patients or to the wearer; aprons and gowns protect clothing and should be changed between patients; eye protection should be used when there is a risk of splashing or risk from respiratory spray. Hands should be cleaned after removing PPE.

Hand hygiene and environmental cleaning

Contact transmission is best counteracted by hand hygiene, before and after patient contact (either hand washing with soap and water or using an alcohol hand rub if hands are visibly clean) and frequent environmental cleaning, particularly of frequently touched items and surfaces, generally using water and detergent.

Surgical face masks (SFMs)

SFMs were originally introduced to be worn during surgery to protect the sterile field (the patient) but they can also be used to protect a wearer from splashes or from infections spread by respiratory droplets. They provide a barrier to the nose and mouth, and also act to reduce touching of the face.

Respiratory hygiene

Respiratory hygiene includes using tissues for covering mouths and noses and to catch coughs and sneezes which are disposed of promptly and hands then cleaned. It also includes the wearing of masks by patients when in communal areas or when being moved from place to place. The use of antiviral tissues (containing antiviral agents, usually citric acid) has been shown to be effective in reducing the transmission of 'colds' when compared with cotton handkerchiefs.

Counteracting aerosol transmission

Respirators

Respirators are designed to protect the wearer from airborne particles including droplet nuclei. They have a higher filtering specification than SFMs and should be used when the risk of exposure to aerosols carries a significant risk of disease transmission. Respirators are categorized according to their filtering efficiency; the European standard EN149:2001 covers FFP1, FFP2 and FFP3 respirators. FFP3 (filtering face piece 3) respirators have the highest filtering efficiency and are broadly similar to the US-standard N99 respirator; the next highest filtering respirator available is the FFP2, broadly similar to the US N95 respirator. To be effective respirators need to be fit-tested for every individual and then fit-checked with each wearing.

Engineering controls

Engineering controls can also be used to counteract aerosol transmission. For example negative pressure isolation rooms can be used but availability may be limited. Ultraviolet light has also been used to counteract transmission by sterilizing infectious aerosols.

8.6 The Evidence for Infection Control Precautions for Influenza

Prospective studies have enrolled participants (from individuals to families or households) into randomized intervention trials and followed them over a period of time during which influenza activity was likely to be high. Studies have been performed in both community (homes, schools, university residences) and healthcare settings; in the latter the effectiveness of SFMs and respirators has been compared. There are indications that some of the interventions deployed in community studies may have had some benefit in certain situations, though only one study (involving hand hygiene) has shown positive results with regard to primary study objectives. Challenges with these studies have included low rates of compliance with interventions and the fact that interventions in secondary prevention studies are often only deployed after symptoms begin and so miss periods of possible transmission when an index case has initial symptoms or is pre-symptomatic.

The evidence for face mask or respirator use

A systematic review of the evidence that masks (SFMs or respirators) can prevent influenza transmission concluded that there is some evidence to support the use of either an SFM or respirator by an infected person to protect others, but fewer data to support the wearing of an SFM or respirator to prevent the wearer from becoming infected.

A primary prevention study took place amongst young adults in university accommodation. Volunteers were assigned to SFM use, SFM plus hand hygiene (HH) or a control arm for 6 weeks during an influenza season. Neither intervention resulted in a significant reduction in influenza-like illness (ILI) over the entire study period but during weeks 4–6 there was a significant reduction (46%) in ILI in the SFM plus HH group and during weeks 4 and 5 there was a significant reduction in ILI (31%) in the SFM only group. Compliance was poor with the average use of a SFM each day being only 3.5 h.

In a secondary prevention study household contacts of an index case were randomized to interventions to reduce transmission. Interventions were: (i) control; (ii) HH; and (iii) HH plus SFM. The primary outcome was laboratory-confirmed influenza in household contacts. The secondary attack rate in the study was low (8%) and no differences were seen across the intervention arms. In a subgroup of households who implemented the interventions within 36 h of symptom onset, transmission was significantly reduced in the HH plus SFM group. Another secondary prevention study involved households where a child was unwell with a respiratory illness. Household members were randomized to interventions that consisted of: (i) SFM; (ii) respirator (FFP2 mask, not fit-tested); and (iii) control. No statistically significant differences in ILI were observed between the groups. In a subgroup of adults who reported good compliance with mask use over a 5-day period (i.e. wearing one most or all of the time) use of either mask reduced their risk for ILI by between 60 and 80%.

Two randomized studies have reported data on the use of masks to reduce influenza transmission by studying nosocomial transmission between patients and healthcare workers who attend them.

A study compared SFMs with (fit-tested) respirators (FFP2) to protect healthcare workers from influenza. Nurses working in Canadian emergency departments were randomized to a mask and asked to wear it whilst caring for patients with febrile respiratory illnesses during an influenza season. No significant difference between outcomes was seen. A study conducted in China also compared SFMs with respirators (N95), both fit-tested and non-fit-tested. Masks were worn during all work hours for 4 consecutive weeks. Over a range of clinical and laboratory-based outcomes, respirators were associated with an approximate halving of risk compared with SFMs. However, after adjustment for clustering, the only significant finding was that respirators were more protective against symptomatic respiratory infection compared with SFMs.

In summary, the effectiveness of SFMs and respirators to prevent the transmission of influenza remains uncertain.

Evidence for hand hygiene

Contaminated hands undoubtedly play a part in the transfer of infections in general. Hand hygiene has been shown to be particularly effective in young children in reducing respiratory virus infections. A study carried out in schoolchildren in Cairo found that implementing a hand hygiene regime of hand washing twice a day had a significant effect on reducing absences from school, as well as decreasing the incidence of influenza by 50%. A different study used a hand hygiene and respiratory hygiene intervention with children and found that whilst there was no overall decrease in total influenza, there was a decrease in the incidence of influenza A and a reduction in school absence.

Evidence for environmental cleaning

Data demonstrating the effectiveness of environmental cleaning in healthcare or community settings specific to reducing *transmission* of influenza is sparse, but there is evidence that the influenza virus is rapidly killed by many agents including soap and water, detergent, other readily available household cleaning agents, and even household products such as dilute (10%) vinegar. There is also evidence that the virus can survive for periods of several hours, depending on the surface type; thus environmental cleaning is important in settings where

either the risk of transmission to susceptible people or the likelihood of frequent re-contamination is high.

Evidence for respiratory hygiene

Respiratory hygiene incorporates a number of measures including hand hygiene, mask wearing by those with a respiratory infection and the use of tissues; where evidence is lacking, common sense dictates these will reduce direct and indirect contact spread. When used as an intervention alongside hand hygiene, respiratory hygiene has been shown to decrease influenza A and school absences.

8.7 Translating Evidence on Influenza Transmission into Practical Advice

In the healthcare setting a variety of measures can be put in place to reduce transmission between patients, from patient to healthcare worker, and from healthcare worker to patient. Standard and droplet precautions are required to reduce the transmission of influenza (these will also cover the *contact* route as standard precautions embrace the requirement for gloves and PPE when in contact with respiratory secretions), and under some circumstances at least, precautions against aerosol transmission will be required. In addition environmental cleaning and good respiratory hygiene are important.

Some infection control measures are administrative and include advising ill staff not to come to work, separating patients with and without influenza, and having separate staff caring for each group. For example, patients can be nursed in single rooms, or patients on a ward or in a nursing home can be placed together (cohorted) and looked after by staff who do not move between them and patients without influenza. In primary care settings waiting areas can be split so that patients with respiratory symptoms do not mix with patients without respiratory symptoms. Patients who can tolerate it could be asked to wear an SFM when in communal areas, or when moving from one area to another. Healthcare workers should wear SFMs when in close contact with patients – these provide a barrier to the nose and mouth and should also help reduce contact transmission by discouraging the wearer from touching their face.

In brief, limiting *droplet and contact* transmission of influenza in the healthcare setting involves:

- instructing staff with respiratory symptoms not to come to work;
- segregating patients with and without influenza as soon as possible;
- separating staff into those who look after patients with influenza and those who do not;
- restricting access to visitors who are symptomatic;
- implementing precautions including SFM use, good hand hygiene and appropriate use of PPE (including careful removal and disposal to prevent contamination);
- frequent environmental cleaning with water and detergent;
- offering patients an SFM when being moved;
- encouraging good respiratory hygiene – with access to tissues and means of disposal; and
- cleaning hands with soap and water or an alcohol hand rub before and after patient contact, or contact with the patient's environment.

8.8 Minimizing Aerosol Transmission of Influenza in the Healthcare Setting

Uncertainty about the modes of transmission fuels the debate about whether it might be appropriate to use respirators for all close patient contact, instead of SFMs, i.e. if the risk from short-range aerosols is significant. Patients can be placed in negative pressure rooms if these are available. Some medical procedures lead to the production aerosols (see below) and respirators are recommended in these circumstances.

Aerosol-generating procedures (AGPs) in healthcare settings

Some AGPs, such as intubation, cardiopulmonary resuscitation and bronchoscopy, have been categorized by the World Health Organization (WHO) as being associated with an 'increased risk of disease transmission'. During the 2009 pandemic, in the absence of evidence specific to influenza, UK pandemic infection control guidance took a precautionary approach and advised the use of FFP3 respirators when such procedures were carried out. For some other procedures, categorized by WHO as having a 'controversial/possible' increase in risk of transmission (non-invasive positive pressure ventilation, high-frequency oscillating ventilation and nebulization), FFP3 respirators were also recommended in the absence of a clear assessment of risk.

The 2009 pandemic offered the opportunity to evaluate AGPs specifically for risk of influenza transmission. One such air sampling study was able to conclude that healthcare workers were exposed to potentially infectious aerosols in hospital, although the aerosols could not be confidently linked to all so-called AGPs. This result notwithstanding, excess risks seem likely for bronchoscopy and airway suctioning. Whilst work is on-going looking at the risk from AGPs, there is currently insufficient evidence to draw a firm conclusion on the risk of transmission of influenza to healthcare workers during AGPs and the WHO list of potential AGPs should be adopted as part of a sensible precautionary stance.

8.9 Experience of Infection Control Measures during the 2009 Pandemic

Since the end of the 2009 pandemic there have been few published studies with a significant focus on infection control and the use of SFMs, respirators and other PPE. One simulation exercise carried out prior to the pandemic assessed UK pandemic infection control guidance. The exercise found that tasks took longer than usual when wearing PPE and that face masks hampered communication. Others have reported more frequent headaches when wearing face masks. It is also accepted that healthcare workers are not always particularly compliant with infection control precautions, particularly the use of respiratory protection. These factors, the personal experience of those who used them during the pandemic, and their perceived usefulness may affect views about their use during a future pandemic.

Infection control advice for public settings and the family home

The results of community studies looking at interventions such as hand hygiene and mask wearing suggest that the public are generally poor at complying with infection control advice. In the event of another pandemic, compliance may only be improved if the 'fear factor' is high. Advice for families during a pandemic needs to be simple, pragmatic and justified to increase the likelihood of compliance.

Prior to the 2009 pandemic, advice to the public in the UK included recommendations that anyone ill with influenza-like symptoms should stay at home and that social/family contact should be minimized until their symptoms have resolved. It is also suggested that those without influenza could reduce their risk of catching it by avoiding unnecessary close contact with others and by adopting high standards of hygiene including hand hygiene, respiratory hygiene and cleaning in the home.

There is little evidence that generalized widespread use of masks by the public would be useful, therefore most authorities do not advocate stockpiling masks for general use (Chapter 16). However, it might be prudent for a household member who is acting as the principal caregiver to wear an SFM when in close contact (e.g. in the same room) as the patient. Or cases could consider wearing an SFM to protect others, particularly if leaving the home whilst symptomatic. In addition, masks may be considered in specific occupational settings after a thorough risk assessment.

8.10   Unresolved Infection Control Questions

There are a number of important gaps in our knowledge concerning influenza transmission (Table 8.1), many of which particularly impact on infection control: the importance of pre-symptomatic and asymptomatic transmission is not clear; it is not known which AGPs carry a significant risk of transmission; the effectiveness and efficacy of SFMs and how this compares with respirators; the distance from a patient that SFMs should be employed (assuming droplet transmission proves important); how readily contact with contaminated surfaces results in infection; whether ventilation (including simple measures such as opening windows) has a role in reducing transmission. All these questions are important but complex (and expensive) in terms of designing research studies to specifically address them. Some of the unanswered questions might be best approached via human challenge studies, such as the effectiveness of SFMs and how readily contact with contaminated surfaces results in infection, as conditions can be much more readily controlled than in community or hospital settings. Other questions will be best answered by studies in natural settings such as studies exploring shedding and infectiousness. Addressing these unanswered questions should be a priority for all those concerned with transmission and control of pandemic influenza, so that the evidence base underpinning infection control advice for both healthcare settings and to the public is significantly improved in advance of the next pandemic.

- Many factors could influence the likelihood and routes of influenza transmission in a given setting. These include: environmental factors (e.g. temperature, humidity and ventilation); virus properties; the setting for human interactions (e.g. home, school, workplace, healthcare); symptoms, virus shedding and social behaviour of infected people; and the age and immune status of those exposed.
- Whilst there is strong evidence for virus survival on touched surfaces, the evidence proving that this is a potent means of influenza transmission is lacking. The evidence for droplet and aerosol transmission is incomplete; both may play important roles but evidence is lacking to establish a clear hierarchy of importance between the two. It seems clear that influenza is spread by short-distance transmission (3–6 ft); there is little evidence to support long-distance transmission.
- Until more data become available, sensible practical measures that can be recommended for reducing influenza in healthcare are: isolation; cohorted care for larger numbers of patients; 'standard' and 'droplet precautions' for close patient contact; and respirators for known or suspected aerosol-generating procedures.
- The evidence that face mask or respirators work to prevent influenza transmission remains inconclusive. This does not mean they should not be used in healthcare settings as precautionary measures. However in general settings, there is more evidence to support masking of the infected person (to prevent spread to others) than for masking to protect the wearer.

Further Reading

Aiello, A.E., Coulborn, R.M., Aragon, T.J., Baker, M.G., Burrus, B.B., Cowling, B.J., Duncan, A., Enanoria, W., Fabian, M.P., Ferng, Y.H., Larson, E.L., Leung, G.M., Markel, H., Milton, D.K., Monto, A.S., Morse, S.S.,

Navarro, J.A., Park, S.Y., Priest, P., Stebbins, S., Stern, A.M., Uddin, M., Wetterhall, S.F. and Vukotich, C.J. Jr (2010) Research findings from nonpharmaceutical intervention studies for pandemic influenza and current gaps in the research. *American Journal of Infection Control* 38(4), 251–258.

Brankston, G., Gitterman, L., Hirji, Z., Lemieux, C. and Gardam, M. (2007) Transmission of influenza A in human beings. *Lancet Infectious Diseases* 7(4), 257–265.

Centers for Disease Control and Prevention (2012) Infection control in healthcare settings. Available at: http://www.cdc.gov/flu/professionals/infectioncontrol/ (accessed 1 April 2012)

Cowling, B.J., Zhou, Y., Ip, D.K., Leung, G.M. and Aiello, A.E. (2010) Facemasks to prevent transmission of influenza virus: a systematic review. *Epidemiology and Infection* 138(4), 449–456.

Department of Health (2011) Evidence base underpinning the UK influenza pandemic preparedness strategy. Available at: http://www.dh.gov.uk/en/Publicationsand-statistics/Publications/PublicationsPolicyAndGuidance/DH_125318 (accessed 1 April 2012).

Killingley, B., Enstone, J., Booy, R., Hayward, A., Oxford, J., Ferguson, N., Van-Tam, J.N. and Influenza Transmission Strategy Development Group (2011) Potential role of human challenge studies for investigation of influenza transmission. *Lancet Infectious Diseases* 11(11), 879–886.

Lindsley, W.G., Blachere, F.M., Thewlis, R.E., Vishnu, A., Davis, K.A., Cao, G., Palmer, J.E., Clark, K.E., Fisher, M.A., Khakoo, R. and Beezhold, D.H. (2010) Measurements of airborne influenza virus in aerosol particles from human coughs. *PLoS One* 5(11), e15100.

Loeb, M., Dafoe, N., Mahony, J., John, M., Sarabia, A., Glavin, V., Webby, R., Smieja, D.J., Chong, S., Webb, A. and Walter, S.D. (2009) Surgical mask vs N95 respirator for preventing influenza among health care workers: a randomized trial. *Journal of the American Medical Association* 302 (17), 1865–1871.

Talaat, M., Afifi, S., Dueger, E., El-Ashry, N., Marfin, A., Kandeel, A., Mohareb, E. and El-Sayed, N. (2010) Effects of hand hygiene campaigns on incidence of laboratory-confirmed influenza and absenteeism in schoolchildren, Cairo, Egypt. *Emerging Infectious Diseases* 17, 619–625.

Tellier, R. (2009) Aerosol transmission of influenza A virus: a review of new studies. *Journal of the Royal Society/Interface the Royal Society* 6(Suppl 6), S783–S790.

Weber, T.P. and Stilianakis, N.I. (2008) Inactivation of influenza A viruses in the environment and modes of transmission: a critical review. *Journal of Infection* 57(5), 361–373.

9 Pandemic Preparedness

Caroline S. Brown and Michala Hegermann-Lindencrone

WHO Regional Office for Europe, Copenhagen, Denmark

- What are the most important features of national pandemic preparedness planning?
- Did preparedness activities improve our response to the 2009 pandemic?
- Which areas of pandemic preparedness need to be improved?

9.1 Preparing for a Complex Global Public Health Threat

For more than 10 years, countries and the global community have invested considerably in pandemic preparedness. This is due to an increased awareness of the need for coordinated action to respond to cross-border health threats including the threat of bioterrorism, the possibility that the avian influenza virus A(H5N1) that first emerged in humans in 1997 followed by a resurgence in late 2003 could cause a future pandemic; and the outbreak of severe acute respiratory syndrome (SARS) in early 2003. In June 2007, the new International Health Regulations (2005) (IHR) came into force; they are legally binding to all Member States (MSs) and describe the obligations of both MSs and the World Health Organization (WHO) in responding to cross-border public health threats (Chapter 17). In 2006, WHO published a document stating that MSs must first focus on pandemic preparedness.

Although many countries have generic plans covering response to a variety of disasters or hazards, the need for a specific plan addressing an influenza pandemic was recognized due to the unpredictability, complexity and potential impact of the latter on the global population, health services and other essential sectors. One particularly obvious and important difference between a pandemic and many other forms of disasters and hazards is that a pandemic represents what is known as a 'rising tide' incident, played out over many months, where sustainability becomes a key issue; in contrast many other emergency situations are known as 'big bang' incidents, which reach a rapid crescendo and require a response lasting only days or weeks (Chapter 10).

What is known is that an influenza pandemic will last for months and perhaps years and that even a relatively mild pandemic will cause disease in a large portion of the population and disruption of health services due to workplace absenteeism. A severe pandemic is also likely to impact essential services, such as water and power plants, police, firefighters and logistics companies involved in delivery of food and medicines (whose continued operation during a pandemic is essential) (Chapter 18).

Although influenza vaccine is a widely recognized public health tool to prevent infection, using current technology it will take about 6 months to develop a vaccine once the pandemic virus has been detected and characterized (Chapter 15). It is therefore necessary to plan and prepare for the use of public health measures to prevent spread of the disease as well as provision for the medical treatment of cases, particularly for the period before pandemic vaccine is widely available and for longer in settings where access to vaccine will always be limited.

The sustained response involving health and other essential sectors over a long period of time distinguishes a pandemic from other health emergencies, and is a key reason why countries and international organizations undertake pandemic preparedness planning and develop pandemic preparedness plans.

In this chapter, pandemic preparedness is considered to be a collection of activities defined as follows:

pandemic preparedness in a country. It should be established at the inter-ministerial level (e.g. cabinet of ministers) but usually with the Ministry of Health leading. The committee should have clear terms of reference, be formally endorsed by the government to develop the national pandemic plan and have sufficient resources to perform the task. These resources include manpower (technical and secretarial) to write the plan, organize meetings and coordinate with relevant stakeholders, and organize training and exercises.

The committee will decide on the components of the pandemic plan and planning process. The committee will usually be comprised of a core planning group, which is responsible for writing the plan and for involving and coordinating additional stakeholders that need to contribute to the planning process by developing specific chapters of the plan and/or strategies (e.g. the pandemic vaccination strategy) or setting up certain systems (e.g. enhanced surveillance capacity). Wherever possible, the committee should be supported by high-level technical expertise; for example virologists, epidemiologists, infectious disease physicians and logisticians (for vaccine and antiviral drug distribution). The full range of stakeholders that should be involved in pandemic planning would typically be as listed in Table 9.1.

The group should ideally meet frequently throughout the planning process. In the beginning of the planning process, the timeline for the writing process and for the implementation of the plan based their pandemic plans on the 2005 guidance, which described the actions that countries and WHO should take to prepare for, and respond to, a pandemic. It divided pandemic planning into a number of core areas:

- command and control systems and public health measures;
- surveillance systems to monitor the spread and characteristics of the pandemic;
- healthcare provision preparation (including surge capacity);
- vaccination strategy;
- antiviral stockpiles;
- public health measures (non-pharmaceutical);
- maintaining essential services and businesses – business continuity planning;
- legal issues;
- ethical issues;

When the pandemic planning committee starts to develop the national plan, it first defines the specific aims of pandemic preparedness. For most countries, the broad aims of pandemic preparedness planning are to mitigate the negative impact an influenza pandemic will have on society by:

- reducing morbidity and mortality;
- maintaining essential services;
- reducing short- and long-term socio-economic consequences (Chapter 18).

Planning to achieve these aims requires an assessment of the anticipated threat (severity and impact) of a pandemic. Since the exact features of a future pandemic are not known, pandemic preparedness plans are best based on a range of scenarios, such as mild, moderate and severe. These scenarios are developed by extrapolating the potential number of cases (mild and severe), and deaths, from the characteristics of previous pandemics and seasonal influenza epidemics. This allows estimates of possible clinical attack rates, incubation periods and infectiousness (R_0), number of severe cases and case fatality rate (CFR) for a future pandemic. Such estimates or planning assumptions can be used to plan interventions but not to predict the precise impact of a future pandemic. The pandemic planning guidance published by WHO in 2005 included global estimates of approximately 233 million outpatient visits, 5.2 million hospital admissions and 7.4 million deaths due to a pandemic. A number of national pandemic plans developed before the problems that may be prioritized over pandemic influenza in national health budgets (Chapter 25). For this reason, the degree of preparedness will vary among countries and many rely on international donors and organizations like WHO to support their pandemic preparedness planning and activities.

Pandemic planning committee

A national pandemic plan describes what a country will do in response to a pandemic, and what needs to be prepared in order to be able to do this. Once the government has committed itself to this process, the first step is to establish a national pandemic planning committee to oversee and coordinate the writing and implementation of the plan. The national pandemic planning committee, or working group, should be multi-sectoral, multidisciplinary, and responsible for organizing and coordinating

C.S. Brown and M. Hegermann-Lindencrone

symptomatic cases, hospitalization rates of up to 4% and CFR of between 0.4% and 2.5% were assumed. A CFR of 2.5% was based on the global CFR estimated from the 1918 A(H1N1) pandemic, which was considered to be very severe. The 2009 A(H1N1) pdm09 pandemic has taught us that planning assumptions need to include far milder scenarios. In 2007 the US Department of Health and Human Services proposed a simple 'hurricane style' severity rating scale for pandemic influenza (PSI) based on CFR with categories from 1 (very mild) to 5 (very severe), designed to inform the proportional use of non-pharmaceutical measures (Chapter 16). However given that the 2009 was very mild, rated Category 1 according to the PSI, yet quite disruptive in other ways, for example in relation to the demand for intensive care, it has been widely recognized that a more sophisticated multidimensional tool is needed for the future.

Based on planning assumptions and country characteristics such as health system development, vulnerable populations, climate (which affects seasonality), trade links and tourism, the potential impact on health and society can be anticipated. This in turn will allow the specific aims of the national pandemic plan to be defined, as well as how these aims will be achieved. The main aims of pandemic preparedness as well as the range of possible scenarios should be described in the national plan.

Flexibility in planning

Although the pandemic plan will guide the response during a pandemic, it should be clearly stated in the plan that during a pandemic, the actual situation 'on the ground' in country should dictate which response measures are implemented as well as the triggers for both scaling up and scaling down the response, rather than what has been written in the plan or what is happening at the global level. This is an important lesson learned from the 2009 A(H1N1)pdm09 pandemic, as many countries based their response on global phases declared by WHO which did not relate to the local situation. This is because the timing of the spread of the pandemic to a country, the time between the detection of the first cases and the period during which there is sustained transmission in the community and thus many cases (a proportion of which will be severe), will differ between countries, as will the impact on healthcare services and the whole of society. As soon as a new influenza virus with pandemic potential emerges, each country should conduct a risk assessment of the situation, which will be continuously updated as the pandemic unfolds. The risk assessment is informed by national early warning and surveillance systems, information from WHO and other international organizations, neighbouring countries, from regional platforms and cooperations, information on flights to and from affected countries, from the board of tourism, etc.

By applying a flexible approach in the planning phase and planning for more than one scenario, countries will be able to adjust their response to the actual situation by adapting the measures implemented at the national and local level according to severity and impact. This means that some strategies and systems developed during the preparedness phase may not be implemented, whilst others may need to be modified, or enhanced.

The planning cycle: endorsement, exercising and revision

Once completed, pandemic plans should be formally endorsed by the national authorities. They should also be regularly exercised using scenarios and simulations as this will strengthen the existing capacity and help identify the shortcomings and areas of pandemic preparedness that need further attention. Exercises are mostly addressing command and control and coordination in a pandemic. Pandemic exercises may be held at national, subnational and international levels and are described in detail in Chapter 11.

Pandemic plans at all administrative levels and in all sectors should be reviewed and updated when necessary. This can be whenever an exercise has been undertaken, if there are new scientific developments, changes in country health systems or communicable diseases legislation (national or international, such as the IHR) or other important events, such as the re-emergence of A(H5N1) avian influenza in 2003 and the 2009 A(H1N1)pdm09 pandemic. When revised, the plan should again be disseminated to all stakeholders and the changes should be highlighted and explained. Major changes should be disseminated and may require a new round of training of healthcare workers and other relevant groups. If changes are made in national plans, all other pandemic plans in the country should be revised accordingly to ensure that the plans are in line with the national plan. The revised national plan can then be formally endorsed by the government and published.

C.S. Brown and M. Hegermann-Lindencrone

Focus Box 9.1. UK preparations for an influenza pandemic.

Professor Lindsey Davies CBE FFPH FRCP, President, Faculty of Public Health, London, UK

The UK has a population of approximately 61 million. Its four component countries (England, Scotland, Wales and Northern Ireland) have differing levels of devolved responsibility for health matters and increasingly divergent health and public health systems. Coordinated planning to protect the UK's population was challenging but was, ultimately, successful.

The UK government has taken pandemic influenza planning seriously for many years, publishing its first national plan in 1997. In 2005 this was revised and updated to provide a more detailed 'Influenza Pandemic Contingency Plan'. Written by the UK's four departments of health, advised by their health protection agencies, the plan drew attention to the potential impact of a pandemic and the risks it could pose. Although it acknowledged the need for all organizations to be ready to respond, the plan itself focused primarily on health service preparedness, emphasizing the importance of national stockpiles of vaccines, antiviral drugs, antibiotics and face masks in order to build resilience – an approach described as 'defence in depth'. The 2005 plan played an important role in raising awareness of the potential impact of a pandemic and of the need to prepare; it also enabled national officials to begin the complicated process of developing business cases, negotiating funding and procuring and storing the necessary supplies; and it stimulated the development of a suite of national communication materials to provide public information during a pandemic. It was clear, however, that implementation of the policy would not be straightforward: the resources required were substantial; prominent scientists and clinicians continued to challenge the underpinning evidence base and the conclusions drawn from it; health services had many other priorities; and the population was, largely, unconcerned. Recognizing that a dedicated national focus with strong leadership was required, the Department of Health for England appointed a National Director of Pandemic Influenza Preparedness (DPIP) to lead work across all four nations to develop and implement a revised strategy.

In 2006, a pandemic influenza preparedness programme, led by the DPIP, was set up to take the work forward. This was acknowledged to be one of the UK government's most complex programmes at the time, with work streams addressing science, policy development, implementation and procurement. The programme team expanded rapidly to a core of around 50 people from a range of disciplines and backgrounds including civil servants, management consultants, health and social care professionals and experts in information technology, communications and procurement. This systematic programme management approach enabled progress to be reviewed regularly and remedial action taken quickly when needed; it also enabled the strategy to be adapted in the light of experience and emerging evidence.

As robust national preparedness would require the active involvement of a wide range of interests, it was agreed that the existing 'health' strategy should be expanded to provide a framework for an integrated national response across all sectors, complemented by more detailed operational guidance where necessary. Lead officials from each relevant government department met regularly to review the developing strategy and to monitor national and local progress. The officials' group reported to a cross-government ministerial committee, ensuring that the strategic approach to influenza was integrated with other government policies. The active and explicit involvement, at every stage and in each work stream, of the Health Protection Agency, other professionals, managers and – where appropriate – the public, was key to the programme's success. The importance of engaging the voluntary and commercial sectors sector was also recognized: workshops and working groups were established to ensure that the new strategy addressed their concerns and enabled them to make their unique contributions to the response; and representatives from both sectors were involved in the programme's formal work programme.

Discussions with hospitals which had already made good progress with preparedness identified a number of ethical issues which they felt would be better resolved in advance than left to the judgement of individual clinicians and managers at a time of stress. Rather than leave these entirely for local resolution, with a risk of conflicting ethical advice from different organizations serving the same communities, a national Committee on the Ethical Aspects of Pandemic Influenza was established to develop ethical guidance to accompany the new strategy.

Consensus on the science was essential. Early agreement on the most contentious issues was achieved at a high-level colloquium, chaired by the Secretary of State for Health and involving leading national and international scientists and clinicians. New evidence and emerging scientific issues were addressed subsequently in the Scientific Pandemic Influenza committee

Continued

Focus Box 9.1. Continued.

(SPI) set up for that purpose. Once in place, SPI served as a forum for scientific debate and an independent, authoritative source of expert advice, stimulating research and openly acknowledging uncertainty where necessary. This encouraged professional and public confidence in the strategy itself. Similarly, a national clinical committee was established to consider and advise upon issues related to diagnosis, treatment and patient safety; and an expert surveillance group ensured plans for early identification and monitoring were developed and tested.

Careful attention was paid to ensuring that the plans would work in practice. The delivery of antiviral drugs to patients within 48 h of symptoms first arising was a key plank of the strategic response – but a way had to be found to achieve this without patients leaving their homes and infecting others. The 2005 proposal that a healthcare professional should visit every symptomatic patient at home, assess their condition and give them drugs if appropriate was quickly dismissed as impractical by those who would have to implement it. After detailed consultation, an innovative solution was proposed involving web- or telephone-based assessment for patients and designated distribution centres from which 'flu friends' would collect the necessary drugs. This added a further level of complexity to the programme, but resulted in a new system which can in the future be adapted for use in a range of emergency situations.

Robust preparedness relies upon every family and every organization, large or small, taking the pandemic threat seriously and making proportionate preparations. Nationally, a series of exercises was used to test the emerging plans and raise awareness in key players. Perhaps the most powerful of these was one held at an early stage in the development of the new strategy, when senior decision makers were asked to make real-time decisions based on existing resources and response capacity, rather than assuming an 'ideal' situation. The fragility of existing resilience quickly became apparent and preparations received a welcome new impetus – and in due course increased investment. The unexpected arrival in 2006 of a dead swan found to be infected with A(H5N1) in Scotland, on a day when there were no other notable media events, was also helpful in raising awareness: an influenza virus known to have the potential to kill humans had found its way to the UK and others could, presumably, follow.

In 2007, after wide national and international consultation, the UK's new National Framework for Pandemic Influenza Preparedness was finally published and implementation began in earnest. Detailed operational guidance was developed for individual countries, sectors and settings. Each local authority and NHS organization was required to develop its own plans, in line with the strategy and based on realistic – rather than idealistic – assumptions of the resources that would be available should a pandemic strike. The strong regional infrastructure then in place in England, complementing the well-established networks in the other three countries, enabled progress to be reviewed, experience shared and a national consensus reached on areas needing closer attention. Meanwhile, stockpiles of countermeasures were built and the technology to support the National Pandemic Flu Service (the 'Flu Line') was developed. Communication materials were refined and in 2008 a national campaign supported local activity to make good respiratory hygiene a habit.

What did we learn? Robust preparedness takes time, resources, diplomacy and determination. The active engagement of those who will have to implement the plans is essential. And openness and honesty – especially when there are no clear 'answers' – pay real dividends.

Sub-national planning

In general, national pandemic plans provide outlines of the different strategies that will be applied in a pandemic, e.g. for vaccination or the healthcare response, with the details being incorporated in separate, more operational, plans. Depending on how a country is organized administratively, operational plans may be developed at the national or sub-national level, e.g. by regional, local or municipal authorities, by different sectors and settings. National and sub-national operational plans should be based on the national pandemic plan and strategy.

The provision of planning templates or frameworks and planning assumptions by national authorities will facilitate sub-national planning, which will provide the details on how the healthcare services will be organized as well as details on business continuity of essential services outside the health sector, ranging from the provision of food and energy to funeral services and refuse collection. Local government plans should be developed in cooperation with private businesses where these are responsible for supplying essential services.

C.S. Brown and M. Hegermann-Lindencrone

Although the main policy decisions in the response to a pandemic are made by the central government, sub-national authorities will be implementing the decisions and may need to activate certain parts of the response earlier than in other parts of the country, as the pandemic may evolve at different rates in different parts of a country. Therefore, planning at sub-national level is fundamental to a successful response and these plans, too, need to be flexible to enable response to pandemics of varying severity. Sharing plans and collaboration on pandemic preparedness across regions and municipalities is important to streamline approaches as much as possible. Ideally, sub-national pandemic plans are formally audited against the national pandemic plan to make sure actions and strategies have been implemented and are in line with those defined at national level. Obligatory timelines and progress audits help ensure that planned sub-national responses do not vary or conflict and that no regions are significantly underprepared compared with their neighbours.

Members of the national planning committee have an important role in supporting sub-national pandemic planners, by providing technical assistance for the actual development of the plan and by providing training and exercises. In turn, inclusion of sub-national planners in national preparedness planning and in national exercises will improve the quality and feasibility of implementation of the national pandemic plan.

Communication and coordination

As described, pandemic preparedness involves a broad range of experts, stakeholders and sectors. Planning needs to be coordinated across these parties, as well as within stakeholder organizations at the national, sub-national and local levels; this requires robust communication mechanisms between governmental tiers (national, sub-national, local), between agencies, between sectors (e.g. human health and animal health), with healthcare workers and the public. Everyone must be aware of their roles and responsibilities in a pandemic and should be briefed on the content of the national pandemic plan as well as relevant sub-national plans. National pandemic plans should also be communicated to the international community, through publication on a ministry website, communication to WHO and through other international professional organizations for health.

Pandemic plans should describe how the pandemic plan will be activated if a pandemic is declared. During a pandemic, relevant ministries and sub-national governments will need situation updates (epidemiological, virological, impact on healthcare services' capacities, etc.) in order to take informed decisions regarding the interventions to be implemented. To prevent dissonance between technical epidemiological and virological risk assessments and the political aspects of risk management, it should be decided beforehand which means of communication will be used and which meetings of which stakeholders will be held during a pandemic.

Businesses and employee organizations should also be informed about the evolving situation and receive up-to-date guidance from the national level, e.g. on how to best protect employees.

The media needs to be involved in the pandemic planning process, to ensure they will be briefed as to the strategies that are planned to be implemented as well as the challenges that governments will face. This also allows them to ask any questions they may have about the national pandemic preparedness strategy. Countries should designate a national spokesperson for the media and hold regular press conferences during the pandemic. This ensures that the national authorities are the first to deliver messages and news about the pandemic. Communication channels should have the flexibility to scale up or down, depending on the situation; e.g. press conferences may be daily at the start of a pandemic and weekly later on, or ad hoc to announce the launch of measures such as the pandemic vaccination campaign. Last but not least, the opinions and concerns of the public and professionals should be monitored during a pandemic and responded to rapidly.

Command and control

The pandemic plan should describe the response that will be mounted at different stages of the pandemic, as this will be different according to whether cases have been detected in the country, whether the virus is spreading in the population, when pandemic activity peaks (by individual wave), whether healthcare services have become saturated, when the pandemic has passed its peak, or has been declared over. These stages may occur at different times within a country and pandemic plans must allow for the possibility to implement different measures at different times in different parts of the same country. This will increase the flexibility of the response.

The roles and responsibilities of all involved stakeholders at all levels, both in the planning process and in the response, need to be explicit in the national plan. It is important to decide beforehand which ministry or other authority will lead the response at national and sub-national levels and this may differ between countries and may also be influenced by the severity and impact of the pandemic. For example, the Ministry of Health may be in charge as long as the impact is restricted to the health sector but the Ministry of Emergencies or even the military may take overall leadership if there is widespread impact on non-health essential services. Typically, generic preparedness plans describe which command and control structures will be used. For pandemic preparedness, it should be considered whether the usual levels of autonomy of e.g. regions, cantons and municipalities will be allowed or overridden by central government. For example, if a certain region is affected by the pandemic worse than others, should decisions about response measures in that region (e.g. school closures) be autonomous or remain nationally coordinated?

Capacity and expertise

Capacity building is fundamental to good preparedness for a pandemic, or for any threat to public health. Education and training of staff to increase knowledge about pandemic influenza and raise awareness about pandemic preparedness and response is essential to effective pandemic preparedness planning. National and sub-national work can be supported at the international level by WHO and regional organizations, e.g. through country visits to assess pandemic preparedness and identify gaps (Fig. 9.1).

It is important to know the capacity of the healthcare sector, for example the number of hospital beds (adult, paediatric and intensive care unit), staff, stockpiles of medicines, essential equipment and personal protective equipment, and to have means to dynamically monitor these. Within each healthcare facility it has to be determined what the existing capacity can deal with and how additional capacity can be created, should it be necessary. Ways to raise capacity in a pandemic should be considered (staff, freeing up beds by cancelling elective surgery, stockpiling essential medicines, etc.). Appropriate channels also need to be in place for local tiers to feed back to regional and/or national levels when there are strains on capacity in healthcare facilities.

Planning for surge capacity is required at the national level but also at all levels of implementing pandemic plans across all sectors. Many services will need to operate on a 24/7 basis at least in the early stages of a pandemic. Doing this for many months is extremely demanding on the staff so possible solutions should be planned for in advance, e.g. working in extended shifts, recruiting on-call staff, etc. Surge capacity planning for staffing is required because of the increased number of persons requiring care and because of significant staff absenteeism, which can be expected in all sectors.

Evaluating the response to a pandemic

Evaluation of the response to a pandemic and subsequent pandemic plan revision should be an integral and mandatory part of any national pandemic plan. Research protocols to study the effectiveness of specific measures and interventions need to be prepared, agreed and funded beforehand for immediate re-activation during a pandemic. A methodology to evaluate the overall response should be developed and included as part of the national plan. Findings from national studies of the effectiveness of specific response measures should be shared internationally as soon as they become available for other countries to benefit from the findings. Likewise, national evaluations of the overall response to a pandemic are also useful for other countries to learn from.

9.3 International Cooperation and Coordination

An influenza pandemic is a global health event with even a mild pandemic having a negative impact on health and world economies. It is therefore an event of global as well as national concern. The IHR specifically mention a new subtype of influenza as being notifiable by a country to WHO (Article 6 Notification). For these reasons, pandemic preparedness requires international support and the response to a pandemic requires international coordination amongst global agencies including the WHO, United Nations Children's Fund (UNICEF), United Nations System Influenza Coordination (UNSIC), the Food and Agriculture Organization of the United Nations (FAO) and the World Organization for Animal Health (OIE). These organizations, as well as regional organizations such as the EU and its associated technical agencies (notably the European Centre for Disease

C.S. Brown and M. Hegermann-Lindencrone

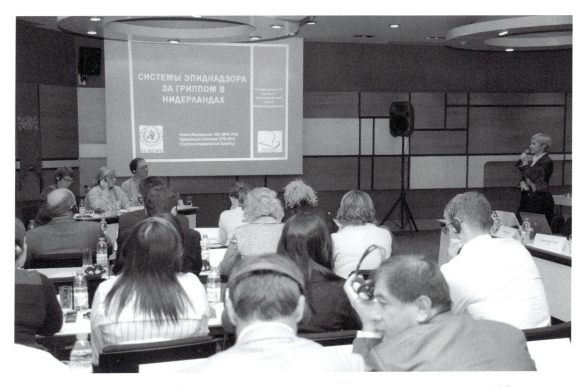

Fig. 9.1. From 2004 onwards the WHO has placed major emphasis on capacity building for pandemic influenza through international workshops and training events.

Prevention and Control (ECDC)) and the Association of Southeast Asian Nations (ASEAN), and donors such as the World Bank, the Bill & Melinda Gates Foundation, the United States Agency for International Development (USAID), the Asian Development Bank (ADB) and national development corporations, all have a role in supporting countries' pandemic planning and coordinating this support.

Before the 2009 pandemic, most countries based their pandemic plans on WHO guidance. Some consulted plans of neighbouring countries, or countries with similar social and economic development and structures. Countries, often facilitated by WHO and other international organizations, shared good practice and experience in pandemic preparedness planning with other countries and conducted inter-country exercises. These common activities contribute to the interoperability of pandemic plans. Knowing what a neighbouring country will implement in the response to a pandemic is also important if a different strategy will be employed compared to your own. An example is vaccination strategy: one country may plan to vaccinate the whole population while its neighbour decides to vaccinate risk groups, and another has resources to vaccinate only healthcare workers. Such policy differences can give rise to major problems if the borders between countries are relatively permeable. Knowledge and forewarning helps countries prepare their communication strategies, which will be needed to explain these differences to the public and other stakeholders.

In response to the 2009 pandemic, WHO took advice from the Emergency Committee established according to procedures under the IHR, from the Strategic Advisory Group of Experts (SAGE) on Immunization and from consultation with international networks of experts (in the field of public health, epidemiology, virology, clinical treatment, etc.), vaccine manufacturers, non-governmental organizations (NGOs), regional organizations and other stakeholders. Surveillance data and data on the impact of the pandemic were collected through notifications under IHR, and through the Global Influenza Surveillance and Response System (GISRS). In the 2009 pandemic, the GISRS proved to be crucial as only weeks after the pandemic A(H1N1)-pdm09 virus was identified and characterized, the WHO Collaborating Centre (CC) at the US Centers for Disease Prevention and Control (CDC), Atlanta, distributed rapid detection kits to all National Influenza Centres (NICs) globally. Throughout the pandemic, NICs continued to share viruses and data with the WHO CCs and WHO. Based on the above, recommendations and guidance were issued on surveillance, laboratory detection, clinical management of patients, deployment and use of vaccines, how to prevent spread of the disease, etc.

9.4 Pandemic Preparedness in the Next Interpandemic Period

The 2009 A(H1N1)pdm09 pandemic occurred between June 2009 and August 2010 and was the first for more than 40 years. Although it was mild in the majority of cases, the healthcare sector became overloaded in many countries, especially critical care facilities. Respiratory patients, severe cases and deaths were seen in different groups of the population compared with seasonal influenza, namely children, healthy adults, pregnant women and those with morbid obesity. Due to modern technology and the existence of well-developed health systems across the globe, the emergence, spread, severity and impact of the pandemic A(H1N1)pdm09 virus was tracked and studied in a detail that was not possible during previous pandemics. It gave the global community the opportunity to test pandemic plans and

to show how well prepared it was to respond to a pandemic.

Numerous evaluations at the country, regional and global level were undertaken following the pandemic and they showed that countries in general planned and prepared for the right things. An evaluation undertaken in the WHO European Region showed that pandemic preparedness activities were worthwhile and that they improved the response to the pandemic in 2009, 'the broad range of tasks and work streams undertaken as pandemic preparedness activities (e.g. exercises, capacity planning) being ultimately more important and influential than the Plan itself'. This indicates that while pandemic preparedness plans and supporting documents are important, the real advantage of pandemic preparedness planning is the broad involvement of stakeholders who become familiar with each other and with the required steps in pandemic response.

Notwithstanding, countries had in general prepared for a more severe pandemic than that in 2009, many having avian influenza A(H5N1) uppermost in mind; subsequently, scaling down of the response was needed. However some plans had been very detailed in describing the scenario and which measures would be implemented, and ultimately were not considered flexible enough.

When considering the level of preparedness at the global level required to respond to a severe pandemic, the review of the functioning of the IHR and WHO during the 2009 pandemic concluded that the world is ill prepared to respond to a more severe influenza pandemic. The need for specific plans addressing preparedness and response to an influenza pandemic and further strengthening pandemic preparedness thus remains.

- Key elements of national pandemic preparedness planning include: leadership; a coordinating framework (usually via a national multi-agency committee); flexibility and adaptability of arrangements; providing guidance and support for sub-national planning; communication and coordination; command and control; building capacity and expertise from national down to local level; exercises and simulations; evaluation of response.
- Although revealing problems and issues, national and international evaluations of the response to the 2009 pandemic overall suggest that the intensive pandemic planning undertaken since 2004 proved worthwhile.
- Areas of pandemic planning specifically identifiable as in need of improvement in the post-pandemic period include: increasing flexibility and adaptability of response at national level; planning for intensive care provision; communication with the public and healthcare workers, especially with regard to uncertainty and pandemic vaccines; and logistic arrangements for antiviral drugs and vaccines.

C.S. Brown and M. Hegermann-Lindencrone

Further Reading

Hashim, A., Jean-Gilles, L., Hegermann-Lindencrone, M., Shaw, I., Brown, C., Nguyen-Van-Tam, J.S. (2012) Did pandemic preparedness aid the response to pandemic (H1N1) 2009? A qualitative analysis in seven countries within the WHO European Region. *Journal of Infection and Public Health* 5(4), 286–296.

Nicoll, A. and Sprenger M. (2011) Learning lessons from the 2009 pandemic: putting infections in their proper place. *European Journal of Epidemiology* 26(3), 191–194.

World Health Organization (2005) International Health Regulations. Available at: http://www.who.int/ihr/9789241596664/en/index.html (accessed 9 April 2012).

World Health Organization (2011) Implementation of the International Health Regulations (2005) Report of the Review Committee on the Functioning of the International Health Regulations (2005) in relation to Pandemic (H1N1). Available at http://apps.who.int/gb/ebwha/pdf_files/WHA64/A64_10-en.pdf (accessed 9 April 2012).

World Health Organization and University of Nottingham (2011) Recommendations for good practice in pandemic preparedness: identified through evaluation of the response to pandemic (H1N1) 2009. Available at: http://www.euro.who.int/__data/assets/pdf_file/0017/128060/e94534.pdf (accessed 21 September 2012).

World Health Organization (2011) Two countries in the WHO European Region publish revised pandemic preparedness plans. Available at: http://www.euro.who.int/en/what-we-do/health-topics/communicable-diseases/influenza/news/news/2011/12/two-countries-in-the-who-european-region-publish-revised-pandemic-preparedness-plans (accessed 9 April 2012).

10 Emergency Preparedness and Business Continuity

Andy Wapling and Chloe Sellwood

NHS London, London, UK

- How does pandemic influenza preparedness differ from more standard emergency preparedness?
- What is the key aspect of pandemic preparedness planning?
- What is the biggest challenge to the health sector in planning for and responding to a pandemic?
- What is the role of business continuity planning (BCP) in pandemic preparedness?

10.1 Introduction

This chapter concerns emergency preparedness and business continuity in relation to pandemic influenza and answers the key questions 'why do we need to plan?' and 'why can't we just use existing systems and processes to manage the next pandemic?' Despite the recent 2009 pandemic, at the time of writing pandemic influenza remains the UK's highest risk on its National Risk Register. Planning for unique, rare or extreme events such as a pandemic provides a host of benefits to responders, organizations and patients. This chapter explains those benefits and provides a generic structure for planning.

In order to respond to a pandemic it is important that there is a structured and coordinated framework within which responders can operate safely and effectively. Critically this framework should reflect existing day-to-day systems. Improvising the response to a pandemic will only lead to a disorganized response and in turn people will suffer and lives may be lost. Additionally, without a framework to operate within, staff will face unnecessary stress and resources will be wasted as people and organizations try to serve their communities in an uncoordinated or haphazard way. It is therefore important that there is a concept of operations for organizations to follow in order to provide the best possible care for the most people during such events.

It is also important to ensure there is flexibility in the plan to allow for a number of variations in response. To be too prescriptive will mean that the plan doesn't quite match the incident and the responders will either feel constrained in their approach or the plan will be discarded, and there will be reversion to an improvised response. The skill therefore is to ensure that planning provides a suitably flexible framework that suits a range of scenarios whilst still providing the security of a structure in which to respond. Finally, it is important that technical information is available so that those who are making the decisions are informed and can apply scientific knowledge and rationale to the situation and the response as both evolve over time.

One of the greatest benefits of the planning process is not always the plan itself, but the journey taken and the exploration made in arriving at the plan. During the early days of pandemic planning, in the UK, the process was conceptually described as starting in a corridor with lots of doors leading off. Opening the first door led into another corridor full of even more doors; and one by one each door was opened and the challenges behind it understood and addressed before moving on to the next. The process of 'opening each door' or considering each aspect of planning (such as human resources (HR) issues, communicating with the public, clinical pathways, vaccine production and delivery) meant that organizations and above them whole governments travelled through a great learning experience which in turn provided a robust basis when responding to the challenge of a pandemic.

One of the largest challenges for the health sector in planning and responding to a pandemic is that effectively two types of incident must be managed concurrently. Not only is there an increase in patients with influenza and associated complications, but there may be fewer healthcare staff available to care for these patients, due to increased sickness absence. In addition, the same quantity of usual emergency cases (e.g. cardiac patients, road traffic injuries, obstetric patients, etc.) must still be managed with potentially fewer staff. No public service worker is immune from catching pandemic influenza at the start of the outbreak (unless they have received a pre-pandemic vaccine of the same strain; Chapter 15); therefore staff will be affected at the same or higher attack rate as the communities in which they live. With all these points in mind planning in the health sector should include details of responding to the increase in patients as well as incorporating business continuity plans to maintain critical services in the face of reduced staff. Both aspects are explored within this chapter.

10.2   Response Planning

The analogy of the corridor of doors goes some way to explaining the need for a structured process, as planning for a pandemic covers a vast spectrum of topics, everything from critical care to community pharmacies, communications to legal and ethical issues, and immunization during pregnancy to excess deaths; with each domain there may be multiple challenges to solve. Furthermore, with such a wide diversity of subjects to cover, a structured process is necessary to avoid becoming overwhelmed.

There are a few different planning models available but all incorporate some common key principles. These include the need for risk-based planning and proportionality; integration with existing systems and processes, and with partner organizations; and a mechanism of verifying the plan.

One of the most effective planning models is that espoused by the UK Cabinet Office (the UK government department responsible for managing the Government's function and cross-departmental policy), which, in line with the concept of integrated emergency management, provides a continual cycle of planning, review and revision. Good practice in emergency planning follows a continual eight-point

emergency preparedness cycle, which is repeated at intervals. There is one addition that is often made to this model and that is an initial action to 'assess'. It is important to fully understand the scientific and technical information about the scenario before a specific risk assessment can be undertaken. For pandemic influenza this is about understanding the nature of the virus, its virulence, how it is transmitted, how it presents as an illness, etc. A common planning cycle format is therefore shown in Fig. 10.1 and covered in detail in the following sections.

Assess

In order to accurately assess the risk and impact of a pandemic a good baseline knowledge of the hazard is required. A naïve understanding may over- or under-assess the impact and will result in either the planning being insufficient or an overreaction. Planners don't need to be an expert in every scenario but a good basic understanding as to the impact that each scenario is likely to have is important.

This is especially true with pandemic influenza as there are still many myths and misconceptions that could impede effective planning and response. Understanding how the virus is spread will affect delivery of interventions such as antiviral medication and vaccines, while an understanding of the likely clinical presentations will affect which part of the health service will require bolstering and can facilitate directed planning in advance. This research enables planners to fully understand what they are dealing with so that they can accurately assess the potential impact and plan accordingly. This process should be included in the cycle and revisited on a regular basis as science and evidence change and it is important that understanding of the hazard is reviewed and current. Individuals may undertake this research by consulting with other organizations that provide expert advice on infectious diseases such as pandemic influenza; which will provide a sense check to the planner, as we don't always know what we don't know.

Risk assessment

Assessing the risk of a potential hazard is a fundamental aspect of emergency preparedness and response. Risk assessment needs to be

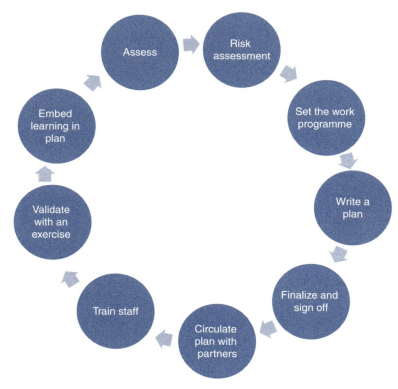

Fig. 10.1. The emergency planning cycle.

proactive and reactive, systematic and dynamic, and this section serves to describe the basic principles.

At its most basic, risk assessment is the process of assessing the impact of a specific scenario on the health of a population against the likelihood of it occurring. For example a meteor hitting the earth will have a huge impact on health, but the likelihood is very slim. Conversely, the impact of the common cold on population heath is minimal but the likelihood is substantial. A common matrix format can be used to assess and score the impact and likelihood from 1 to 5 as below:

Impact	Likelihood
1. Insignificant	1. Negligible
2. Minor	2. Rare
3. Moderate	3. Unlikely
4. Significant	4. Possible
5. Catastrophic	5. Probable

Working on a matrix of these scores, the two numbers can be multiplied to give an overall risk rating (Fig. 10.2). These overall risk ratings can then be prioritized; the greater the score the higher the risk, the more urgent attention required.

Note that although this approach encourages a somewhat mathematical approach to risk assessment within a broadly scientific framework, pandemic preparedness requires high-level political support (Chapter 9). The final risk assessment made at senior government level may also encompass risk assessments from both political and societal (public opinion) perspectives.

Set a work programme

A good understanding of the hazards and a comprehensive risk assessment will give the priority order for addressing the challenges. Thus the greatest risks should be given the most urgent attention and lower risks the least attention. For example,

A. Wapling and C. Sellwood

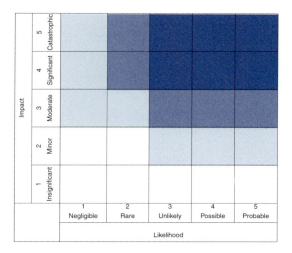

Fig. 10.2. Risk impact × likelihood matrix.

the risk of nursing staff being unavailable during a pandemic might be assessed as higher than the risk of running out of supplies of non-pharmaceutical countermeasures and so should be tackled first. However planning should not be a linear process and it may be necessary to have a number of projects under way in parallel; indeed this will be the best way to approach interrelated risks.

This is especially true for pandemic influenza planning as there are a number of high- and moderately high-risk areas of planning that need to be developed at the same time. This includes the need to work out how to distribute antiviral drugs to the eligible population, as well as vaccine once available. While they sound similar in delivery, operationally each of those areas will need a different delivery strategy.

It is therefore important that a comprehensive and realistic programme of planning activity is developed using the information gained from the 'assess' and 'risk assessment' processes. This programme should be agreed in association with partner organizations; planning together will make responding easier and more productive.

Write a plan

With a full and comprehensive work programme in place it is time to commit actions to paper and develop the plan. However, writing the plan is not always as easy as it sounds as it needs to have the right balance of structure, logic and practical information. The first rule is to write a document that anyone can pick up and use, without needing the author to decipher it. The plan also needs to be presented in a way that is easy to use in the real event. Few people are as interested in the details of the plan as its author and even when staff are engaged in the process, few will actually pick it up and read it from cover to cover in advance of the emergency.

The strength of a good plan is that it is structured, succinct, brief, easy to navigate and provides sufficient operational information to be workable in the event of the emergency. For example to simply state that the response will need the setting up of Antiviral Collection Points (ACPs), as were used in England in 2009/10, would be too little information for the users of the plan to understand operationally what is needed. Instead, there needs to be a section on ACPs, which would include some practical information on what is needed – for example, dedicated staff, physical security, Internet access, the need for a reordering process, documentation, etc.

The temptation can be to 'over plan', to try and structure the response too tightly. However experience shows that it is virtually impossible to accurately predict the exact course of events for each emergency. The plan needs to provide the right level of detail for the responders to inform their response, but not too much that the actual response does not fit with the emergency. There needs to be enough flexibility in the plan to allow users to deliver the response that is required for the emergency. Many organizations learnt this during the 2009 pandemic where plans had been based around a severe scenario (perhaps 1918-like or due to avian influenza A(H5N1)). The reality was somewhat different and where some had kept their plans suitably flexible, others hadn't, which meant that their plans were abandoned and users improvised the response as they went along.

A practical solution to this is that the emergency plan should contain a framework for response. There should be enough background information so that the responders have sufficient science to make informed decisions. It should include a command and control framework to manage the response, and a sufficient amount of operational options so that the responders can choose which to use depending on the incident and the issues it presents.

Finalize with executive-level sign off

It is important that there is top-level sign off and organizational ownership for the plan. It is right that the plan is owned by the organization and its senior officials, and not just the emergency planner or plan writer. This means that the executive team of the organization takes responsibility for the plan and should be taken to the Board for organizational sign off.

Circulate the plan with partners

No one organization will be able to respond to a pandemic in isolation. The impact of a pandemic is far reaching into all communities and in turn requires the response from a number of community-facing organizations. Plans from each organization should be shared so that all partners know what each other is planning to do and when, so as to inform their own response. Areas of potential conflict are also identified quickly.

This could be taken a step further through the development of joint inter-agency plans as was the case for London prior to the 2009 pandemic. At a local community level (each covering 200,000–250,000 residents), Influenza Pandemic Committees (IPCs) were convened under the chair of the local Director of Public Health. Membership included organizations such as the local authority, police, hospitals, mental health organizations, ambulance service, voluntary organizations and more. These committees developed local community plans which were truly inter-agency plans for inter-agency response. This approach was considered highly successful during the response to the A(H1N1)-pdm09 pandemic.

Train staff

Training people to respond to incidents and emergencies is of fundamental importance. Many organizations are geared to responding to routine, everyday challenges by following usual business practices; yet very few respond to major emergencies on a frequent basis. There is however an expectation that employees and teams will be able to pick up the pace and respond effectively to a challenging event. This demands practice. If staff are to respond to an emergency in a safe and effective manner they require the tools and skills to do so.

Once the plan is complete there is a need to undertake a training needs analysis to ensure that all relevant staff have the skills and abilities to undertake their role in an emergency. It would be negligent to place people in a position that they were not trained for in an emergency, not just to that member of staff but to the communities that they serve. For pandemic influenza this could be the need for more staff to have the skills to deliver vaccines, therefore it will be necessary to ensure that enough staff are trained in this technique and that these skills are maintained. Another may be that of media training. During the 2009 pandemic the media regularly sought interviews that the health service wanted to deliver as it was an excellent resource for reassuring the public and sharing key messages. Therefore maintaining a pool of media-trained staff is important. There are, however, many other examples of training needs for pandemic influenza.

Training should be ongoing, to ensure that skills are maintained. Not only do staff change jobs and organizations, but if the skills are not used on a regular basis then they are soon forgotten. Therefore an accurate list of who has had what training and when must be kept and a cycle of regular updates must form part of the training strategy. Without such monitoring, there is a substantial risk of loss of corporate memory and experience over time.

Validate the plan with an exercise

The plan needs some form of validation to ensure that it is fit for purpose and has been tested. To unleash an untested plan and newly trained staff on to the community in an emergency would be careless and neither the plan nor the response would stand up to any formal scrutiny, such as a public enquiry, following an emergency.

One of the best ways to validate a plan is through an exercise. An exercise also provides the ability to test possible concepts, strategies and solutions in an environment that is safe to make mistakes, without participants feeling scrutinized or threatened. The concept of exercises is discussed in detail in Chapter 11.

Ensure that the learning from the exercise is incorporated back into the plan

Before starting over, the last part of the cycle is embedding the learning from issues identified in the exercise back into the plan to inform practice. After every exercise, and indeed every time a plan is used for a real incident, there is a responsibility to ensure that those lessons identified are embedded back into the plan and training so that the lessons are learnt. Experience has shown that following significant incidents and subsequent legal processes, organizations will be asked if lessons identified in exercises informed the plan and response. Many organizations have been found wanting when the lessons have not been embedded into their plan and thus their response; and legal processes have in turn ruled these to be forms of corporate negligence.

Closing the loop

Emergency preparedness is a continual cyclical process, not simply writing the plan and leaving it until it is needed. It is important that the planning process is kept alive and always moving. Knowledge of a hazard will change, especially with things like pandemic influenza as we learn more or new potential pandemic threats emerge from the animal and bird kingdoms. Organizations change, people change and indeed populations change. Therefore planning must follow the cyclical process described and return to the first point and start over, to ensure organizational plans remain robust and current.

10.3 Business and Service Continuity

As identified at the start of this chapter, responding to a pandemic presents two challenges, that of responding to the incident in the management of increased numbers of sick people, but also to manage a response where organizations see an increase in staff absenteeism and potential disruption to services. Business continuity planning (BCP) is an essential business activity and should be a part of routine corporate responsibility for all types of commercial and public sector organizations. The basic principles of business continuity are outlined in this section and as with emergency planning follow a cyclical process.

The terms business continuity and service continuity can be used interchangeably. Business continuity

has traditionally been seen as a commercial function; however health and public sector organizations have a requirement to protect and ensure that critical services are maintained during disruptive events.

The UK national model for business continuity (BS25999) sits as part of a suite of British Standards and information on this is readily available online. This standard applies to all types of organization, including healthcare providers. The cyclical process follows four steps, which are described in detail over the following paragraphs:

1. Understanding your business.
2. Determining your business/service continuity strategy.
3. Developing and implementing business/service continuity management response.
4. Exercising, maintaining and reviewing.

Understanding your business

Some would argue that this is the most important aspect of business continuity management as it really drills down into the details of the organization. This process helps to make overt the interdependencies and core functions and services of organizations.

This aspect starts by identifying the organization's objectives, purpose and vision; the stakeholders and the organization's obligations to these; and any statutory functions and duties. Basically, what does the organization do and for whom? What is essential for the delivery of the organization? The second part in this action is to look at the services of the organization in relation to the above and identify the assets, staff and resources required to deliver these, including those external interdependencies. This is to identify what is needed in staff, buildings and hardware to deliver core functions and services.

As with emergency planning, a risk assessment needs to take place. In addition to identifying hazards related to the delivery of service (e.g. risk of flooding and risk of IT failure), the risks associated with the loss of one or all of these services needs to be assessed. If a disruptive event occurred, what services need to be bought back online sooner than others? Where should efforts be directed first? For example in the health service, emergency surgery should receive more attention for restoration than non-urgent outpatient activity.

For some organizations the greatest risk could be that of loss of reputation or confidence, which is just as important for healthcare organizations as it is for finance and retail. For the health service, this could be the risk of failure to provide emergency and life-saving services. Following the business continuity process will help to identify and assess the impact and consequences of a failure to deliver services. It will also help to identify the risks associated with a geographical location as well as the risk to reputation should an organization fail to deliver a core service.

All this information is then used to undertake a business impact assessment (BIA) which prioritizes the core or key services which need to be restored or protected from disruption. A competent BIA will also provide the recommended restoration time-frames for each key service so that during a disruptive challenge, those working to bring about normality will know at a glance which services should be brought back by when and what resources this will require. This can be broken down into timeframes, for example those in Table 10.1. It also provides a list of those services that are of lesser priority from where staff and resources can be diverted to maintain key services. This process also provides the framework to identify those services which cannot be disrupted under any circumstance, such as critical care, thereby providing the evidence base for the organization to invest time and resources to ensure disruption does not occur, within reasonably foreseeable circumstances.

Determining your business/ service continuity strategy

Once critical services have been determined, it is important to identify if there is a way to reduce or mitigate the risks associated with this service. An example could be a function that is very IT dependent, such as medical imaging; therefore

measures to ensure continuation of IT networks and computers would be a priority. Provision of uninterrupted power supplies on key equipment may be a less expensive solution compared to the risk of outright power failure. Another example would be a staff-intensive process that requires a number of specifically trained staff. This may necessitate the training of additional staff in advance so as to create a wider pool of people to call upon if there are sickness-induced shortages. An example of this is staff who can vaccinate. A larger pool of trained vaccinators will prove valuable in a pandemic in order to be able to deliver the population vaccine while coping with an increase in staff sickness. Any mitigating actions should then be reflected in the risk assessment as this could decrease the likelihood and will most certainly reduce the impact.

For a business/service continuity strategy to be effective it requires a structure and governance arrangement that ensures that the organization owns and accepts the risks to service delivery and the mitigating actions for this. Additionally, senior-level support will allow funds to be directed to preserve those business critical areas. In healthcare organizations an effective way to achieve this is through nominating an executive director to hold the business continuity portfolio and represent this on the organization's board. This provides top-level buy in and a mechanism to get the strategy and mitigation actions on to the board agenda.

Developing and implementing business/ service continuity management response

A management plan for the response to a disruptive event is a key part of the business continuity management strategy. Having understood the business and taken mitigating actions, it is important that arrangements are in place for responding to and effectively managing the restoration to normality from a disruptive event.

This plan clearly needs to be led by the BIA to identify which services need to maintained throughout or be restored most promptly, in which order, with which staff and what equipment/hardware is required. A framework to manage the response can then be produced with this information that identifies who will lead the response and how communication with service users and stakeholders will be maintained.

Many organizations have local service-level recovery plans, which provide practical information on

Table 10.1. Business impact assessment template.

Recovery time	Service	Staff	Hardware
1 hour			
1 day			
1 week			
1 month			
6 months			
1 year and over			

how the local service will be maintained or restored in a disruptive event. These are then pulled together with an overarching strategic organizational plan, which sets out how the organization as a whole will manage its recovery and restoration. This is likely to be run by an executive incident team, which is there to provide the strategic leadership and prioritization, and to support local service teams in their recovery.

Exercising, maintaining and reviewing

As discussed in the first part of this chapter there is a need to validate plans and test the response. One of the most effective methods to do this is through exercises. These help staff and organizations to walk through the plans and identify any issues that require solutions. These useful activities help identify all the little things that are not thought about in the planning stage, but which come to light when the system is tested. Exercises need to be held regularly so that plans are up to date, relevant and alive to the organization.

Once exercised and validated the business continuity strategy and response plan needs to be signed off by the executive board so that it is owned by the organization at the most senior level. As with emergency planning it is then important to go back to the beginning and start the process again by reviewing the organizational aims, purpose and key activities – to ensure that the plan reflects the organizations and hazards.

10.4 Summary

Pandemic influenza presents a global public health emergency that, if severe, will impact on most organizations and businesses. Robust and embedded emergency preparedness and business/service continuity management processes are essential components of an organization's ability to respond to a range of challenges from flooded premises, industrial action and loss of IT networks, through to global incidents such as a pandemic. Through thoroughly understanding the hazard and undertaking the process of reviewing and writing plans, coupled with training, testing and exercising (Chapter 11), organizations are able to respond to the best of their ability, with the best possible outcome for their population, partners and other stakeholders.

- Pandemic preparedness addresses a 'rising tide' event that lasts over an extended period of time with little scope for mutual aid, whereas more standard emergency plans are aimed at 'big bang' events where the duration of the incident is likely to be short-lived and mutual aid is more likely to be available.
- Flexibility in planning a response is the most important aspect of pandemic preparedness to ensure that responders can meet the challenges of the real event.
- Pandemic preparedness and response in the health sector effectively considers two types of incident that must be managed concurrently. Not only is there an increase in patients with influenza and associated complications, but there may be fewer staff available due to increased sickness absence. The same number of emergency cases (e.g. cardiac patients, road traffic injuries, obstetric patients, etc.) must still be managed, with potentially fewer staff.
- An influenza pandemic will affect all sectors of society over an extended period of time. The impact of such extended interruption should be considered through generic BCP in the first instance. Issues that cannot be addressed through BCP should then be considered individually.

Further Reading

British Standards Institution (2012) BS25999/BS ISO22301: Business Continuity. Available at: http://shop.bsigroup.com/en/Browse-by-Subject/Business-Continuity/?t=r (accessed 21 September 2012).

Cabinet Office (2006) Chapter 5 Emergency Planning. Available at: http://www.cabinetoffice.gov.uk/sites/default/files/resources/ep_chap_05.pdf (accessed 1 April 2012).

Cabinet Office (2006) Chapter 6 Business Continuity Management. Available at: http://www.cabinetoffice.gov.uk/sites/default/files/resources/ep_chap_06.pdf (accessed 1 April 2012).

Kuster, S.P., Shah, P.S., Coleman, B.L., Lam, P.P., Tong, A., Wormsbecker, A. and McGeer, A. (2011) Incidence of influenza in healthy adults and healthcare workers: a systematic review and meta-analysis. PLoS One 6(10), e26239.

London Emergency Services Liaison Panel (2012) LESLP Manual – Eighth Edition. Available at: http://www.leslp.gov.uk/docs/major_incident_procedure_manual_8th_ed.pdf (accessed 21 September 2012).

NHS London (2010) Review of the London health system response to the 2009/10 influenza A/H1N1 pandemic. Available at: http://www.london.nhs.uk/webfiles/Emergency%20planning%20docs/NHSL_FLU_REPORT_WEB.pdf (accessed 1 April 2012).

A. Wapling and C. Sellwood

11 The Role of Exercises in Pandemic Preparedness

JOHN SIMPSON

Health Protection Agency, Porton Down, UK

- What are the main types of exercises that can be used in pandemic influenza preparedness?
- Why is it important that health sector pandemic influenza exercises involve partner organizations?
- Why is time a problem in the design of pandemic influenza exercises?
- Why has the development of 'off-the-shelf' exercises been important in pandemic influenza preparedness?

11.1 Background to the Role of Exercises in Pandemic Preparedness

The UK has been very prominent internationally in using exercises to test and develop pandemic preparedness. It is therefore impossible to avoid such emphasis in this section; however the underlying principles of exercises and exercise design are similar for all jurisdictions and their value in pandemic preparedness has been firmly established. Nevertheless, the way services in the health sector and in related government departments operate and relate to each other may vary considerably from country to country. This section is not a detailed discussion of the operational aspects of running pandemic influenza exercises but is intended to give the reader an understanding of how exercise methodologies can be used to develop and improve pandemic response.

For centuries military doctrine has stated that exercises (the use of simulated battle situations where troops and material are deployed on 'practice' manoeuvres) are a crucial part of the training and development of a military force. Philip of Macedon (reign: 359–336 BC), father of Alexander the Great, was a keen advocate of this system, and his considerable military success is partially attributed to the thorough training of his armies. Military exercises can be used to test the operational aspects of a military unit but almost as importantly they can be used to test operational planning status and the command and control structure of a force.

Today the military and some other front-line responding services such as Fire and Rescue Services spend a considerable amount of time (over 50% in some services) exercising and training, and this has become an accepted and funded part of their work pattern. One of the main reasons for this is that through exercising activities repeatedly, staff can follow protocols and operate equipment in high-pressure, real-event situations in an efficient and effective manner. Exercises are an important part of the emergency planning cycle (Chapter 10 and Fig. 10.1), being an important tool to assess what has been learnt from training and to identify components of a response that can be rectified by amending plans or service configuration.

In the healthcare sector the concept of specifically designing and running exercises to examine and explore the plans drawn up for and the responses to emergency situations, either manmade (e.g. deliberate release of a toxic material) or natural (e.g. an influenza pandemic), is relatively recent. In the UK most exercises prior to 2001 were small scale and conducted within hospitals or ambulance services, which have a statutory responsibility to exercise annually. In general, healthcare services (apart from the ambulance services) were not routinely involved in large-scale multi-agency civil response exercises held up until the late 1990s.

After the events of 9/11 and the anthrax letters of autumn 2001 in the USA, there was a significant shift in thinking as it became apparent that a well-trained and practised healthcare service response would be crucial to optimizing the response to a deliberately released biological organism, noxious chemical or an explosive device containing the above. Therefore further funding was made available in the UK for the design and running of exercises to develop healthcare responses to deliberate release incidents. The early exercises were successful, although some work was needed to convince clinicians and healthcare managers that these activities were a good use of staff time. When severe acute respiratory syndrome (SARS) appeared in 2003, exercises were requested to assess how healthcare systems could respond to this threat. The success of exercises has made them an increasing part of the emergency preparedness and response culture in the UK healthcare system. Designing exercises to explore the operation of pandemic influenza plans began in 2003, coinciding with an increase in the pace of pandemic preparedness activities, as influenza A(H5N1) re-emerged in South-east Asia.

The underpinning rationale for performing exercises in a healthcare context is to:

- create multi-agency links with relevant non-healthcare organizations;
- clarify roles and responsibilities between agencies and between tiers within organizations (e.g. primary and secondary care);
- identify lessons and gaps in capability that can then be rectified;
- improve preparedness and response to health protection emergencies;
- reinforce training and identify training gaps.

Pandemic preparedness addresses a 'rising tide' event that lasts over an extended period of time with little scope for mutual aid, whereas more standard emergency preparedness plans are aimed at 'big bang' events where the duration of the incident is likely to be short lived (although the full response may take longer); in the latter case, mutual aid is more likely to be available and is indeed considered to be a normal part of the UK healthcare response.

Although healthcare exercises are clearly a vital part of pandemic preparedness, it would be incorrect to suggest that these should occur in isolation of other sectors. Pandemic influenza is rightly regarded as a whole-of-society emergency that generates many non-health issues (e.g. business continuity and maintenance of essential services) and it requires a coordinated multi-sectoral approach (Chapters 9 and 10).

11.2 Types of Exercise

There are three main types of exercise design that can be used in healthcare settings and examples of each with respect to pandemic influenza are discussed in this chapter. Rather like the three main types of epidemiological study, where each in turn is more appropriate for answering some types of questions than others, these three exercise designs are each best suited for testing different elements of pandemic response. They also vary in the resources needed to run them and the choice of exercise is important: it should provide the most appropriate and cost-effective way of achieving its aim and objectives.

One of the most important issues when organizing an exercise is to be very sure of the aims and objectives of the activity, i.e. what responses or functions are to be tested? This then allows the design of an appropriate and targeted exercise. A poorly designed and run exercise represents an expensive mistake that is often avoidable, and one of the commonest mistakes is not having clear aims and objectives.

Desktop exercises

'Desktop exercises' (DTXs), or 'table top exercises' (TTXs) as they are also known, are a very cost-effective and efficient method of testing plans, procedures and people; they are so named because they can literally be played sitting around a desk or table. Players from the participating agencies assemble in one place for a typical period of one or two days and play out in theory what would happen in practice, using specially designed scenarios. They are difficult to run with large numbers (150 people is a sensible maximum), but those players who are involved are provided with an excellent opportunity to interact with, and understand, the roles and responsibilities of the other teams and agencies taking part. A DTX can engage players imaginatively and generate high levels of realism. Participants will gain familiarity with key procedures along with the people with whom they may be working in an emergency, in a realistic fashion. Those who have exercised together and know each other will provide a much more effective response than those who come together for the first time when an incident occurs. An element of 'media play' (rehearsing under pressure, what would be communicated to the media) can be introduced under controlled conditions, and this creates a lot of interest and realism, as well as pressure on participants.

The aims and objectives of many pandemic influenza exercises have concerned not only testing plans at various healthcare service command and control levels, but also looking at how healthcare plans integrate with partner agencies' plans, and consequently DTXs are often the most appropriate format of exercise to use. Depending on the complexity of the plans being tested and the number of agencies involved, some pandemic influenza DTXs have a complex structure of inter-agency relationships between organizational teams (called 'syndicates' in exercise terminology) and require careful planning and skilled facilitation. Where multiple agencies are involved, a multi-room venue is often best; this allows space for individual agencies to debate and formulate decisions in private, yet the proximity to other syndicates to facilitate 'exercise play'. An example is given in Fig. 11.1.

Because demand for pandemic influenza DTXs rapidly outstripped the number of skilled exercise facilitators available, 'off-the-shelf' packages have now been produced. These packages have instructions on how to design and manage a simple DTX, sets of injects (questions to be answered or situations to be introduced during the course of the exercise) and DVD clips to introduce and move on the exercise play. These allow organizations to adopt a 'do-it-yourself' approach, and have proven very popular; one such package in the UK has been used by over 70 healthcare organizations. Some of these packages are freely available from the World Health Organization (WHO).

Command post exercises

In a command post exercise (denoted CPX), the organizations or teams (including communications teams) from each participating organization are positioned at the actual command post locations or 'duty stations' they would use during a real incident. This tests communication arrangements and, more importantly, information flows between remotely positioned teams within participating organizations. A CPX is usually more realistic than a DTX because flaws in communications and information technology are readily exposed.

CPXs are also especially good at examining how geographically distant organizations will communicate with each other (particularly important in pandemic response); they are also very useful in

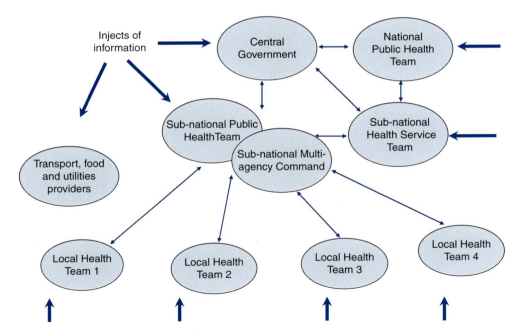

Fig. 11.1. Example of a desktop exercise (DTX) syndicate structure (note that an inject is a piece of information deliberately given to some or all exercise participants (players) to stimulate activity or force decisions to be made).

testing data flows and the assembly of information for surveillance and reporting, although this requires considerable work in preparing 'dummy' data to test the systems. There have been a large number of international CPXs that have explored cross-jurisdiction communication, especially in the early stages of a pandemic, and with further refinement of pandemic phases this may need re-examination.

Live exercises

Live exercises (or LiveEx) involve deploying staff and assets in live play, and range from a small-scale test of one component of a response, e.g. evacuation (ranging from a building or 'incident' site to an affected community), through to a full-scale test of the whole organization's response to an incident, e.g. pandemic influenza. Live exercises provide the best means of confirming the satisfactory operation of emergency communications, and the use of 'casualties' can add to the realism.

Whilst large-scale live exercises to test the response to an avian influenza incident might be possible, testing a response to pandemic influenza in this way is not practical. However, live tests of individual components of the overall response have been undertaken in many countries. Examples of live exercises undertaken include looking at how hospital infection control procedures would work during an influenza pandemic, how a port health system would operate at an airport, and assessing the most efficient mode of distributing antiviral medication through a mass prophylaxis centre.

'Complex' exercises

Because of the severe societal issues raised by an influenza pandemic, many countries have held large, complex exercises to test their national influenza pandemic plan, using two or even all three of the above modalities to test the plan's operability on a nationwide basis (looking at the coordination of local, regional and national response). Such exercises are difficult and expensive to design and run, but are valuable in showing players including senior officials and government ministers how a pandemic might be managed and some of the complexities and nuances of the response needed. They are probably not the best starting option for governments and organizations who are new to or inexperienced in conducting exercise.

One such exercise held in the UK in 2007, called Exercise Winter Willow, was the largest healthcare response exercise in the UK since the end of the Cold War. With over 5000 participants from the local healthcare providers to the ministerial level, this exercise tested the command and control structures in the UK and helped identify areas for further planning. Operation Cumpston 06 took place in Australia in 2006 to test pandemic response, and was the largest civil exercise undertaken in that country. Examples (and note that these are illustrative examples and not an exhaustive list) of major pandemic specific issues that can be explored using exercises are:

- command, control and decision making by officials and ministers;
- healthcare system response;
- use of public health measures;
- ports and border issues;
- pharmaceutical countermeasures, including supply chain issues;
- vaccine availability and prioritization;
- simultaneous high-level sickness absence in all employment sectors;
- loss of key staff;
- food, fuel and power shortages/outages;
- infection control measures and use of protective equipment;
- civil disorder and panic;
- loss of mass transportation systems; and
- assistance to 'home' citizens stranded overseas.

11.3 Potential Problems in the Design of Pandemic Influenza Exercises

Interaction with expert advice

Pandemic influenza is a complex subject and most people who are involved in exercise planning and design are generally more experienced in scenario writing and developing exercises that look at the response to major acute events and are not usually influenza experts. It is therefore important to obtain advice and work closely with subject matter experts to provide relevant and challenging scenarios for the exercises; policy makers are often best placed to point out the areas of known concern and highlight areas where testing is most needed. Likewise, technical experts in pandemic influenza must engage with exercise design teams to make the best of their specialist skills to create realistic scenarios. For example, without an expert understanding of the medical science and policy aspects of human A(H5N1) vaccines, a generic exercise planner would have great difficulty in designing an exercise that tested critical decision making points regarding their potential deployment; and an exercise scenario based on a theoretical A(H7N3) pandemic virus would by definition rule out exercise play involving A(H5N1) vaccines. This example reinforces the need for careful definition of the aims and objectives.

Time dimensions

An influenza pandemic wave may last 3–4 months in any given country and in general exercises can only be run in a healthcare setting for one or two days due to staff availability. This (and the impossibility of providing meaningful exercise play lasting several months) means running an exercise exploring the whole pandemic response in real time is not an option. When exercises were first designed to look at pandemic influenza response in the UK in 2006, there was a great emphasis on pre-pandemic to early pandemic activity. As confidence in the response to these phases increased, exercises progressed to focus on peak activity, with an emphasis on business continuity, or on the recovery phase. There was also more emphasis on how certain parts of the system would respond in detail, for example exercises to test the pharmaceutical supply chain. Therefore various different designs have been developed so response across a pandemic wave can be explored. Three of these are discussed in detail as follows.

The time block method

In this design the exercise is broken into three or more time blocks, each of which looks at issues that need to be addressed on a single day in the pandemic response. Often in a three-block design there have been blocks looking at: the early stages of the pandemic; the peak of the pandemic; and the recovery phase. Each block usually lasts 2–3 h and it is important that before each block starts all players are certain where they are in respect to the pandemic timeline. This requires careful 'pre-loading' (i.e. building up the scenario or the story) using written materials and the use of pre-recorded DVD footage; for example, using simulated news broadcasts to 'set' players' minds to the correct time. The majority of DTXs looking at pandemic influenza response use this methodology.

Running for half a day or 1 day per week over multiple weeks

In this methodology each session explores a half-day or whole day in the pandemic response each week for say 8 to 12 weeks. This gives a very good sense of the protracted length of the response needed with respect to pandemic influenza and is achievable in a CPX format. It does however require considerable resources to design and run; also considerable commitment from participating organizations because of the need to release staff from their normal duties to play the exercise for such an extended period.

Running for 2 to 4 days in real time, playing out part of 1 week of the response

This again is suitable for CPX format and was the methodology for Exercise Winter Willow in 2007. It gives some idea of the intensity, complexity and need for sustainability in the response to an influenza pandemic and is more easily achievable than 1 day per week for up to 3 months.

Scene setting

Pandemic influenza exercises need data on attack rates, morbidity and mortality rates, sickness absence and hospitalization, etc. in order to make the exercise scenarios plausible and challenging. Many pandemic influenza exercises are therefore built around a mathematical model, which can provide these data. In the UK the model often used is a simplified model with a single pandemic wave, which gives a good approximation of real data but is easy and quick to run (most 'full function' planning models are difficult to use and take a significant time to produce data).

11.4   Lessons Identified

One of the major reasons for running an exercise is to identify gaps in plans and capabilities that can then be reported to the relevant organizations and authorities for remedies to be devised, thus allowing continuation of the emergency planning cycle (Fig. 10.1). It is important that any exercise is evaluated fully and a report written and disseminated; there are many detailed methodologies for analysing the outcome of exercises, but these lie outside the scope of this book. It is important that the lessons are reported against the aims and objectives as the aims in a large CPX will be very different from those of a small live exercise looking at infection control on a ward. This is one of the reasons why setting accurate, realistic and achievable aims and objectives is so important in exercise design. It is also important to have follow-up activity after exercises (6 months later) to ascertain whether lesson identified have been followed up by changes in policy and procedure.

Some generic lessons from pandemic influenza exercises performed by the Health Protection Agency in the UK and overseas that informed planning and response during the A(H1N1)pdm09 pandemic include:

- Increased communication between healthcare and non-health agencies at all levels is essential. Regular contact between the sectors at local, regional, national and international levels will facilitate better working in an emergency.
- The cooperation within and between local, regional and national organizations should be developed and improved. There should be a clear chain of command and communication from top down (national to local level) and bottom up (local to national level).
- Further consideration is needed on the burial of the dead and school closures during a pandemic.
- International cooperation towards rapid development and production of a pandemic strain vaccine and its dissemination is key.
- There is a lack of detailed guidance available on the recovery phase of a pandemic; plans focus primarily on the preparedness and response phases of a pandemic without much consideration to how 'a return to normality' might be achieved. Many organizations are unclear about their

priorities at the end of a pandemic. This is not surprising, as it is difficult to predict what position they will be in or what resources will be available. The impact on business continuity, particularly of the healthcare service, is likely to be prolonged and severe. However, the demand for services to return to normal as quickly as possible following a pandemic is likely to be considerable.

11.5 Testing Revised Pandemic Plans in the Post-pandemic Period

During the 2009 pandemic, pandemic influenza plans were put into operation at national, regional, local and service level. Many lessons have been identified within these levels as well as at international level (e.g. European Commission). These have fed into a 'second generation' of revised pandemic plans; for example, in late 2011 the UK published an updated plan incorporating lessons from the pandemic. Such new plans (especially areas encompassing a major change of strategy or approach) now need to be tested using exercises.

11.6 Summary

A future influenza pandemic poses one of the greatest infectious disease threats to mankind, especially if severe.

Planning for the response to pandemic influenza has been important in the evolution of civil exercises. Such exercises are now considered an integral and acceptable element of pandemic preparedness in many countries. Novel methodologies have been developed to cope with the particular scientific challenges of the pandemic response.

- There are three main types of exercises that can be used towards pandemic preparedness: desktop or table top exercises, command post exercises and live exercises.
- Pandemic influenza could generate many non-health issues (e.g. business continuity issues due to high levels of staff absence). The whole-of-society effect means exercises are much more valuable when they explore a coordinated, multi-agency approach.
- The extended length of time of an influenza pandemic wave means real-time exercising is appropriate only for exploring issues over a small part of the pandemic event. To address this, methodologies have been developed to allow coherent play across the time span of a pandemic wave such as the time block methodology.
- There has been a great demand for exercises to explore pandemic influenza responses. The limited number of expert staff available cannot design and run exercises for every organization that wishes to run them, and have needed to concentrate on designing the more complex exercises with a wide scope. An 'off-the-shelf' package, designed by a specialist unit, allows organizations to run a more simple exercise design using their own staff resources and expertise.

Further Reading

Australian Government Department of Health and Ageing (2007) National Pandemic Influenza Exercise. Exercise Cumpston 06 Report. Available at: http://www.flupandemic.gov.au/internet/panflu/publishing.nsf/Content/cumpston-report-1 (accessed 21 September 2012).

British Standards Institution (2012) BS ISO 22398 Societal security – Guidelines for exercising and testing. Available at http://shop.bsigroup.com/en/ProductDetail/?pid=000000000030242445 (accessed 1 April 2012).

Cabinet Office (2007) Exercise Winter Willow Lessons Identified. Available at: www.cabinetoffice.gov.uk/ukresilience/pandemicflu/exercises.aspx (accessed 1 April 2012).

European Commission (2006) Exercise Common Ground, Final Report. Available at: http://ec.europa.eu/health/ph_threats/com/common.pdf (accessed 1 April 2012).

European Commission (2010) Assessment Report on the EU-wide Response to Pandemic (H1N1) 2009 Covering the period 24 April 2009 – 31 August 2009 (excluding vaccine policy issues). Available at: http://ec.europa.eu/health/communicable_diseases/docs/assessment_response_en.pdf (accessed 1 April 2012).

Phin, N.F., Rylands, A.J., Allan, J., Edwards, C., Enstone, J.E. and Nguyen-Van-Tam, J.S. (2009) Personal protective equipment in an influenza pandemic: a UK simulation exercise. *Journal of Hospital Infection* 71(1), 15–21.

12 Local Health Service Responses to A(H1N1)pdm09 Pandemic Influenza

Martyn Regan[1] and Chris Packham[2]

[1]Health Protection Agency (East Midlands), Nottingham, UK;
[2]Nottingham City Primary Care Trust, Nottingham, UK

- What are the challenges to a local pandemic response?
- What were the key local functions of the initial response phase in the UK?
- What were the key aspects of the UK's treatment phase?
- How was primary and community care supported during the pandemic?

12.1 Introduction

The A(H1N1)pdm09 pandemic virus emerged in Mexico in early 2009 and rapidly spread globally, causing mild or asymptomatic disease in the majority of cases in Europe, but severe illness and death in a small proportion (Chapter 7). In the UK, the first cases were confirmed on 27 April and over the subsequent 10 months until the UK response was stood down in February 2010, an estimated 330 deaths and almost 2 million clinical cases had occurred, with 1.2 million doses of antiviral medication and 5.5 million doses of vaccine administered over the same period. In August 2010 the World Health Organization (WHO) officially declared the A(H1N1)pdm09 pandemic over.

In describing the course of the pandemic response at a local level (the East Midlands region of the UK) (Fig. 12.1), we have divided the sections to describe what actually had to be done in different parts of the health service, reflecting underlying differences in health service structure across the region. This is likely to be the case in almost all health services worldwide, demonstrating that pandemic response 'on the ground' needs to be tailored not only to the characteristics of the infectious agent and the population's response to it, but also the realities of health service delivery – who actually interacts with who, where this takes place and when.

12.2 A Local Response: City of Nottingham, UK

Healthcare systems worldwide will have variable preparedness for emergency and untoward incidents or prolonged events. In the UK, there is a long-standing well-developed health protection planning process in the context of a national health service (NHS) that is state-funded, and, for citizens, free of significant charges at points of delivery; furthermore, responses to major infectious disease challenges are regularly planned (Chapter 10) and rehearsed through exercises (Chapter 11). As such, when the 2009 pandemic commenced, most health organizations were ready to respond, and existing emergency plans made it possible to mobilize additional staff and providers rapidly. The local response was always operationally focused – concerned with how things actually got done. The strategy regarding what was required in terms of antiviral drugs, vaccination schedules, risk groups, and reporting and surveillance, was nationally defined. Local services were responsible for enacting the response throughout the two phases in the UK.

Assessment, surveillance and containment phase

At the onset of the pandemic in the UK, there was little evidence about the severity and impact of the virus, so the initial focus was on treating affected individuals and reducing the spread of the disease.

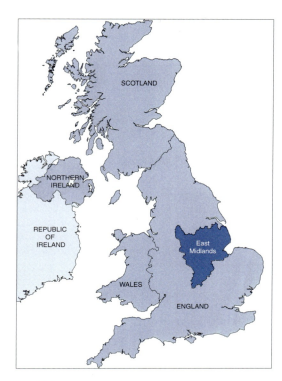

Fig. 12.1. Map of the United Kingdom of Great Britain and Northern Ireland showing the East Midlands region. (Kindly provided by Bruce McKenzie.)

An additional priority was data collection to assist in national epidemiological and clinical assessment. At a local level, this phase also saw the NHS prepare intensively for handling potential surges in primary care and hospital demand later in the year. By late June 2009, sustained community transmission of the A(H1N1)pdm09 virus was clearly established with an initial epidemic wave peaking in late July 2009, then declining once school summer holidays started. Clinically, the infection appeared to cause a mild illness in most cases, but with higher-risk groups emerging, and in contrast to patterns of morbidity and mortality seen with seasonal influenza, evidence of protective immunity in older groups (those born before 1957). The UK Health Protection Agency (HPA) (the UK's public health authority, with around 5000 personnel) played a key role during this phase, with the heaviest NHS impact falling on primary care services. The key aims during this phase were to rapidly detect and respond to suspected cases and prevent further transmission within the community using antiviral drug treatment and prophylaxis for close

family contacts, using nationally defined guidance and case management algorithms. Alongside this focus there was clearly an opportunity, and a need, to capture and share intelligence on the clinical epidemiology of A(H1N1)pdm09 to guide and inform further local and nationally coordinated actions, and policy response to the new virus. Attempts at containment therefore were conducted 'hand-in-glove' with rapid response research and development (R&D) activities to evaluate the emerging epidemiology and related public health interventions.

As virus activity became more widespread, extraordinary local responses were triggered in several 'hotspots' where it was clear that disease activity was especially intense, necessitating a change in health service response away from attempted containment towards 'treatment' (only), deliberately 'out of sync' with the wider national response. This meant that local health protection teams had to be very alert to respond ahead of a single national trigger point, reflecting the realities of the passage of the virus across the country. Hotspot activity is inevitable, and may mean that locally tailored action has to be taken when national guidance is not ready. Some actions that are initiated in hotspots may have to be refined at a later date following subsequent national advice.

Locally, the 'containment phase', as it became known in the UK, was also accompanied by intensive planning activity in anticipation of the next phase in the UK national response, and by constant local communication activity, with sustained media pressure for updates. Uncertainty about antiviral stocks, delivery and protocols for use meant local planning had to remain flexible and responsive. Antiviral distribution sites were agreed and planned. Ahead of national solutions, clinical anxiety and sometimes genuine demand also saw local telephone and triage systems being devised and in some cases being enacted ahead of national solutions. A key element of the nationally coordinated response during this phase was the establishment of a national network of ten sub-national 'Flu Response Centres' (FRCs), which were the focal point for joint local action by the HPA supported by NHS colleagues. FRCs coordinated the response to individual suspected cases, as well as clusters of community cases, working closely with primary care services. In the HPA, this was a time of intense pressure in moving fluidly between planning and response to A(H1N1)pdm09 while maintaining continuity of response to the full range of other high-priority infectious disease and environmental health protection threats that did not cease just because a pandemic was under way.

Treatment phase

Some 3 months after the initial UK cases had first been confirmed, a national decision was made on 2 July 2009 to move to a 'treatment phase', in particular signalling an ending of attempts to delay transmission through the use of antiviral drugs for post-exposure prophylaxis in households. This initially involved putting in place services to offer antiviral medication to the whole population for the treatment of suspected A(H1N1)pdm09 if they met the pre-defined clinical criteria, based on symptoms and signs. The National Pandemic Flu Service (NPFS), which was activated in England on 23 July (Focus Box 9.1), provided an online and telephone self-assessment service, enabling large numbers of people to be assessed and authorized to receive antiviral medicines from local Antiviral Collection Points (ACPs). The major part of the NHS response from this time onwards was to ensure that antiviral drugs were accessible to all who were eligible for them. ACPs in Nottingham and elsewhere across East Midlands opened in late June 2009 and closed in early April 2010.

The NPFS was designed to assist existing healthcare services, mainly primary care, in coping with surges in demand for advice and treatment during peak influenza clinical activity, and speeding access to antiviral treatment for influenza patients whilst maintaining capacity for other non-influenza related workload. It provided a telephone and web-based triage system for any patient with suspected pandemic influenza to check symptoms and determine eligibility for antiviral medication, using pre-set algorithms without the direct involvement of a healthcare worker.

Local ACPs were set up to distribute antiviral medication to eligible groups that had been triaged by the NPFS or by local telephone or primary care triage systems. Wherever possible these were sited to avoid interference with normal primary care, community or hospital buildings, and were typically located in the community. The use of non-symptomatic relatives or friends ('flu friends') to collect antivirals on behalf of the patient was a cornerstone of the NPFS model, to avoid increasing the likelihood of transmission, but this sometimes caused problems due to lack of transport or simply because some people did not have local close friends they could ask to collect their medication, an especially common problem for inner city residents. Professional and voluntary support was planned to address this gap and was in part successful.

Locally, in Nottingham, this phase was relatively smooth, but with unpredictable surges in demand putting pressure on primary care and on ACPs, typically located in community pharmacies. The use of routine healthcare staff, particularly community pharmacy staff, to service these sites gradually had a detrimental effect on mainstream community services but this was containable within the 2 to 3 month timeframe of the peak pandemic surge during autumn 2009. Coordination between healthcare planners in adjacent health areas was essential to avoid duplication or worse, gaps, in coverage for distribution of antivirals to the public and other supplies such as face masks, gloves and gowns to hospitals.

The A(H1N1)pdm09 pandemic presented itself in the UK in two 'waves', one closely following the other. It is believed that the closure of schools for the summer holidays in late July 2009 led to a reduction in contact rates in children and thus an interruption of the first 'wave' at the beginning of the school holidays; this might also have been assisted by the effect of summer weather conditions on influenza transmission. Once schools re-opened in September, the rate of infections grew again until mid-October, possibly due to the start of half-term school holidays. The second wave peaked between September and November 2009 in different UK regions, and ended in early January 2010.

12.3 Primary Care

A major risk of the pandemic was the overwhelming of normal primary care services. This risked increased morbidity and mortality not just in patients with A(H1N1)pdm09, but also all patients with existing or newly presenting medical conditions who rely on general practitioners (GPs) and community nurses to provide life-saving healthcare interventions. The NPFS was conceived partially to mitigate this pressure by handling the majority of suspected influenza-related calls from the public and from symptomatic patients. It was determined that only moderately or severely ill patients and certain high-risk groups should seek medical consultation for influenza in the first instance.

Plans developed in the months leading up to activation of the NPFS involved primary care in three ways. First, information was provided about national, regional and local support services.

The establishment of the NPFS was made known to all the GPs, health centres and community clinics on a systematic basis so all staff were aware of the system for dealing with patients with suspected A(H1N1)pdm09. Second, clinical and epidemiological information was supplied to primary care staff including GPs. This ensured they were able to inform patients and know what to do to assess, diagnose and treat patients who presented to them, especially those who were not eligible for assessment via the NPFS (patients who were moderately or severely unwell, children under 5 years of age and pregnant women). Third, resilience and business continuity planning required robust planning between groups of GPs, including 'buddy' arrangements to cover sickness in medical and support staff, vaccine and antiviral access and storage issues and local discussions about arrangements for the potential challenge of visiting very sick patients in their own homes when general workload was overwhelming. In general, local solutions were required as this level of detail was not provided nationally. In addition, the potential to support and 'buddy' neighbouring GP practices was for the first time rehearsed via real-time exercises. This level of cooperation between potentially rival business units broke down many previously long-standing barriers, but required very strong leadership from local professional leaders and service commissioners. Practical support was also offered for stockpiling of clinical materials such as gowns and gloves.

12.4 Vaccination

Vaccines became available in the UK from 21 October 2009. The health service response to the challenge of vaccination was to deliver this primarily via GPs; however in the planning before the pandemic, it had been envisaged that public mass vaccination would be delivered via large vaccination centres. Local health services used national modelling to estimate the scale of the immunization task and this helped plan the eventual response. The vaccination programme initially targeted people in the normal risk groups for seasonal influenza in the UK, with the addition of pregnant women. All children under 5 years of age were then added as more vaccine became available and the excess risk of hospitalization in young children became apparent from surveillance data. Antiviral medication remained available for eligible symptomatic patients throughout the vaccination programme.

12.5 Secondary Care

Secondary care facilities prepared business continuity plans covering a wide range of issues including surges in demand at hospital emergency departments and related triage issues, staff sickness (including cohort nursing plans), utilities and supply chain robustness, intensive care capacity, plans to stop elective care if needed, and communication challenges. The UK capacity for extracorporeal membrane oxygenation (ECMO) was also increased to provide greater capacity for this treatment at a national level.

12.6 Multi-agency Working

At the time of the pandemic, each county district in England had a Local Resilience Forum (LRF) generally covering a geographic area with a population of about 1 million residents. For the City and County of Nottingham this provided the key focus for multi-agency working across health, social care, councils, emergency services, water and power companies, and private and voluntary sector interests, led by the civil police services. The county fora were further supported and coordinated by Regional Resilience Teams (covering areas of about 4 to 5 million residents) who linked nationally, and acted on issues that crossed county boundaries and functions, including:

- **Social care:** planning for the response to social care challenges required close work by health and social care organizations (statutory, private and voluntary sector) to align staff support as well as the positioning of ACPs to complement and support local services. There were additional unforeseen political and cultural pressures in the locating of ACPs, taking into account issues of cultural diversity, perceptions of fair access for disadvantaged groups, and even gang territory issues common in many larger Westernized cities. Close working with council colleagues was essential to resolve these issues.
- **Voluntary sector:** utilizing this sector was encouraged nationally to support individuals requiring transport to ACPs or additional home care; but it was found that during the peak time, the peer or friend support capacity of the voluntary sector was not able to meet promised levels of activity. Smaller community organizations often found it difficult to maintain business continuity.
- **Other agencies:** a variety of advice and planning was needed on a wide range of fronts such as

Table 12.1. Local pandemic response: some key indicators of activity in Nottingham City, East Midlands, UK.

Indicator	Eligibility and capacity	Actual activity (between July 2009 and February 2010)
Population of Nottingham City	325,000	n/a
Number of people receiving antiviral medication via local ACPs	Potentially eligible population 90,000 based on an attack rate of 30%	21,000 (including 6000 children)
Number of people receiving A(H1N1)pdm09 immunization to end August 2010	Eligible population estimated at 70,000 (20% of population)	47,000 (95% immunized in primary care)
Capacity of ACPs[a]	Capacity designed to be around 20–40 people per hour per site	Six people per hour per site[b]

[a]Because antiviral medication was not readily available except via the Antiviral Collection Points (ACPs), these data captured almost all that was used. A small additional amount of hospital-prescribed medication was provided to inpatients. [b]Two ACPs open at any one time.

maintaining business continuity with regard to utilities (electricity and water), food supplies, waste and environmental services, mortuary storage, public safety and public order. These were coordinated by the LRF.

The work involved in local pandemic response for a population of 325,000 is summarized in Table 12.1. One of the most striking and unexpected aspects of local planning was the extent to which people living in outlying areas tended to gravitate towards the city, increasing pressure on centrally sited ACPs and health facilities.

12.7 Major Challenges for Local Responses to Pandemic Situations

A number of key challenges face any team dealing with a pandemic situation at a local level.

- **Communication:** in rapidly changing pandemic situations, and with advice to patients, the public and to health professionals being amended almost on a daily basis, one of the greatest challenges faced was that of ensuring everybody was able to access the latest advice. Leadership and clear responsibility, strict channels of communication and 'version control' were key factors.
- **Coordination:** in a situation where smooth logistics for the supply and distribution of initially antivirals and later vaccines to eligible population groups were needed, this required scrupulous and intensive day-to-day coordination.
- **Consistency between responders:** ensuring all partners worked together and gave consistent

and coordinated messages and took consistent and coordinated actions was a constant challenge. While detailed plans were in flux, a 'concept of operations' approach was critical in providing a framework of mutual understanding and trust to enable agencies to work together consistently and effectively despite the lack of detail and a rapidly changing planning and response environment. This was achieved by familiarity with working together, achieved via pre-pandemic exercises.

- **Capacity:** planning so that enough staff, beds and supplies would be available to maintain key health and social care functions was central to ensuring resilience.
- **Confusion:** changing advice on screening for suspected cases, case containment, then later infection control and treatment confused both patients and professionals. Added to that was the problem of changing target and at-risk groups as the epidemiology of the pandemic unfolded, and changes in delivery models from those initially proposed: for example, the decision to deliver vaccination via normal primary care services and not via specially convened mass vaccination centres.

12.8 Reflections and Lessons Learnt from Local Health and Social Care Responses in a Pandemic

As described in Chapter 10, a key part of the planning process involves identifying lessons and incorporating these into ongoing planning.

The following points were identified in the East Midlands through the response to A(H1N1)pdm09.

Tactical and operational coordination

- Do act to address immediate gaps if no national solution is forthcoming and patient need demands action.
- Do liaise closely with all partners and ensure robust leadership of local planning.
- Do adjust the frequency of meetings and reports to reflect the natural speed or progress of the incident – in this case a slow-burn pandemic allowed a relaxation in emergency planning meeting frequency. In situations such as an influenza pandemic it is critically important to pace the response, recognizing that such situations are more akin to a 'marathon' than a 'sprint'.

- Do liaise very early on with clinical providers so antiviral and vaccination plans are deliverable and acceptable to the clinical community.
- Do ensure there is a well-appointed central coordination room with all necessary emergency planning support functions.
- Don't try to set up local arrangements that are out of line with definite national plans (such as telephone lines).
- Don't keep groups or planning structures operating if they duplicate activity already going on or if they don't deliver advantages.

National guidance

- Do accept that national guidance will change rapidly and local communications that seek to capture, summarize and distribute the latest advice require obsessional version control and simple communication channels.

Communications

- Do make sure locally produced information passes via a single coordination point to check consistency, clarity and distribution, especially advice to patients and clinical professionals.
- Do date and time stamp all communications to public, patients and professionals alike – things go out of date very quickly.

Reporting and performance management

- Do make sure a dedicated resource is available to do this at the required frequency.
- Do make sure reporting 'up' to regional and government command structures is well organized – government wants and needs 'one single version of the truth'.

Antiviral Collection Points

- Do make sure high-quality catchment area planning is undertaken or risk confusion and inefficiency in terms of sensible coverage, opening times, staffing and support services.

Protecting workers

- Antiviral and vaccination programmes need to be robustly coordinated between staff in different health and social care providers.

12.9   Summary

Organizing and delivering a local response to a pandemic situation was challenging, and the length and complexity of the response meant that pre-existing plans and protocols were only partially suitable for the actual situations faced on the ground. Clear leadership was vital within the framework provided by a 'concept of operations' and a focus on logistics, as was a responsive and pragmatic approach. As former US President Dwight D. Eisenhower once said: 'in planning for battle I have always found that plans are useless, but planning is indispensable'.

One of the most difficult aspects of the local response was the duration of the pandemic and the healthcare response to it. Maintaining the necessary response in the face of staff absence was difficult, even in this pandemic where the clinical illness was, for the most part, mild. It was surprising that only a few months after the pandemic ceased, recall about the exact sequence of events and learning points began to fade. However, there was substantial learning from the event, and in any such local situation, it is very important to carefully document what took place. Finally, a strong national, regional and local public health system that provides technical support and advice for civil authorities is vital to an effective response to a pandemic or other population-wide major infectious disease challenge.

- The local pandemic response needs to be tailored to the characteristics of the virus, the local population's response to it, and the realities of health service delivery in a given locality. National strategy defines what is required regarding antiviral drugs, vaccination schedules, risk groups, and reporting and surveillance; but the local response is operationally focused – concerned with how things actually get done.
- The initial local response phase saw activities aimed at assessment, surveillance and containment. This included rapidly detecting and responding to suspected cases and attempting to prevent community transmission through antiviral treatment and prophylaxis. Clinical epidemiological information was collated and shared to inform local and national actions and policy. There was intense planning in anticipation of the next phase, and constant local communication.
- The UK treatment phase saw the establishment of services to offer treatment antivirals to patients who met pre-defined symptomatic clinical criteria. The National Pandemic Flu Service (NPFS) was activated in England on 23 July 2009 to provide an online and telephone self-assessment service and local Antiviral Collection Points (ACPs). By the time of its closure on 11 February 2010, NPFS had supplied antiviral drugs to 1.2 million people.
- Primary care was supported through the provision of information about national, regional and local support services; provision of clinical and epidemiological information; and resilience and business continuity planning. Secondary care was supported through business continuity planning to address surges in demand at hospital emergency departments, staff sickness, utilities and supply chain robustness, intensive care capacity, plans to stop elective care if needed. All of this was supported through multi-agency partnership working at local and regional levels.

M. Regan and C. Packham

Further Reading

Bell, D.M., Weisfuse, I.B., Hernandez-Avila, M., Del Rio, C., Bustamante, X. and Rodier, G. (2009) Pandemic influenza as 21st century urban public health crisis. *Emerging Infectious Diseases* 15(12), 1963–1969.

Lessler, J., Reich, N.G., Cummings, D.A.; New York City Department of Health and Mental Hygiene Swine Influenza Investigation Team, Nair, H.P., Jordan, H.T. and Thompson, N. (2009) Outbreak of 2009 Pandemic Influenza A (H1N1) at a New York City School. *New England Journal of Medicine* 361(27), 2628–2636.

NHS London (2010) Review of the London health system response to the 2009/10 influenza A/H1N1v pandemic. Available at: http://www.london.nhs.uk/webfiles/Emergency%20planning%20docs/NHSL_FLU_REPORT_WEB.pdf (accessed 1 April 2012).

US Department of Health and Human Services (2012) Department of Health and Human Services Concept of Operations (CONOPS). Available at: http://www.phe.gov/Preparedness/support/conops/Pages/default.aspx (accessed 1 April 2012).

VanVactor, J.D. (2011) Health care logistics: who has the ball during disaster? *Emerging Health Threats Journal* 4, 7167.

13 Bio-mathematical Modelling and Pandemic Preparedness

PETER G. GROVE

Department of Health, London, UK

- What is modelling and what is its role in pandemic preparedness?
- What can modelling tell us, and what can't it tell us?
- How does modelling actually work?
- What did modelling contribute towards the 2009 pandemic response?

13.1　What is Modelling?

The word 'modelling' is used to describe many diverse activities even within the scientific disciplines. However, the essence is to use one's broad knowledge of whatever system is under consideration to construct a simplified or idealized version, the 'model'. The model can then be analysed in detail, often and in practice most usefully, using complex mathematical techniques.

Why build a model? There are basically two reasons. The first is that broad knowledge of a given system is not sufficient to describe the detail that needs to be considered. The second is that even if every detail were known, the very amount of information would make it hard to handle and impractical to work out what was going on. Of course it is necessary to include 'significant detail', and the choice of what is 'significant' in this respect is a matter of judgement based on our broad knowledge of the system in question.

Modelling is thus not an alternative to having knowledge about a system; rather it is a way of sorting knowledge to determine the relative importance of various factors and re-ordering the information to provide answers which are not always immediately obvious. For example, and grossly oversimplifying, infectious disease modelling involves attempting to predict the total number of people who will be infected by a disease from the number of people one person infects and how quickly that infection takes place.

As the 'significant' detail will, in general, depend on the question being asked, different questions will require different simplifications. Hence many different models are usually required to capture the different aspects of a complicated problem. Thus knowledge of how a particular model fails to capture all the aspects of the real situation is at least as important as the model itself.

A large component of the 'broad knowledge' required for biomedical modelling is, of course, the germ theory of disease; in particular, medical knowledge of how the disease is passed from one person to another, along with our knowledge of the effects on that person and the results of treatment of various kinds. Of course, in relation to influenza, many of the details of how the infection is transmitted are poorly understood (Chapter 8), posing additional challenges. The other important component is information on how people interact, how often do they meet and how often do they travel from place to place?

A corollary of all this is that modelling can only be as good as the data fed into the models and the assumptions made in the design of the models. As earlier chapters have indicated, in the case of dealing with a future pandemic influenza virus, there are few specific data and a wide range of plausible assumptions. Therefore, the role of modelling prior to a pandemic cannot be to make definitive forecasts of what will happen. If this is the case, why is modelling essential to planning for a pandemic?

©CAB International 2013. *Pandemic Influenza,* 2nd Edition (eds J. Van-Tam and C. Sellwood)

What modelling can do is: help map out the range of possible risks; and, more importantly, suggest which responses or interventions appear robust over the range of uncertainty. Put another way, modelling can help determine how bad a pandemic might be and see which interventions have a reasonable chance of improving the situation. Indeed, it is essentially the only way of seeing which interventions (or combinations of interventions) will have any chance of working across the range of uncertainty.

13.2   How Bad Might a Pandemic Be?

Modelling helps map out the range of possible risks by providing a description of how quickly a pandemic would move across the world and what would happen if a pandemic arrived in, say, the UK, assuming no interventions. The modelling is based on empirical information from past pandemics and seasonal influenza of the kind described in earlier chapters. The objective of this kind of analysis is to indicate the scale of the problems involved in dealing with a pandemic.

It would be wrong to think that the assessment of how severe a pandemic might be comes solely from modelling. The real value of modelling in this aspect of planning is to cross-check and to integrate various different sources of information. For example, the rate of increase of the number of clinical cases of influenza in the second wave of the 1918 pandemic in both the UK and the USA suggests that one person infected about two others (a figure called R_0). Modelling then tells us that in a fully susceptible population, 80% of the population might become infected (the infection attack rate). Information from seasonal influenza suggests that between 50 and 66% of the cases might show significant clinical symptoms, which combined with the 80% infection attack rate gives a resultant clinical attack rate of up to 50%. On the other hand, information from the 20th century pandemics suggests clinical attack rates in the general community of up to 40%. Thus the various ways of looking at past data suggest that it would be reasonable to plan for 'reasonable worst case' clinical attack rates in the range of 40–50%.

One can also use empirical information from past pandemics and seasonal influenza to estimate the case fatality and hospitalization rates. This is

often difficult owing to the way the data were originally collected. Another use of modelling is to construct a model of the community from which the data came in order to help understand if the way in which the data were collected may have either inflated or deflated the estimates. Once estimates of case fatality and hospitalization are obtained, these can be combined with the clinical attack rate to see if services would be overcome by the demand.

The next step is to look at the disease spread. There are three aspects:

- How quickly would it arrive, say, in Europe or the UK?
- How quickly would it spread though a given land mass, for example the UK or mainland Europe?
- What would be the timing of the epidemic both nationally and locally?

Again empirical data exist from previous pandemics (seasonal flu data are less useful because of the low susceptibility of the population, i.e. high levels of immunity); however, they are not definitive. The pandemic of 2009 was generally mild and it seems likely that large numbers of cases built up, in countries affected early in the pandemic, before an international health emergency was recognized. The 2009 pandemic is also, arguably, a poor model of the kind of pandemic requiring special precautions because of the levels of immunity in older adults. Considering the more severe pandemics of the 20th century, of the kind which generate most concern for planners, transport and communications, especially international transport, have changed greatly since even the 1968 pandemic and do not in themselves provide a good guide. The models can accommodate these changes in travel patterns and indicate what would have happened in 1918 or 1957 had there been modern-day patterns of travel.

We have stressed that modelling does not replace knowledge but rather allows it to be used more efficiently. Modelling the worldwide spread of a pandemic can be done, but a fundamental lack of understanding means that there is an important aspect of a pandemic for which modelling currently cannot provide answers. This is the question of pandemic 'waves' (Chapter 5).

Modellers can generate pandemics with waves; for example, by assuming a seasonal effect on the transmission of influenza either due to, say, the effect of humidity or ultraviolet light on the virus or the changing ways in which people interact in different seasons of the year (e.g. due to school holidays). The 'double peaked' UK epidemic in 2009 has been successfully modelled taking account of the effect of summer, especially school, holidays. However, more generally none of the suggested mechanisms can explain all the observations in historical pandemics. Fortunately, for most planning purposes a single wave is the 'worst case' with the greatest number of people becoming sick or requiring hospitalization at any one time.

13.3 What Might Work?

The second role of modelling is to help find 'robust' packages of interventions. There are two stages to this. The first is to separate those interventions that are expected to have some useful impact across the range of uncertainty from those that would have an insignificant impact and/or an impact only in very specific circumstances. Only modelling can do this. One reason for this is that many of the most important interventions such as antiviral drugs and vaccines have not been available in previous pandemics. The exception is of course 2009; however in this case the mild nature of the outbreak and hence the limited proportion of those ill who actually presented for treatment makes the interpretation of the evidence difficult. Similarly, the context of interventions such as travel restrictions has changed significantly since the last significant pandemic in 1968, while the interpretation of the spread in 2009 is problematic. Modelling is also needed to disentangle the effects of interventions used in combination in the past and use this information to assess the different combinations one would wish to use in a future pandemic. Equally important is the fact that only modelling allows consideration of the effects of the interventions for pandemics of different severity.

Some interventions can be shown to be essentially worthless at any practical level of implementation – in particular travel restrictions and attempts to 'contain' the virus outside the country of origin. Others can be shown to be more effective than one might imagine; for example, a poorly matched prepandemic vaccine which reduced transmission (by reducing the probability of being infected) by only 20% would have a significant impact on a pandemic, particularly if targeted at schoolchildren and those most at risk of severe illness.

A close relative of the epidemiological modelling we have been considering so far is 'operational' modelling. This kind of modelling investigates if there are practical ways of implementing the countermeasures that are shown to be effective in conventional epidemiological studies. Only if some practical route of implementation exists (i.e. the intervention can be properly delivered at the 'coal face') can a countermeasure be considered to 'work'.

Some interventions, such as some kinds of social distancing measures, tend to be effective only at low values of R_0 and hence they do not in themselves turn out to be robust measures though they may be very effective in such circumstances, for example school closures combined with seasonal holidays in 2009. Some (again, for example, school closures) have in themselves generally limited impact across the range of possible pandemics, but seem to offer important adjunct effects when used alongside other measures such as household post-exposure prophylaxis using antiviral drugs (Chapters 14 and 16). This indicates one particularly important feature of modelling: it allows us to consider several measures in combination. We can therefore consider packages of measures in which we can not only consider the situation where they all work as expected, but also where some measures fail. Reasons for possible failure include:

- antiviral prophylaxis failing to have the anticipated effect because drugs do not get to people quickly enough;
- antiviral treatment failing due to the emergence of drug resistance; or
- antibiotic treatment failing because most complications are not bacterial.

Packages can therefore be designed to be robust not only because each individual measure has a reasonable possibility of working across the range of uncertainty, but also because if one measure fails the other parts of the package should still have a significant impact on the epidemic of pandemic influenza.

However, it should be strongly re-emphasized that these calculations do not constitute forecasts of what will happen. Rather they indicate the kinds of effects the different measures might be expected to produce and hence the ways in which they are best included in the package. The point of the exercise is to come up with combinations that will probably work despite the fact that we cannot accurately estimate the effect of each element.

13.4 What Do the Models Look Like?

The simplest epidemiological model that reproduces the most important qualitative features of epidemics is the deterministic homogeneous mixing SIA or SIR model (Fig. 13.1). The population is broken down into three groups: those susceptible (S) who have not been infected or are not yet infectious; an infectious group (I); and an attacked (A) group who have either recovered (R) or died. As it is most likely to be the case with pandemic influenza that most people recover, this is often called an SIR model (as shown in Fig. 13.1). Often the attacked group is referred to as 'removed', that is recovered or dead. Members of the susceptible population have an equal chance of being infected by a member of the infectious population and in turn becoming infectious. The average flows between the groups are described by 'non-linear differential' equations, which essentially means that people are treated as a kind of 'fluid' that moves between the groups and the calculations are analogous to the 'bath filling problems' of secondary school calculus courses. The mathematically inclined reader may have been alerted to the 'non-linear' description of the differential equations; the implications of this will be discussed later.

Given its simplicity, the basic SIA model gives a remarkable degree of insight into how epidemics behave, but it is easily extendable to give more realistic representations. The S, I and A groups can be broken down by, say, age or geographical region, and members of each group then meet and/or infect people of different ages and regions at different rates. Additional groups can also be introduced, such as those infected or ill but not (so) infectious. It is possible to get away from treating people as a fluid, but instead as individuals introducing a probability of infection – creating a so-called 'stochastic model'. Such stochastic models

are particularly important in considering the early evolution of an epidemic.

One common approach to infectious disease modelling is to build up from an SIA model of the kind described to a level of complexity that captures the problem at hand.

An alternative approach is to start not at the level of a population group but of the individual, an approach pioneered in the UK by Ferguson and colleagues at Imperial College London. Here a model is constructed of each person who travels from home to work or school, or across or out of the country by delivering goods or going on holiday. Because of the limitations of data the individuals are (at least conceptually) bunched into groups with similar behaviour. Additional complexity is introduced into this model by adding more groups with a wider range of different behaviours.

Which approach is better? The simple answer is that we need both approaches. The individual-level approach is much more flexible than the SIA-based approach. It is much easier to test out strategies such as the post-exposure prophylaxis of households or the isolation and/or quarantine of cases in a model that considers individuals. On the other hand, the sheer complexity of an individual-based model makes it difficult to see the implications of the large number of assumptions that have had to be made in the construction of the model. In an SIA approach the implications of the few necessary assumptions are clear.

The need to understand the impact of the assumptions of the model is particularly important because of the 'non-linear' nature of the models mentioned earlier. This has two implications. The first is that it is impossible to write down an explicit formula for, say, the number of people who will become ill on any given day, even for the very simplest SIA model. A computer can approximate the curve for a specific case but this is very different from knowing what will happen in general (particularly important when dealing with a new virus). The second is that small changes in the parameters (i.e. the numbers which describe the model like R_0) do not just produce small quantitative changes in

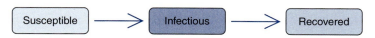

Fig. 13.1. SIR model (the SIA model where all recover).

the results, but can change the entire qualitative behaviour of the model. Such changes can be tested for, and explored, by investigating the effects of changing the parameters (so-called 'sensitivity analysis'). More seriously, small differences in assumptions of the structure of the model can have similarly large qualitative effects and there is no systematic method analogous to 'sensitivity analysis' to test for such effects.

This critical dependence on assumptions impacts on the two families of models in different ways. In the SIA type of approach the 'significant detail' may not be obvious and small effects that have a significant effect on the results may have been ignored. Fortunately, SIA models seem to be relatively robust against small changes in parameter and/or assumption. On the other hand, in the individual approach there are so many implicit assumptions there is a considerable chance of implicitly making one which changes the results significantly. The structural stability of such models in the epidemiological sphere is currently poorly understood.

These considerations mean that it is, at least initially, essential to compare the results of many models to draw any conclusions from epidemiological modelling. Only after obtaining a consensus that a particular approach, or set of approaches, is appropriate is it possible to construct a model that can be used to produce results similar to the consensus view over a limited range. Even then, some divergence in views is possible if there is no agreement on the parameters of the model. This is especially the case if parameters have been derived by seeing which parameters allow models to describe historical epidemics. On the other hand, different models may suggest very different parameters for historical epidemics but agree on the impact of countermeasures in a future pandemic because the difference in parameters compensates for the different assumptions in building the models.

From a policy maker's perspective, if SIA and 'individual' modelling approaches offer the same general conclusions, this increases confidence about making the correct decision in critical areas, although it does not guarantee the eventual outcome. Thus pandemic policy making needs to be based on the expert consensus of results from a number of different models. In the UK a modelling group reporting to the Cabinet Office has been set up for this purpose.

13.5 Economic Models

This chapter has been concerned mainly with epidemiological modelling. We have mentioned briefly the operational modelling required to see if countermeasures are practical in the sense that if, for example, the epidemiological modelling assumes everyone who is ill will be treated with antivirals, it is via some means possible to treat everyone. Another measure of practicality is economic impact. Outputs of the epidemiological modelling are the numbers of deaths, hospitalizations and cases both with and without intervention. These can be placed in standard economics frameworks to assess the cost–benefit of packages of intervention.

Health interventions are usually measured by the cost-effectiveness ratio of the cost to gain a quality-adjusted life year (QALY). If the cost is much in excess of £30,000 per QALY an intervention is highly likely to be rejected. However, the impact of a pandemic is more than simply the health impact measured in QALYs. Instead, attempts are made to produce money estimates of health impacts which can be added to, say, estimates of production lost due to those at home ill or looking after sick children. Precisely what can be estimated and/or should be included differs from one analysis to another, but it is clear that if the annual probability of a significant pandemic is in the range of 1–3% then the standard UK cross-government estimates for the money value of deaths, hospitalizations and lost output would make the use of antivirals, pre-pandemic vaccine and antibiotics strongly cost beneficial in any significant pandemic such as those of the 20th century.

13.6 Real-time Modelling

This chapter has so far emphasized that, before the next pandemic arrives, one cannot attempt forecasting because there is simply too wide a range of possibilities as to how the pandemic will evolve. As information becomes available in a pandemic, however, such forecasting and nowcasting should become possible as the pandemic progresses. This is fortunate, because for some of the (otherwise robust) interventions, there are aspects of their use which can only be decided on the basis of the actual behaviour of the particular pandemic. Examples are the selection of antiviral policy (i.e.

treatment or prophylaxis) given a limited antiviral stockpile and whether or not schools should be closed to reduce transmission. To manage these aspects of the response to an epidemic effectively it will be necessary to both understand what is happening at the time (in terms of cases, deaths, hospitalizations, etc.) and be able to predict the total numbers expected over the course of the epidemic. This knowledge will need to be based on 'within-pandemic' or 'real-time' modelling using timely and accurate surveillance data.

In the particular case of antivirals policy, the largest impact is gained by, in the first instance, the most widespread distribution policy possible with the antiviral stockpile available (e.g. household prophylaxis for stockpiles greater than 50% of the population, or universal treatment for stockpiles less than 50%) and then reverting to more restrictive policies if supplies become limited. The decision to restrict use will need to be taken on the basis of the nowcasts and forecasts available at critical points in the pandemic showing how many antiviral courses will be required and to whom they are most usefully targeted.

Similarly, closing schools may produce large levels of absenteeism as parents need to stay at home to look after their children. Estimates made by the UK government (based on the country's social and occupational structure) suggest that peak workforce absenteeism could be doubled if schools are closed and that this policy is best used either to support antiviral prophylaxis (which would compensate for the additional absenteeism by reducing absenteeism due to illness), with antiviral treatment if children are particularly badly affected, or in a severe epidemic with a low transmissibility (R_0). The actual effects on children can hence only be determined in the pandemic as a result of nowcasts.

Thus, to support both decisions, real-time modelling producing both: (i) nowcasts (reflecting the best estimate of the current situation); and (ii) long-term forecasts of the epidemic will be required. As has been described, nowcasts will provide the best picture of the progress of the epidemic and provide information on the details of, say, who is most badly affected and hence the best targeting of antiviral treatment and whether schools should be closed. On the other hand, the essential information to inform policy decisions on antiviral policy (e.g. if targeting will be

required) within an epidemic will come from long-term forecasts of cases and antiviral usage. The importance of having accurate forecasts is indicated by the fact that making the 'wrong' choice on antiviral policy might lead to a 50% increase in the number of deaths.

In the early stages of a pandemic in the UK it has always been clear that there will still be very few data to use in real-time modelling. This will include some data from abroad along with epidemiological and serological information from contact tracing of the first few hundred UK cases and detailed analysis of the initial outbreaks (Chapter 2). As the epidemic continues, aggregate data, principally from the telephone-based antiviral assessment system, will begin to emerge. It will, however, be a challenge to extract the essential parameters even from the aggregate data until relatively late.

For some time into the pandemic, therefore, the long-term forecasts will predict a considerable range of outcomes and decision making will need to be made in 'windows' when the available information becomes just sufficient to inform the necessary decisions at that stage of the epidemic. In real-time modelling, just as in pre-pandemic modelling, it is important to have alternative models and to compare and discuss the results.

Less severe pandemics present particular challenges for real-time modelling as was shown in the 2009 pandemic (Focus Box 13.1). As most cases are mild, the proportion of those ill seeking healthcare is likely to be low, making estimation of the total numbers ill at any given time difficult. More importantly, this proportion is very likely to vary with time as public concern about the outbreak lessens. This makes it difficult to derive the rate of change of those infected from the change in the numbers seeking healthcare. A mild pandemic might, as was the case in 2009, have a limited size (measured by clinical or infection attack rate) because of significant immunity in some sections of the population. This makes forecasting difficult without serological data, particularly estimates of the background levels of immunity to the pandemic virus (that is, before a significant number of cases or vaccination).

It might be argued that because of the mild nature of such an outbreak the need for real-time modelling is limited. It is certainly true that the critical decisions described above, required to manage a severe pandemic, will not be required in a mild one. However public and governmental expectations of forecasters are likely to be high. If forecasts are to be made in such circumstances it is essential that timely behavioural data on the propensity to consult, and the take up of antiviral treatment and vaccination, are available in real time throughout the outbreak. In addition arrangements need to be in place to rapidly develop a serological assay to allow a rapid survey of background immunity (across age groups) and follow changes in immunity throughout the outbreak.

The development of the consensus view, at the various stages of the outbreak, of the UK modelling group SPI-M which advised senior decision makers in the 2009 pandemic can be followed at http://www.dh.gov.uk/ab/SPI/DH_118862. Real-time modelling was also used to guide decision making on the prioritization of vaccine although these reports are not currently generally available.

Focus Box 13.1. UK real-time modelling in 2009.

Real-time modelling was used to follow the 2009 pandemic in the UK. However special features of the 2009 pandemic made this more difficult than had been expected. As the symptoms were mild, few of those infected presented for healthcare, probably something in the range of 5–10%. This is believed to have differed between the two waves separated by the summer holidays and probably within them. Serological studies of background immunity indicated that there was significant immunity in adults, and particularly in older adults who may have been exposed to the pre-1957 A(H1N1) virus. None of this was known at beginning of the UK outbreak and reports of severity from abroad initially suggested a 1957-like severity. Within 6 weeks, however, estimates of severity had fallen more in line with post-pandemic estimates. Modelling suggested the steeply rising immunity age profile early in the outbreak, but it was considered too optimistic to believe this without serological confirmation.

Following the arrival of serological confirmation of the immunity profile in September, as well as data from the southern hemisphere epidemics, it became possible to construct forecasts for the second wave. As can be seen from the table below, these forecasts turned out to be generally accurate.

The lower and higher estimates represent the expected range of outcomes, with the 'reasonable worst case' indicating the highest credible estimate.

Temporal forecasts were also produced. A typical example, produced by the Health Protection Agency (HPA), is the forecast from late 2009 shown in Fig.13.2. The points indicate the HPA 'case estimates' scaled by ten, the shaded area the range of various individual forecasts. As can be seen, the forecast accurately predicted the end of the second wave in late January 2010.

Predicted second wave estimates versus actual counts (England) from September 2009. (Department of Health SPI-M.)

	Predicted second wave lower estimate	Predicted second wave higher estimate	Predicted second wave reasonable worst case	Actual second wave	Total: first and second waves
GP consultations	270,000	800,000	1,300,000	299,081	687,147
Hospitalizations	5,900	16,800	29,300	17,390	No consistently based series of hospitalizations over both waves
Critical care admissions	900	2,500	4,400	1,857	1,934
Deaths	70	420	840	242	309

Continued

P.G. Grove

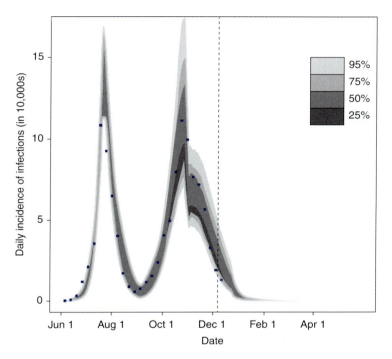

Fig. 13.2. Real-time modelling forecast of the final stages of the 2009 pandemic showing model fit over the preceding months. As described in the text, the points indicate the HPA 'case estimates' scaled by ten, the shaded area the range of various individual forecasts. The forecast accurately predicted the end of the second wave in late January 2010.

Reproduced from Baguelin *et al.* (2010) Vaccination against pandemic influenza A/H1N1v in England: a real-time economic evaluation. *Vaccine* 28, 2370–2384 with permission from Elsevier.

13.7 How Much Confidence Should We Have in Modelling?

There are two basic errors in considering modelling results. The first is to believe them; the second is not to believe them. Even in the most complicated non-linear system, good data and lots of trial and error will eventually produce a model that is predictive most of the time. A good example of this is weather forecasting, where decades of effort and a new trial every day have led to remarkably good short-term forecasting. A vast amount of time and effort, however, has been required to get weather forecasting to this condition, and even now forecast accuracy deteriorates rapidly over a short period of days into the future. On the other hand, simple models that do not take account of the true complexity of a non-linear system are likely to be totally misleading and even more dangerous in public health terms.

Models are most believable if they have resulted from a process in which different models have been compared and improved on the basis of the comparison – and if they are based on a sufficiently good set of data. To determine a 'good' model, one thus needs to be able to talk to the modeller who developed it. In this respect, simple Internet-based 'modelling toolkits' are fraught with problems (even if derived from reputable sources) and can give only the most superficial indication of what might happen.

As we have seen, there are currently few data to put into pandemic models and one should believe only those results that are couched in very general terms – 'this might do some good', 'this will not'. It is an equally safe assumption that any detailed predictions will prove to be wrong. However, if the models have been put together carefully, and their results compared systematically, then these general predictions are likely to be a good guide to what will happen. Good 'within-pandemic' or 'real-time' modelling will be based on models that not only make predictions but also estimate the uncertainty of their predictions, again by the comparison with the results of different models. If the models agree, and their estimated uncertainties fall as real data become available, they can be expected to give a reasonable forecast of what will happen.

13.8 Summary

Because we have limited experience of pandemics, and because we cannot predict with accuracy the behaviour of a future pandemic influenza virus, our preparations must depend partially on modelling results. These results can tell us which preparations are likely to work and which are likely to be of little value. On the other hand, modelling cannot make detailed forecasts of what will happen and plans need to be flexible to take account of this uncertainty.

- Mathematical epidemiological 'modelling' is the construction of a simplified description of the transmission of disease in a population which can be analysed mathematically.
- Modelling can only be as good as the assumptions made in constructing the model and the parameters used in the numerical description. For a pandemic virus there are few data and a large range of plausible assumptions. We cannot, therefore, make forecasts of what *will* happen in a pandemic. The role of modelling before a pandemic is to tell us how bad a pandemic *might* be, and what countermeasures have a realistic possibility of having a significant effect across the large range of uncertainty about the nature and behaviours of the pandemic virus.
- Modelling is not about simply building a model and then 'running it' to find the answer. Reliable results need to be based on a consensus of the views of different modellers using different models. Off-the-shelf (or 'off-the-Internet' models) should be treated with caution.
- Modelling was used extensively during the 2009 pandemic response. Although it was not possible to be precise in the early stages, as more information became available to feed into the models (e.g. serology data, and data from the southern hemisphere first wave) the accuracy with which the size of second wave in the northern hemisphere could be predicted improved dramatically.

Further Reading and Key Papers

This section summarizes a selection of the most influential books and papers on pandemic influenza modelling.

Containment

Ferguson, N.M., Cummings, D.A., Cauchemez, S., Fraser, C., Riley, S., Meeyai, A., Iamsirithaworn, S. and Burke, D.S. (2005) Strategies for containing an emerging influenza pandemic in Southeast Asia. *Nature* 437(7056), 209–214.
Longini, I.M., Halloran, M.E., Nizam, A. and Yang, Y. (2004) Containing pandemic influenza with antiviral agents. *American Journal of Epidemiology* 159, 623–633.

Using individual-based models, these papers indicate that if the first incipient pandemic cases are in a rural part of South-east Asia, stringent social distancing measures, the use of area quarantine and the implementation of a geographically based, large-scale, antiviral prophylaxis policy could contain an outbreak with up to 3 million courses of antivirals for R_0 of up to about 2. Even if the strategy fails to contain the disease, it might delay its progress by around a month.

International spread

Cooper, B.S., Pitman, R.J., Edmunds, W.J. and Gay, N.J. (2006) Delaying the international spread of pandemic influenza. *PLoS Medicine* 3(6), e212.

Cooper and co-workers show that having taken 2 to 4 weeks to build up in the country of origin, pandemic flu could take as little as 2 to 4 weeks to spread from Asia to the UK, with the peak of the UK epidemic following about 50 days later. Imposing a 90% restriction on *all* air travel to the UK would delay the peak of a pandemic wave by only 1 to 2 weeks. On the other hand, a 99.9% travel restriction might delay a pandemic wave by 2 months but is probably impractical. The model is based on an SIA model of each major city with infectious people being moved between cities according to the airline timetables.

Mitigation

Ferguson, N.M., Cummings, D.A., Fraser, C., Cajka, J.C., Cooley, P.C. and Burke, D.S. (2006) Strategies for mitigating an influenza pandemic. *Nature* 442, 448–452.

This paper is a portmanteau of numerous results for an epidemic based on the Imperial College individual-based model. The results have been generally confirmed by other approaches but the Ferguson *et al.* paper remains a good summary. The most important results are that uncontained, a flu outbreak would be expected to spread to all major UK centres of population within 1 to 2 weeks. Because of the probable multiple importations of pandemic influenza, and the concentration of the population in cities, attempts at containment by targeted antiviral prophylaxis and practical social distancing measures are very unlikely to succeed. Mass treatment of clinical cases with antivirals would flatten the temporal profile, lowering the peak and lengthening the base. Although the main purpose of antiviral treatment is to reduce the severity of the disease, treating all clinical cases with antivirals might also decrease the overall attack rate. To obtain a substantial effect the drug must be administered within 24 h of the start of symptoms. Post-exposure antiviral prophylaxis of the household contacts of cases could have a more marked impact on the disease than simply treatment of cases. Prior vaccination with a poorly matched (pre-pandemic) vaccine and antibiotic treatment of those with complications would also be important in controlling the overall impact on hospitalizations and deaths.

School closures

Cauchemez, S., Valleron, A.J., Boëlle, P.Y., Flahault, A. and Ferguson, N.M. (2008) Estimating the impact of school closure on influenza transmission from Sentinal data. *Nature* 452(7188), 750–754.

The impact of closing schools, especially without any antiviral intervention, depends critically on the mixing between children and adults. Different plausible models give different results. This paper based on the evidence from the closure of French schools during seasonal influenza suggests a maximum possible reduction in the peak incidence of one half and rather less in practice. In any case the reduction in the total number of cases is rather less, at most 20%.

The UK Scientific Pandemic Influenza Committee Modelling Sub-group – Modelling Summary

Government preparations for a pandemic cannot await the publication of results in the academic literature. A great deal of unpublished modelling has been considered by the UK Scientific Pandemic Influenza Committee Modelling Sub-group. A summary of these modelling results is available at http://webarchive.nationalarchives.gov.uk/+/www.dh.gov.uk/ab/SPI/index.htm (accessed 21 September 2012).

Introductions to epidemiological modelling

Anderson, R.M. and May, R.M. (1991) *Infectious Diseases of Humans.* Oxford University Press, Oxford, UK.
Daley, D.J. and Gani, J. (1999) *Epidemic Modelling.* Cambridge University Press, Cambridge, UK.

Real-time modelling during the 2009 pandemic

Baguelin, M., Hoek, A.J., Jit, M., Flasche, S., White, P.J. and Edmunds, W.J. (2010) Vaccination against pandemic influenza A/H1N1v in England: a real-time economic evaluation. *Vaccine* 28, 2370–2384.

14 Pharmaceutical Interventions

Jonathan Van-Tam[1] and Wei Shen Lim[2]

[1]University of Nottingham and Health Protection Agency (East Midlands), Nottingham, UK; [2]Nottingham University Hospitals NHS Trust, Nottingham, UK

- What antiviral drugs are available to treat influenza?
- What will be their most likely public health benefits during a pandemic?
- Which antiviral drugs should be stockpiled?
- Is there a role for antibiotics in pandemic preparedness?

14.1 Introduction

One planning assumption made before the 2009 pandemic, which was borne out, was that pandemic-specific influenza vaccine would be unavailable for 6 months after the emergence of a pandemic virus. In 2009, although the A(H1N1)-pdm09 virus began to circulate widely in March 2009, the World Health Organization recommendation to initiate pandemic vaccine production came in late May and most vaccine manufacturers commenced deliveries in early October, 4 months later.

Thus, mitigation of early pandemic activity remains likely to be achieved through public health measures, the treatment of the primary virus infection with antiviral drugs (and supportive care) and subsequent bacterial complications, should these occur, with antibiotics. This chapter discusses currently available influenza antiviral drugs, relevant antibiotics, their potential for stockpiling and use in a pandemic, and what happened in 2009/10.

14.2 Antiviral Drugs

Several antiviral drugs are licensed for the treatment of influenza (Table 14.1). All of these drugs work by blocking a step in the replication cycle of the influenza virus, either at the point where the virus inserts its RNA into the host cell nucleus (M2 channel blockers) or at the point where newly formed viruses are released from the infected host cell (neuraminidase inhibitors) (Fig. 14.1). More

detailed information on the influenza replication cycle is available in Chapter 3.

14.3 M2 Channel Blockers (Adamantanes)

The first influenza-specific antivirals were the M2 ion channel blockers. Amantadine, which has a main indication for the treatment of Parkinson's disease, was licensed for the treatment and prophylaxis of influenza in 1966. This was strain-specific until 1977, when a general licence was granted for influenza A. The initial dosage (100 mg twice daily) has since been reduced to 100 mg daily for use against influenza, which has significantly improved the side-effect profile of the drug. Rimantadine is a newer drug of the same class with an identical mode of action. The two drugs are considered indistinguishable in terms of their effectiveness for treatment and prophylaxis, but rimantadine is associated with fewer central nervous system (CNS) side-effects. Because influenza B does not contain an M2 channel, neither drug is effective against this virus.

Many studies have demonstrated that the M2 channel blockers are efficacious for the treatment and prophylaxis of influenza. There are over 80 clinical trials and observational studies on amantadine, involving over 19,000 patients ranging in age from children (under 1 year) to the very elderly (up to 99 years); however the drug is not licensed in children under 10 years of age. The most common side-effects reported with the use of M2 channel

Table 14.1. Drugs licensed for use against influenza.

Class	M2 channel blockers (adamantanes)		Neuraminidase inhibitors			
Agent	Amantadine	Rimantadine	Zanamivir	Oseltamivir	Peramivir	Laninamivir
Trade name(s)	Lysovir® Symadine®	Flumadine®	Relenza®	Tamiflu®	Rapiacta® Peramiflu®	Inavir®
Influenza activity	A viruses only	A viruses only	A and B viruses	A and B viruses	A and B viruses	A and B viruses
Route of administration	Oral	Oral	Oral inhalation (dry powder)	Oral	Intravenous	Oral inhalation (dry powder)
Use for treatment	Yes	Yes	Yes	Yes	Yes[a]	Yes
Use for prophylaxis	Yes	Yes	Yes	Yes	No	No[b]

[a]Intravenous route of administration makes it most suitable for use in hospital for severely ill patients. [b]Not yet licensed for prophylaxis (April 2012); theoretically likely to be effective for post-exposure prophylaxis.

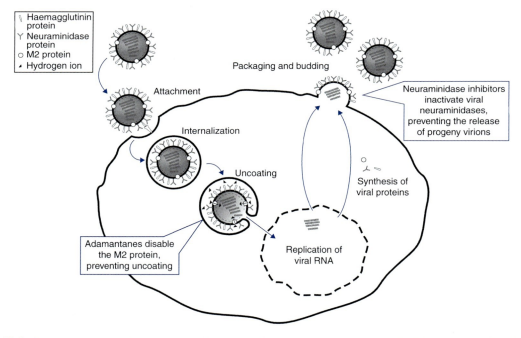

Fig. 14.1. Diagram showing points of action of M2 channel blockers and neuraminidase inhibitors in the replication cycle of influenza virus. (Image kindly supplied by F. Hoffman-La Roche Ltd, Basel, Switzerland.)

blockers involve the CNS: anxiety, concentration difficulty, insomnia, dizziness, headache and jitteriness. In elderly subjects additional undesirable effects include confusion and disorientation.

The biggest concern about the M2 channel blockers in relation to their potential utility as pandemic agents is without doubt the emergence of resistance. There are numerous reports that document the rapid emergence of resistant viruses (within days) after the instigation of therapy; in general this occurs more commonly when the drug is used simultaneously for treatment and prophylaxis in the same setting. Of greater concern is the fact that such viruses appear transmissible and of equivalent virulence to sensitive strains; thus the emergence of resistance does not confer a survival disadvantage to the virus. Aside from reports of the emergence of resistant viruses under pressure from drug usage, routine surveillance of laboratory isolates of influenza suggest that historically the prevalence of adamantane-resistant viruses has been low (<1%); however since about 2000, this proportion has risen sharply, especially with respect to A(H3N2) viruses. By 2006, levels of resistance to A(H3N2) viruses had reached 70% in Hong Kong, 75% in China and about 90% in the USA, prompting the US Centers for Disease Control and Prevention to advise against the use of the adamantanes for the treatment or prevention of seasonal influenza A.

Of the four major clades or sub-clades of avian influenza A(H5N1) associated with human disease (1, 2.1, 2.2, 2.3), 100% of clade 1 viruses and at least 80% of clade 2.1 viruses are already resistant to the adamantanes. Likewise, at the onset of the 2009 pandemic, it was demonstrated very early on that the A(H1N1)pdm09 virus was fully resistant to the adamantanes. These data demonstrate how this class of drugs would have been a totally ineffective stockpiling choice during the 2009 pandemic, and is equally an unsuitable choice for stockpiling for a future pandemic, even if superficially attractive in low-resource settings because of minimal cost. The adamantanes are not discussed further in this chapter.

14.4   Neuraminidase Inhibitors

The development of neuraminidase inhibitors (NAIs) began with the discovery of neuraminidase on the surface of the influenza virus in 1942. A sialic acid analogue capable of inhibiting neuraminidase (2-deoxy-2,3-dehydro-N-acylneuramic acid (DANA)) was identified in 1969 and in 1976, an analogue, FANA (2-deoxy-2,3-dehydro-N-trifluoro-acetylneuraminic acid), was shown to prevent *in vitro* virus replication. However neither DANA nor FANA is an effective therapeutic agent in humans, due to rapid elimination from the body. In 1983 the crystal structure of influenza neuraminidase was described allowing DANA to be modified, which ultimately led to the discovery of zanamivir (Relenza®, GlaxoSmithKline) and oseltamivir (Tamiflu®, F. Hoffmann-La Roche), both licensed in

1999. Both molecules bind to a highly conserved site on the neuraminidase and are highly selective for influenza virus neuraminidase, which strongly reduces the chances of side-effects due to the inadvertent inhibition of human enzyme systems. Newer compounds from the same drug class, namely peramivir (Rapiacta®, Shionogi & Co. Ltd and Peramiflu®, BioCryst Pharmaceuticals Inc.) and laninamivir (Inavir®, Biota/Daiichi Sankyo), have very recently been licensed in parts of the Far East.

Pharmacokinetic differences between zanamivir and oseltamivir

Zanamivir is delivered as a dry powder by oral inhalation through a purposely designed Diskhaler® device, because it is extremely poorly bioavailable via the gastrointestinal tract (<5%). Even when administered by oral inhalation it is relatively poorly bioavailable (10–20%). Whilst drug levels in the respiratory mucosa, at the site of virus replication, are relatively high, patients are not systemically exposed to the drug to any great extent. Zanamivir is excreted almost unchanged in the urine, but because of its wide safety margins, no dose adjustment is necessary in renal impairment. In contrast, oseltamivir is 75% bioavailable by oral administration; the main ingredient is in fact the pro-drug oseltamivir phosphate, which, once ingested, is converted by liver enzymes into its active form, oseltamivir carboxylate, and achieves therapeutic levels in many tissues. Some dose adjustment is necessary in severe renal failure. Both zanamivir and oseltamivir have relatively short serum half-lives, necessitating twice daily administration for treatment.

Treatment effects

The clinical trial programmes of oseltamivir and zanamivir were aimed primarily at gaining licensure for the treatment of influenza symptoms. Whilst this was clearly necessary for commercialization, an unfortunate consequence is that relatively few primary data are available on outcomes (trial end points) of public health significance; the latter have considerably greater relevance to pandemic stockpiling decisions, where the underpinning rationale is to reduce impact through the avoidance of severe complications, hospitalization and death. Another inevitable and unavoidable drawback in the data relates to the fact that the clinical trials have been performed in the setting of 'normal' seasonal influenza (A(H3N2), A(H1N1) and B); it is arguable that these viruses produce milder disease than might be encountered with a future pandemic virus. However, the generally low lethality of A(H1N)pdm09 infections demonstrates that not all pandemics are severe.

From the major pre-licensure trials of both zanamivir and oseltamivir and from subsequent systematic reviews there is strong evidence that both drugs, given within 48 h of symptom onset, deliver fairly consistent yet modest reductions in the duration of major symptoms (headache, myalgia, sore throat, cough, fever or feverishness) and the time taken to return to normal activity is reduced by about 24 to 36 h. These effects have been observed in healthy adults, adults with risk conditions (chronic underlying illnesses that would make such patients candidates for seasonal influenza vaccine), healthy children and the elderly. Evidence suggests that the magnitude of benefit was slightly higher in patients with laboratory-confirmed influenza as opposed to influenza-like illness simply recognized by a doctor; this is entirely to be expected as other respiratory viruses may masquerade as influenza-like illness but would not be responsive to a drug targeted specifically at the influenza virus. Likewise, where treatment was started very rapidly (12 h after symptom onset) the reduction in illness duration was more substantial. Related questions of relevance to pandemic planning are therefore: how quickly can citizens gain access to treatment? and what configuration of healthcare can deliver this effectively?

Public health effects

The evidence of an effect on public health outcomes is of lower quality for both drugs. This shortcoming mainly relates to the relative rarity of severe outcomes for seasonal influenza, particularly hospitalization and death, meaning that studies would need to be very large to have sufficient statistical power to assess these end points; and inevitably this makes them too expensive and logistically complex to undertake. Nevertheless in healthy adults, at-risk adults and healthy children, clinical trial data suggest that both oseltamivir and zanamivir reduce the incidence of antibiotic prescribing for bacterial complications of influenza by about one half. Several observational studies also strongly suggest that the incidence of respiratory complications,

pneumonia, major cardiac events and hospitalization is reduced by oseltamivir treatment in healthy and at-risk adults. Similar data from smaller hospital studies, elderly patients and immune-compromised adult populations suggest that mortality can be reduced by oseltamivir treatment. In children there are data supporting reductions in antibiotic requirements, the incidence of otitis media, pneumonia and hospitalizations with oseltamivir treatment; there are fewer such data for zanamivir but these nevertheless suggest similar conclusions. Modelling data suggest that at a population level, the more rapid the initiation of therapy – ideally within 24 h of symptom onset – the greater the likelihood of public health benefits and, possibly, secondary reductions in community transmission.

New data are available from the widespread deployment of neuraminidase inhibitors during the 2009 pandemic, suggesting that treatment irrespective of timing was associated with reduced mortality and that early treatment (within 48 h of illness onset) substantially reduced mortality by about 60% compared with later or no treatment. Early treatment versus late also reduced the likelihood of severe outcome (intensive care or death). Finally it should be borne in mind that the 2009 pandemic was generally mild and of similar lethality to seasonal influenza. Thus the effects of neuraminidase inhibitors against a severe pandemic virus remain unknown, but can be guessed at from the very limited data on use against avian influenza A(H5N1).

With regard to potential future pandemic threats, limited information is available on the effectiveness of oseltamivir against human cases of avian influenza A(H5N1). In a recent analysis of confirmed cases of A(H5N1) infection taken from a global registry, survival was significantly higher among patients treated with oseltamivir versus those untreated (60% versus 24%); other data suggest a very strongly protective effect of early treatment (within 48 h of illness onset) compared with later. However it is important to remember that these data may not translate directly to a future pandemic virus whose origin is unknown; and that A(H5N1) is presently an avian virus that is non-adapted to humans.

In the context of the overall weaker evidence for public health outcomes, it is important to be clear that studies that are too small to demonstrate a conclusive benefit should not be viewed as providing proof of 'no effect'. It is within this 'vacuum' of emphatic evidence that pandemic policy makers must make decisions 'in the here and now' about whether to insure against a potentially severe future pandemic by stockpiling neuraminidase inhibitors in the belief that, on the balance of imperfect evidence, they are likely to offer meaningful public health benefits. As illustrated by stockpiling decisions made in advance of the 2009 pandemic (Fig. 14.2), many countries have reached such a conclusion.

Prophylaxis

Zanamivir and oseltamivir have both been licensed for use in post-exposure prophylaxis (PEP) – the prevention of influenza in people recently exposed to influenza. In 2009 many countries with large or moderate stockpiles of neuraminidase inhibitors used the drugs in this way to attempt to slow the establishment of sustained community transmission. Such a tactic became widely known as a 'containment strategy' although this was a definite misnomer; no government really expected to contain the disease as much as slow down initial spread and 'buy time'. The evidence in support of this use is very strong. Well-conducted studies show that in households where an index case has influenza, PEP given within 48 h of exposure to close contacts reduces the likelihood of influenza by about 80%. During the 2009 pandemic itself, further data were generated in the UK which suggested that PEP in households reduced secondary cases by over 90%.

Zanamivir and oseltamivir are also licensed for long-term prophylaxis (up to 28 and 42 days, respectively). Zanamivir was evaluated in two studies of long-term prophylaxis with an efficacy of 67% against laboratory-confirmed influenza A in one study and 83% in the other. Long-term prophylaxis with oseltamivir has been shown to be similarly effective in adults and the frail elderly. Whilst impressive, these data are somewhat less relevant to pandemic scenarios where long-term prophylaxis could only be considered for protection of a very small number of individuals until vaccine became available, purely and simply because the amount of drug required to intervene in this way would be massive and the logistic difficulties almost insurmountable.

Adverse events

In clinical trials of zanamivir, the incidence of side-effects was slightly higher in the placebo groups than in the treatment groups (38% versus 33%). All of these were symptoms normally encountered with influenza (e.g. nasal symptoms, diarrhoea, nausea, headache, cough) suggesting that genuine symptoms were reported as adverse events. The only real issue that has arisen with zanamivir is the possibility of induced bronchospasm (sometimes severe) in a small proportion of patients, not necessarily those with underlying lung disease.

The main side-effects encountered with oseltamivir are gastrointestinal, typically nausea and vomiting. The incidence of these side-effects is about 10% (each) at treatment dose, but their severity can be reduced by taking the drug with food and tends to diminish after the first few doses. Few other adverse events are reported. In 2006 the Japanese regulatory authorities issued a warning in relation to the possibility of sudden self-injury or confusion after several reports came to light of teenagers recently treated with oseltamivir, including three deaths that may have been suicides (Focus Box 14.1). In most markets, the drug now carries precautionary advice about the possibility of neuropsychiatric side-effects, especially in children and adolescents.

Resistance

Resistance to zanamivir is hardly described and so far resistant viruses appear less virulent than wild-type viruses. Historically, since launch, the level of resistance reported with oseltamivir has also been low, with resistant viruses being less fit and accounting for <1% of viruses in adults and 4% in children. Some Japanese data reported rates of up to 18% in children treated with oseltamivir; however this may have been due to under-dosing.

In the 2007/08 northern hemisphere winter season, an influenza A(H1N1) virus circulated widely in Europe. A subpopulation of viruses contained a mutation in the neuraminidase gene (NA) denoted H275Y (substitution of tyrosine for histidine at amino acid position 275) that was consistent with very high-level resistance to oseltamivir, which could not be overcome by increasing treatment dosage. The proportion of resistant viruses varied widely from country to country, ranging from 67% to zero. In the following season, although the northern hemisphere winter season was dominated by an A(H3N2) epidemic, the A(H1N1) viruses in circulation in many parts of the world often carried the H275Y mutation. It has become clear that these viruses also carry additional

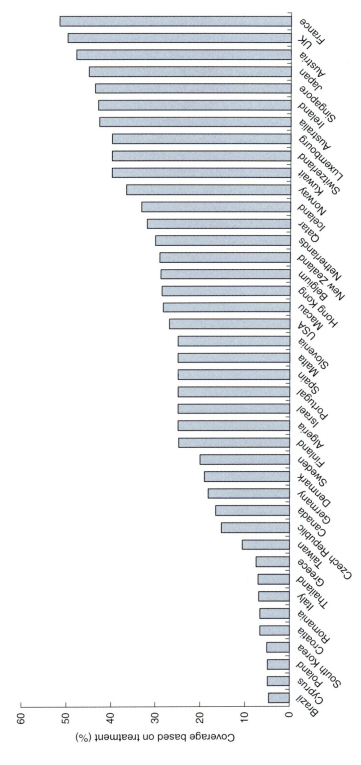

Fig. 14.2. Public domain antiviral stockpiles by country, January 2009, expressed as ability to treat indicated percentage of the population (although a 'treat all' strategy may not have been adopted in the 2009 pandemic in all countries). (Data kindly supplied by F. Hoffmann-La Roche Ltd, Basel, Switzerland (last updated January 2009) and population figures from http://www.geohive.com (January 2007).)

Focus Box 14.1. Use of neuraminidase inhibitors in Japan.

Dr Norio Sugaya MD, Director, Department of Pediatrics, Keiyu Hospital, Yokohama, Japan

Since the approval of zanamivir for the treatment of influenza virus infection in Japan in 1999, followed shortly by oseltamivir in 2000, rapid diagnostic tests have been routinely performed by clinicians in patients who present with influenza-like illness (ILI), and those with positive test results, including otherwise healthy adults and children without underlying illnesses, have usually been treated with neuraminidase inhibitors (NAIs).

It is therefore well-established and widespread clinical practice in Japan to routinely use rapid diagnostic tests for influenza, together with NAI treatment, if indicated. The use of rapid tests is seen as allowing Japanese clinicians to diagnose influenza accurately and prescribe an NAI with confidence. The cost of both the rapid tests and subsequent NAI treatments is largely covered by public health insurance systems.

Even though 20.7 million cases of A(H1N1)pdm09 infection were reported in Japan during the 2009 pandemic, only 198 deaths were reported nationwide. Moreover, not only were there no reports of deaths among pregnant women, who are considered at particularly high risk, neither were there severe cases requiring mechanical ventilation in this group. Japan may well have had the lowest incidence of severe cases worldwide in the 2009 pandemic.

The very low mortality rate due to A(H1N1)pdm09 in Japan was probably attributable to the universal implementation of early treatment with NAIs, which has been the normal standard of care for influenza since 2000. For example, a study of 1000 children hospitalized with A(H1N1)pdm09 infection revealed that over 98% were treated with NAIs, primarily oseltamivir. In 89% of those patients for whom precise timing data were available, treatment with NAIs was initiated within 48 h of symptom onset. Only 12 of the 1000 patients (1.2%) required mechanical ventilation and only one died of A(H1N1)pdm09 infection.

In addition to oseltamivir and zanamivir, the newly approved inhaled drug laninamivir and the newly approved intravenous drug peramivir have been used in Japan since first licensure in time for the 2010/11 winter season, bringing to four the total number of NAIs currently being used in hospitals and clinics nationwide. The Japanese Association for Infectious Diseases recommends that influenza patients who have been hospitalized, especially patients with pneumonia, be treated with oseltamivir or peramivir, and that outpatients without complications be treated with oseltamivir, zanamivir or laninamivir. Peramivir can be used to treat outpatients who cannot be treated with oseltamivir or are unable to inhale zanamivir or laninamivir, especially young children and elderly people.

Although NAI treatment has become routine therapy for seasonal influenza in Japan, neuropsychiatric disorders that were supposedly adverse reactions to oseltamivir became a cause of concern in 2007. In March 2007, the Ministry of Health, Labour and Welfare issued an emergency instruction to suspend the use of oseltamivir for the treatment of patients between the ages of 10 and 19 years; oseltamivir still cannot be prescribed for teenagers in Japan. In a typical case, a 12-year-old boy with ILI who took oseltamivir in the afternoon and in the evening, woke up suddenly at midnight and ran upstairs. He jumped from the first floor of his house, fracturing his leg. He was diagnosed with influenza B virus infection in the emergency department of the hospital, and later explained that he was being chased by a stranger in a dream and was afraid.

In Japan, it is generally thought that abnormal behaviour is caused by influenza virus infection, because a subsequent investigation showed that serious accidents, such as falls from buildings, occurred with influenza patients not only treated with oseltamivir, but also with zanamivir, with laninamivir, or even without treatment. Therefore, it is stressed that children with influenza virus infection should be kept under close observation by parents and guardians until 48 h after the onset of symptoms, irrespective of whether they receive treatment with NAIs.

Sugaya, N., Shinjoh, M., Mitamura, K, and Takahashi, T. (2011) Very low pandemic influenza A (H1N1) 2009 mortality associated with early neuraminidase inhibitor treatment in Japan: analysis of 1000 hospitalized children. *Journal of Infection* 63(4), 288–294.

co-mutations in the NA, which appear to allow the introduction of H275Y without any detrimental impact on fitness *in vivo*; i.e. the virus remains pathogenic and transmissible. A(H1N1) viruses carrying the H275Y mutation remain sensitive to zanamivir.

The phenomenon described above, in which the population of seasonal A(H1N1) viruses became largely resistant to oseltamivir in the space of just a few months, undoubtedly raised concerns that the emergent A(H1N1)pdm09 would also become resistant to oseltamivir. However A(H1N1)pdm09 was sensitive to oseltamivir (and zanamivir) when it emerged, and has largely remained so to date. The prevalence of H275Y mutated viruses detected by surveillance has so far been no greater than 1.5%. However it cannot be assumed that this will always be the case and the situation could change rapidly. A(H5N1) avian influenza viruses carrying the H275Y mutation have also been reported in small numbers, but A(H5N1) may or may not be the cause of the next pandemic. The H275Y mutation does not produce oseltamivir resistance in non-N1 viruses. In the UK and internationally, the vast majority of resistant H275Y mutated A(H1N1)-pdm09 viruses were found in immunocompromised patients or children; and in almost all cases, the detection of resistant clones only occurred after the initiation of antiviral treatment. This has major implications for the correct formulation of antiviral drug prescribing guidelines (especially for immuno-compromised patient groups) and reinforces the need to undertake virological surveillance that incorporates antiviral resistance testing.

Ease of use and suitability for pandemic deployment

Zanamivir suffers from three possible drawbacks compared with oseltamivir regarding ease of use and mass deployment. First, it is an orally inhaled product that requires the use of a Diskhaler® device. One study has raised questions about whether this device can be managed by the elderly or people with poor hand strength/coordination; however the manufacturers have produced oppos-ing data. Second, it must be used cautiously in people with asthma and other chronic pulmonary diseases; and, third, it is not licensed for children under 5 years of age. During the 2009 pandemic, zanamivir capsules were also broken open, the granules mixed with saline and administered (unli-censed) by nebulizer mask to severely ill patients.

In contrast, oseltamivir is licensed from birth (UK Summary of Product Characteristics), is given orally by capsule (three dosage options) and a pae-diatric suspension is also available. Of definite rel-evance to pandemic stockpiling is the fact that oseltamivir is available to governments (only) in magistral formulation, thus providing a lower-cost

stockpiling option. The active pharmaceutical ingredient is a water-soluble dry powder, with a very long shelf-life when stored in sealed drums (Fig. 14.3). When dissolved in water (15 mg/ml) the solution is stable for 3 weeks at 25°C, and for 6 weeks at 5°C. However, this strategy depends upon having sufficient pharmacy infrastructure to cope with large scale reconstitution in the event of a pandemic. The reconstituted mixture is also foul-tasting and a masking flavour is likely to be needed, especially when giving to young children. A com-parison of the main features of zanamivir and oseltamivir is provided in Table 14.2.

Newer neuraminidase inhibitors

Peramivir is a novel neuraminidase inhibitor given via the intravenous route. As such it offers poten-tial advantages in severely ill patients in whom oral or inhalational delivery is difficult, but is clearly only suited for use in hospital. It is licensed in Japan and South Korea, and was granted an Emergency Use Authorization in the USA from 23 October 2009 until 23 June 2010 during the pan-demic. Peramivir is currently undergoing 'fast-track' licensure in the USA. Even though the 2009 pandemic was generally mild, a small proportion of patients became extremely ill and the availability of an intravenous preparation will be of great impor-tance in the future. Intravenous forms of oseltami-vir and zanamivir are also being developed.

Laninamivir is a novel neuraminidase inhibitor delivered as a dry powder for oral inhalation. However, it is long-acting and patients can be treated on a once only ('one and done') basis. This should improve the likelihood of patient compli-ance whilst offering reduced storage and transport cost for pandemic stockpiling and deployment. Some studies suggest that it may be more effective than oseltamivir in children and reduce virus shed-ding faster than oseltamivir in adults and children. At present it is licensed only in Japan, where it has rapidly gained a large market share.

Practicalities relating to pandemic stockpiling and deployment

With regard to pandemic stockpiling, this must always be undertaken against a background of considerable uncertainty about the origin of the next pandemic virus. In this regard it is reassuring that *in vitro* data are available on the efficacy of

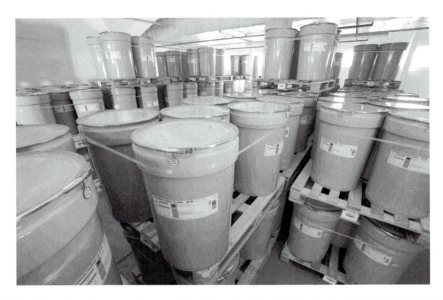

Fig. 14.3. Oseltamivir active pharmaceutical ingredient in sealed barrels. (Kindly supplied by F. Hoffman-La Roche Ltd, Basel, Switzerland.)

Table 14.2. Comparison of main features of zanamivir and oseltamivir.

Feature	Zanamivir (Relenza®)	Oseltamivir (Tamiflu®)
Formulations	Dry powder for oral inhalation	• Dry powder in capsules • Paediatric suspension • Magistral[a]
Age range	≥5 years	From birth
Data on treatment efficacy	Yes	Yes
Data on short-term PEP	Yes	Yes
Data on long-term prophylaxis	Yes	Yes
Drug interactions	Low	Low
Side-effects	Very few	Mainly gastrointestinal (10%)
Specific warnings	Bronchospasm (rare or very rare)	Neuropsychiatric effects (rare)
Bioavailability	10–20%	75%
Treatment dosage	Twice daily (5 days)	Twice daily (5 days)
PEP dosage	Once daily (10 days)	Once daily (10 days)
Long-term prophylaxis dosage	Once daily (up to 28 days)	Once daily (up to 42 days)
Dose adjustment in renal failure	No	Yes (in severe renal failure)
Licensed in pregnancy and lactation	No	No
Significant resistance to date	No	Yes (but pre-pandemic A/H1N1 seasonal virus only)

[a]Available in this form to governments for pandemic stockpiling, but not a 'regular use' licensed formulation

oseltamivir and zanamivir against representative viruses covering all nine neuraminidases. If antiviral drugs are to be considered, the most important questions then relate to their deployment strategy. In practical terms, this can be considered at various levels according to the desired public health objectives. Potential pandemic deployment strategies for antiviral drugs are summarized in Table 14.3.

J. Van-Tam and W.S. Lim

Table 14.3. Possible pandemic deployment strategies for antiviral drugs.

Intended public health objective	Deployment strategy				
	Treatment only for selected groups based on high risk status[a]	Treatment only for selected groups based on employment category/importance of pandemic role[b]	Treatment for whole population[c]	Treatment for whole population plus household PEP	Long-term prophylaxis for selected groups based on employment category/importance of pandemic role[d]
Reduce overall mortality and complications	✓[e]	X	✓✓	✓✓	X
Reduce symptoms and increase speed of return to normal activity	✓	✓	✓	✓	X
Slow rate of occurrence of new cases, buy time and make pandemic's impact flatter and longer (reduce peak incidence), making it easier to cope with	X	X	✓	✓✓[f]	X
Reduce infectiousness and prevent secondary cases occurring	X	X	✓	✓✓	X
Prevent cases almost completely in some groups	X	X	X	X	✓
Reduce impact on CNI and 'essential services'	X	✓	✓	✓✓	✓✓✓
Relative quantity of drugs needed	Medium/ large	Small/ medium	Very large	Extremely large	Medium/ large

PEP, post-exposure prophylaxis; CNI, critical national infrastructure (emergency services, power, fuel, food, etc.). [a]High-risk groups will not be fully known until after the pandemic starts and their identification will depend on high-quality clinico-epidemiological data. [b]Treating selected subgroups will depend upon public, political and ethical acceptability (regarding those excluded). [c]Secondary benefits from 'whole population' strategies depend upon rapid institution of therapy after onset of symptoms (in index case) and adequate logistics to support this. [d]Long-term prophylaxis for selected groups depends upon continuing therapy until pandemic vaccine can be given (i.e. rarely practical). [e]In the 2009 pandemic up to 50% of patients hospitalized did not have underlying high-risk conditions. [f]In the 2009 pandemic, countries which pursued widespread household PEP found this required very intensive human resources, especially when sustained for more than a few weeks.

Focus Box 14.2. Production and supply of antivirals for pandemic influenza: the manufacturers' perspective.

Dr James R. Smith, International Medical Leader: Tamiflu, F. Hoffmann-La Roche Ltd, Basel, Switzerland
Dr Richard South MBChB, Medical Director, Pandemic Centre of Excellence, GlaxoSmithKline, London, UK

The antiviral agents Tamiflu® (oseltamivir) and Relenza® (zanamivir) were important pharmaceutical interventions in the global public health response to the 2009 pandemic. Over several years, many governments and non-governmental organizations (NGOs) around the world built strategic antiviral stockpiles in readiness for a pandemic influenza outbreak. These were deployed to varying degrees during the 2009 pandemic, and were an important element in the first line of defence against the disease.

Nevertheless, Roche and GSK each faced similar challenges in responding to the pandemic, notably in meeting the urgent demand for large quantities of product (even from governments and health authorities who had previously built up emergency stockpiles) and the logistic implications that entailed. Well before the 2009 pandemic, each company had to make its own decisions about establishing and maintaining manufacturing capacity that was not only flexible and responsive enough to meet the annual demands of a normal influenza season, but also capable of being scaled up to produce sufficient stock for building and renewing stockpiles for governments and relevant NGOs, and to supplement those stockpiles during the pandemic response. Although the pandemic has passed, the need to maintain this responsive production capacity continues. Similar challenges face those 'feeder' companies who supply vital raw materials and components for the production of oseltamivir and zanamivir.

The work of rebuilding or maintaining stockpiles of antivirals in readiness for the next pandemic is now under way. Key considerations in this process for public health bodies are that stockpiles should be sufficient to mount an effective response to future outbreaks, be suitable for the widest range of patients and clinical circumstances, consist of more than one antiviral agent to mitigate against the risk of antiviral resistance, and be rapidly deployable. Because of the need for rapid deployment, it is preferable to hold stockpiled material in finished form, even though that may come at the cost of flexibility in meeting the needs of healthcare providers.

The knowledge gained from the 2009 pandemic also suggests other important steps that can be taken by relevant public health bodies (governments and relevant NGOs) to improve preparedness for a future influenza pandemic and the response to it. An important consideration from the viewpoint of antiviral manufacturers is for national pandemic preparedness plans to specify which population groups will be given priority access to antiviral medication and therefore how many people will potentially need antiviral treatment at each stage of the pandemic (initial phase, before pandemic vaccine availability, and following introduction of pandemic vaccination programmes), so that demand during the different phases of a pandemic can be estimated. Pandemic plans should also be clear on how different objectives will be balanced or prioritized with respect to antiviral drug use, e.g. maintaining healthcare service provision versus maintenance of critical national infrastructure (energy, food supply, water, power, security) versus population treatment.

Regulatory authorities should establish procedures for other measures that could help both antiviral manufacturers and health authorities when preparing for, and responding to, future pandemics, such as expedited approvals for additional manufacturing facilities to improve flexibility and for scale-up of existing facilities. Recent regulatory approvals in many countries have increased the shelf-life of approved formulations of Relenza® and Tamiflu® to 7 years for all newly manufactured product, which assists in the maintenance of antiviral stockpiles. Other regulatory approvals allow the compassionate use of their respective intravenous formulations while clinical development is under way.

Manufacturers of newer neuraminidase inhibitors in development will also have a role in planning for future pandemics. If they succeed in gaining worldwide regulatory approval for their drugs, they will share the responsibility for expanding and maintaining total manufacturing capacity to cope with future demand for antivirals.

The rapid emergence of oseltamivir resistance against seasonal influenza A(H1N1) prior to the 2009 pandemic reinforces the need to take a risk-averse approach and consider a mixed stockpile of drugs so that options are available in the event of one drug failing, most likely due to the emergence of resistance. In addition the availability of peramivir for intravenous use and the problems encountered with treating severely ill patients in 2009/10 suggest that this should feature as a minority holding in any future pandemic stockpile.

A difficult issue is what to do when the first outbreak occurs in a country. In some simulation exercises, and in the 2009 pandemic, a number of authorities tried to contain the first outbreaks using conventional measures (such as contact tracing) and distributing large amounts of antiviral drugs to ring-fence the outbreaks by treating patients and giving PEP to their close contacts. The consensus and experience is that these measures treated many people successfully and they may have delayed spread a little, but they failed to contain the infection. In addition, resources were expended and public health staff experienced unprecedented workloads before the pandemic had really started. There were also difficulties in explaining to professionals and the public any policy switch from treatment and prophylaxis in the early stages, to treatment only as the pandemic progressed. These measures will need very careful consideration for a future pandemic.

However, it is not possible to specify for individual countries whether antivirals should be procured nor how they should be deployed. There is no 'one size fits all' approach and what can be achieved depends to a large extent on what can be afforded, governmental priorities and pandemic risk assessment. The larger the stockpile, the greater the options that can be considered for strategic use. Given what is known about clinical attack rates in the pandemics of the 20th century, a stockpile of around 40% of population size is needed before a 'treat-all' strategy can be achieved in practice (unless the clinical attack rate is very low); and at least 60–70% would be needed to be able to consider a strategy of 'treatment plus household PEP'.

The 2009 pandemic has demonstrated clearly that as important as choosing the right national strategy for antiviral drugs, is having the ability to deploy the stockpile effectively. The decision to stockpile antiviral drugs carries with it the necessity to plan a strategy for effective, timely delivery. This needs to take into account the availability of medical and pharmacy staff and the legal basis of prescribing (which may require alteration for a pandemic). If rapid delivery at population level cannot be achieved through conventional physician prescribing, it may be necessary to consider allowing prescribing by non-physician healthcare workers or the use of protocol-driven 'prescribing' by non-healthcare personnel, as practised in the UK in 2009/10 (Focus Box 9.1).

It is almost inevitable that antiviral drugs will need to be administered without diagnostic confirmation of any sort, partly because this service will not be available in sufficient capacity during a pandemic and partly because the emphasis will be on rapid delivery and waiting for diagnostic tests will result in unacceptable delays. Thus a case definition will be required and real-time epidemiological data will be needed to optimize its sensitivity and specificity. Nevertheless, wastage (treating people who do not have pandemic influenza) is an inevitable consequence of mass population-level deployment. It must simply be factored into considerations of stockpile size and the logistic planning of mass treatment.

14.5 Antibiotics

A close interaction between bacterial infections and influenza is well established. Many studies have demonstrated a temporal relationship between seasonal influenza activity and bacterial pneumonia. Rates of pneumococcal infection have been found to be up to three times higher when winter respiratory viruses are circulating and animal studies suggest that influenza infection predisposes individuals to bacterial infections.

This association is also true for the pandemics of the 20th century in which substantial morbidity and mortality were attributed to secondary bacterial infections. Data from these pandemics suggest that bacterial pneumonia developed in 15–20% of patients with influenza. The development and use of antivirals for the management of influenza might reduce the incidence of secondary bacterial infections. However, robust data to demonstrate such benefit are still unavailable. During the 2009 pandemic when antivirals were used widely, secondary bacterial infections were identified in 15–20% of patients hospitalized with A(H1N1)pdm09, and in up to 30% of patients who died.

In addition, in observational studies related to seasonal influenza, mortality was higher in patients with mixed infections (i.e. both influenza- and influenza-related bacterial pneumonia) compared to patients with only influenza-related pneumonia. Data from the 2009 pandemic have been variable; some reports have described an increased mortality and increased need for intensive care in patients with mixed influenza and bacterial infections, while others have not found such associations. The widespread use of antibiotics in the early treatment of patients severely ill with influenza during the 2009 pandemic may account for these apparently conflicting observations.

Given the potential extent and severity of secondary bacterial infections, it is a reasonable assumption that bacterial complications of influenza will occur, and require consideration as part of pandemic preparedness. Patients groups most at risk of secondary bacterial infections include the elderly, persons with chronic illnesses, particularly heart and lung conditions, and those with weak immune systems from disease (e.g. cancer) or treatment (e.g. methotrexate). In countries where HIV/AIDS is more prevalent, rates of bacterial infection may be even higher. Patients with secondary bacterial infections are more likely to require increased medical attention (including hospital care) compared to most patients with uncomplicated influenza infection.

Patients with mild secondary bacterial infections may recover with supportive treatments alone (i.e. bed rest, adequate fluids and antipyretics). However, the mainstay of treatment for bacterial infections, particularly bacterial pneumonia, is antibiotics. In bacterial pneumonia, both delay in administration and inappropriate choice of antibiotics have been associated with poorer outcomes. Modelling data suggest that although antibiotics would have no impact on the incidence of influenza (having no action against a viral agent), as many deaths might be averted through appropriate use of antibiotics as through the use of antiviral drugs. Reductions in hospital referrals and intensive care admissions are other benefits that might be expected from the early, appropriate use of antibiotics. Consideration of methods to increase stocks of selected antibiotics as part of pandemic preparedness is therefore warranted.

14.6 Which Antibiotics Should be Stockpiled?

The choice of antibiotics for the management of secondary bacterial infections in influenza should be guided by the range of likely bacterial pathogens involved. Based on data from the last four pandemics, the spectrum of pathogens implicated is similar to that observed in interpandemic community-acquired pneumonia; the four main groups to consider are *Streptococcus pneumoniae*, *Haemophilus influenzae*, *Staphylococcus aureus* and *Streptococcus pyogenes*. Of these, *S. pneumoniae* is consistently the commonest, accounting for approximately one half of all bacterial pneumonias. This emphasizes the importance of programmes of childhood vaccination against pneumococcal disease with conjugate vaccines, which have reduced the rates of pneumococcal carriage and disease in children in interpandemic years, and the rate of invasive pneumococcal disease in adults through a herd protection effect; modelling suggests that such programmes might also contribute to reductions in bacterial infections during a pandemic.

S. pneumoniae penicillin resistance rates vary widely across the globe; from less than 4% to over 50% of *S. pneumoniae* isolates. Fortunately, high-level penicillin resistance is still uncommon, which means that high-dose oral antibiotics can still achieve therapeutic levels without loss in clinical efficacy. Rates of resistance to macrolide antibiotics (e.g. clarithromycin) and quinolone antibiotics also vary widely. In these instances, using a higher dose of antibiotic does not overcome the resistance. Instead, alternative antibiotics need to be selected.

The emergence of community-acquired methicillin-resistant *S. aureus* (cMRSA) has raised concerns that this could be a significant pathogen in relation to pandemics given the association of increased staphylococcal infections following influenza. The antibiotic susceptibility profile of cMRSA is generally different from hospital-acquired MRSA, and also different from 'typical' methicillin-sensitive *S. aureus* (MSSA). Fortunately during the 2009 pandemic, cMRSA was not a major problem.

Clearly, an understanding of the local epidemiology and resistance profile of likely respiratory pathogens is very important in guiding the choice of antibiotics to stockpile. In the UK where cMRSA remains relatively rare, clinical management guidelines for pandemic influenza recommend co-amoxiclav (amoxicillin + clavulanate) or doxycycline as the preferred first-line oral agent, with oral clarithromycin, erythromycin, levofloxacin or moxifloxacin as alternatives. Drug acceptance, tolerability and licensing in children and pregnant women should be considered in the choice of antibiotic type and formulation.

Use of existing ciprofloxacin stockpiles

A number of countries hold stockpiles of ciprofloxacin as a bioterrorism countermeasure. In the

UK, this quinolone can be expected to be active against most *H. influenzae* and *S. aureus* isolates. However, ciprofloxacin's activity against *S. pneumoniae* is only intermediate and clinical failure with this agent has been reported, especially in more severely ill patients with pneumococcal pneumonia. Therefore, in a pandemic, ciprofloxacin should only be considered as the first-line choice if all other more suitable antibiotic drug supplies are exhausted.

14.7   Strategy for Antibiotic Use

Typically, the symptoms and signs of secondary bacterial pneumonia develop 4 to 5 days from the onset of initial influenza symptoms. However, it is not generally possible to discriminate bacterial complications from viral complications based on clinical features alone. Furthermore, a diagnosis of a bacterial infection may not be microbiologically confirmed for a few days, if at all. Therefore, antibiotic use will of necessity be empirical (i.e. selected without confirmed microbiological test results).

Most clinical management guidelines for pandemic influenza recommend empirical antibiotics based on: (i) clinical severity of illness – e.g. as evidenced by worsening symptoms beyond 3 days or features of pneumonia; and (ii) presence of risk factors for bacterial complications because of chronic illnesses (e.g. chronic obstructive pulmonary disease).

An extension of the above strategy is to offer selected patients an antibiotic prescription at first consultation. The antibiotic prescription should be accompanied by clear instructions that the antibiotics should be collected and used only if the illness is not starting to settle after 2 days, or if there is worsening of symptoms. This strategy of 'delayed prescription' has been shown to reduce primary care reconsultation rates in the management of interpandemic lower respiratory tract infections, without any increase in antibiotic usage. The strategy requires a high degree of openess and trust between patient and the health service, particularly that there are sufficient antibiotic stocks to ensure it will be available if needed and that there is no advantage in 'cashing in' the prescription immediately.

What size of antibiotic stockpile is needed?

The quantity of antibiotics to stockpile is a critical issue for government pandemic planning. The estimated proportion of bacterial infections that might be expected (15–20% of estimated influenza cases, as described above) represents the theoretical minimum. However, as antibiotic use will be empirical, the actual quantity of antibiotics required may be larger. Therefore, this figure should be adjusted according to the chosen strategy for antibiotic use and the population profile of 'at-risk' patients with chronic illness. These estimates do not take account of wastage or a higher rate of secondary bacterial complications than expected.

With an empirical antibiotic strategy based on clinical severity, the proportion of persons who qualify for antibiotics would be higher the more severe the pandemic. On the other hand, in a mild pandemic such as occurred in 2009, antibiotic demand may not exceed levels usually associated with seasonal influenza. This was true in England where antibiotic prescribing for lower respiratory infections in primary care over the last two quarters of 2009 was not distinguishably different compared with the same period in the preceding year.

14.8   Storage and Turnover of Antibiotic Stockpiles

Decisions regarding the composition of pandemic stockpiles, procurements and size depend primarily on financial considerations at a national level. International organizations may also have influence through a variety of mechanisms, from direct financial support to centralized antibiotic stockpiling.

The initial stockpile not only needs to be purchased and stored but also maintained, potentially over a prolonged period of time period. Vaccines for influenza virus subtype A(H5N1) and neuraminidase inhibitors are being stockpiled exclusively for pre-pandemic and pandemic use in many countries. By contrast, antibiotics are widely used every day. Therefore antibiotic stockpiling as part of pandemic preparedness can be approached differently. In most healthcare systems, a 'buffer stock' of antibiotics can be held instead of a true stockpile (conceptually similar to a vendor-managed inventory). Increased stores of antibiotics could be channelled into day-to-day use and replaced through fresh procurement (Fig. 14.4).

A number of benefits may be realized with this system: (i) wastage due to the exceeding of expiry dates can be reduced; (ii) the range of antibiotics can be altered over time in response to the epidemiology of emerging pathogens, antibiotic resistance

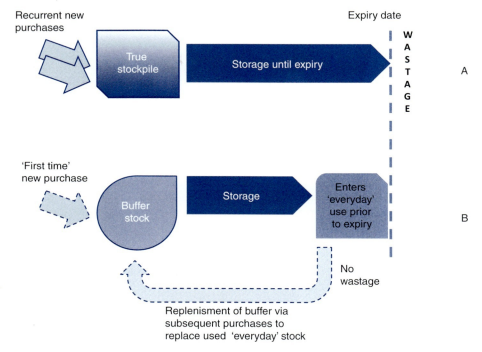

Fig. 14.4. Conceptual illustration of differences between true stockpiling approach (A) and buffer stock approach (B) (in the absence of stock deployment consequent on a pandemic) (note size of shapes is not indicative of quantity).

or availability of new drugs; and (iii) a range of alternative antibiotics can be stocked. Effective storage of such buffer stocks could also be facilitated; whereas antiviral drugs and vaccines essentially need to be held in secure centralized storage (the latter within the cold chain) until eventual deployment, antimicrobial drugs can be held, at least in part, lower down the supply chain by wholesalers and community pharmacies or their equivalent. This would expedite local delivery during a pandemic when services and transport links may be compromised. The adoption of a buffer stock may influence the choice of antibiotic to take account of the range of antibiotics that are in day-to-day use.

14.9 Pneumococcal Vaccines

Pneumococcal polysaccharide vaccines (PPVs) and pneumococcal conjugate vaccines (PCVs) may form part of a coherent pandemic response strategy, most likely achieved through routine immunization programmes and pre-pandemic usage. The introduction of PCVs into childhood immunization schedules has substantially reduced invasive pneumococcal disease (IPD) in children by direct effect, and in adults through its impact on pneumococcal carriage in children. Adult immunization with PPV also offers some protection in adults against IPD, while the value of adult PCV vaccination is under evaluation. Therefore, it seems highly likely that a routine pneumococcal immunization strategy would avert deaths and hospitalizations in a pandemic situation where secondary pneumococcal disease was a prominent feature.

14.10 Summary

Neuraminidase inhibitors reduce both the severity and duration of influenza and are effective against a wide variety of influenza A subtypes and influenza B, especially when treatment is started rapidly. Additional evidence suggests that complications, hospitalizations and deaths may also be reduced. Whilst most data derive from studies of seasonal influenza, newer data from the 2009 pandemic corroborate these findings by suggesting that early treatment reduces mortality and severe outcomes compared with later treatment. Oseltamivir and zanamivir were both widely stockpiled (in advance) and used safely during the 2009 pandemic. It will never be clear in advance if these benefits will be seen against a future pandemic virus, although likely to be the case to some extent. However, on balance, neuraminidase inhibitors offer an important cornerstone of pandemic preparedness in countries that can both afford the financial outlay and implement their chosen policy in a timely and efficient way. A 'mixed stockpile' offers better insurance against possible but unpredictable emergence of resistance.

Secondary bacterial infections are common after influenza infection, resulting in increased healthcare use and increased morbidity and mortality.

The main bacterial pathogens implicated are *Streptococcus pneumoniae, Haemophilus influenzae, Staphylococcus aureus* and *Streptococcus pyogenes*. Antibiotics reduce the complications and mortality related to bacterial infections. Early treatment is more efficacious compared to late treatment. An antibiotic strategy based on clinical severity of illness and risk factors for bacterial complications helps target the populations that would benefit most. Because antibiotics that might be useful in an influenza pandemic are generally also widely used during interpandemic years, a 'buffer stock' of antibiotics can be held thus increasing flexibility and reducing wastage compared to holding a true stockpile.

- M2 channel blockers and neuraminidase inhibitors (NAIs) are available for the treatment and prophylaxis of influenza. NAIs are vastly superior and have far fewer side-effects.
- Although the effectiveness of NAIs against a future pandemic virus cannot be known in advance, it is likely that they will reduce the duration of symptoms, complications, hospitalizations, severe outcomes and mortality. Data from the 2009 pandemic are still being analysed but the advantages of early versus late initiation of therapy are already clear. The 2009 experience has demonstrated that NAIs can be used safely in a widespread fashion, and that they may be the only specific pharmaceutical intervention available for up to 6 months until vaccines are manufactured.
- Although virus resistance to NAIs did not become widespread in 2009/10, this possibility cannot be eliminated for a future pandemic virus; thus, a mixed stockpile of NAIs is recommended, including an intravenous formulation for patients with severe disease.
- Antibiotics should be stockpiled in anticipation of secondary bacterial complications in 15% to 20% of pandemic influenza cases; broadly they should offer cover against *S. pneumoniae, S. aureus* and *H. influenzae* when used empirically. The precise choice of antibiotics should always be decided upon and reviewed regularly in the light of what is known about patterns of antibiotic resistance.

Further Reading on Antiviral Drugs

Adisasmito, W., Chan, P.K., Lee, N., Oner, A.F., Gasimov, V., Aghayev, F., Zaman, M., Bamgboye, E., Dogan, N., Coker, R., Starzyk, K., Dreyer, N.A. and Toovey, S. (2010) Effectiveness of antiviral treatment in human influenza A(H5N1) infections: analysis of a Global Patient Registry. *Journal of Infectious Diseases* 202(8),1154–1160.

Aoki, F.Y., Macleod, M.D., Paggiaro, P., Carewicz, O., El Sawy, A., Wat, C., Griffiths, M., Waalberg, E., Ward, P. and IMPACT Study Group (2003) Early administration of oral oseltamivir increases the benefits of influenza treatment. *Journal of Antimicrobial Chemotherapy* 51, 123–129.

Chan, P.K., Lee, N., Zaman, M., Adisasmito, W., Coker, R., Hanshaoworakul, W., Gasimov, V., Oner, A.F., Dogan, N., Tsang, O., Phommasack, B., Touch, S., Bamgboye, E., Swenson, A., Toovey, S. and Dreyer, N.A. (2012) Determinants of antiviral effectiveness in influenza virus A subtype H5N1. *Journal of Infectious Diseases* (epub ahead of print).

Hsu, J., Santesso, N., Mustafa, R., Brozek, J., Chen, Y.L., Hopkins, J.P., Cheung, A., Hovhannisyan, G., Ivanova, L., Flottorp, S.A., Sæterdal, I., Wong, A.D., Tian, J., Uyeki, T.M., Akl, E.A., Alonso-Coello, P., Smaill, F. and Schünemann, H.J. (2012) Antivirals for treatment of influenza: a systematic review and meta-analysis of observational studies. *Annals of Internal Medicine* 156(7), 512–524. Available at: http://www.annals.org/content/early/2012/02/27/0003-4819-156-7-201204030-00411?aimhp (accessed 31 March 2012).

Kaiser, L., Wat, C., Mills, T., Mahoney, P., Ward, P. and Hayden, F. (2003) Impact of oseltamivir treatment on influenza-related lower respiratory tract complications and hospitalizations. *Archives of Internal Medicine* 163, 1667–1672.

Lee, N., Chan, P.K., Choi, K.W., Lui, G., Wong, B., Cockram, C.S., Hui, D.S., Lai, R., Tang, J.W. and Sung, J.J. (2007) Factors associated with early hospital discharge of adult influenza patients. *Antiviral Therapy* 12(4), 501–508.

Longini, I.M. Jr, Halloran, M.E., Nizam, A. and Yang, Y. (2004) Containing pandemic influenza with antiviral agents. *American Journal of Epidemiology* 159, 623–633.

Louie, J.K., Acosta, M., Jamieson, D.J., Honein, M.A. and California Pandemic (H1N1) Working Group (2010) Severe 2009 H1N1 influenza in pregnant and postpartum women in California. *New England Journal of Medicine* 362, 27–35.

McGeer, A., Green, K.A., Plevneshi, A., Shigayeva, A., Siddiqi, N., Raboud, J., Low, D.E. and Toronto Invasive Bacterial Diseases Network (2007) Antiviral therapy and outcomes of influenza requiring hospitalization in Ontario, Canada. *Clinical Infectious Diseases* 45(12), 1568–1575.

Muthuri, S.G., Myles, P.R., Venkatesan, S., Lenoardi-Bee, J. and Nguyen-Van-Tam, J.S. (2012) Impact of neuraminidase inhibitor treatment on outcomes of public health importance during the 2009/10 influenza A(H1N1) pandemic: a systematic review and meta-analysis in hospitalized patients. *Journal of infectious Diseases* (in press).

Further Reading on Antibiotics

Alpuche, C., Garau, J. and Lim, V. (2007) Global and local variations in antimicrobial susceptibilities and resistance development in the major respiratory pathogens. *International Journal of Antimicrobial Agents* 30 (Suppl 2), S135–S138.

British Infection Society, British Thoracic Society and Health Protection Agency (2007) Pandemic flu: clinical management of patients with an influenza-like illness during an influenza pandemic. Provisional guidelines from the British Infection Society, British Thoracic Society, and Health Protection Agency in collaboration with the Department of Health. *Thorax* 62 (Suppl 1), 1–46. (Erratum in: *Thorax* (2007) 62(6), 474.)

Chien, Y.W., Levin, B.R. and Klugman, K.P. (2012) The anticipated severity of a '1918-like' influenza pandemic in contemporary populations: the contribution of antibacterial interventions. *PLoS One* 7(1), e29219.

Crowe, S., Utley, M., Walker, G., Grove, P. and Pagel, C. (2011) A model to evaluate mass vaccination against pneumococcus as a countermeasure against pandemic influenza. *Vaccine* 29(31), 5065–5077.

Estenssoro, E., Ríos, F.G., Apezteguía, C., Reina, R., Neira, J., Ceraso, D.H., Orlandi, C., Valentini, R., Tiribelli, N., Brizuela, M., Balasini, C., Mare, S., Domeniconi, G., Ilutovich, S., Gómez, A., Giuliani, J., Barrios, C., Valdez, P. and Registry of the Argentinian Society of Intensive Care SATI (2010) Pandemic 2009 influenza A in Argentina: a study of 337 patients on mechanical ventilation. *American Journal of Respiratory and Critical Care Medicine* 182(1), 41–48.

Kuster, S.P., Tuite, A.R., Kwong, J.C., McGeer, A., Toronto Invasive Bacterial Diseases Network Investigators and Fisman, D.N. (2011) Evaluation of coseasonality of influenza and invasive pneumococcal disease: results from prospective surveillance. *PLoS Medicine* 8(6), e1001042.

Little, P., Rumsby, K., Kelly, J., Watson, L., Moore, M., Warner, G., Fahey, T. and Williamson, I. (2005) Information leaflet and antibiotic prescribing strategies for acute lower respiratory tract infection: a randomized controlled trial. *Journal of the American Medical Association* 293(24), 3029–3035.

Morens, D.M., Taubenberger, J.K. and Fauci, A.S. (2008) Predominant role of bacterial pneumonia as a cause of death in pandemic influenza: implications for pandemic influenza preparedness. *Journal of Infectious Diseases* 198(7), 962–970.

Palacios, G., Hornig, M., Cisterna, D., Savji, N., Bussetti, A.V., Kapoor, V., Hui, J., Tokarz, R., Briese, T., Baumeister, E. and Lipkin, W.I. (2009) *Streptococcus pneumoniae* coinfection is correlated with the severity of H1N1 pandemic influenza. *PLoS One* 4(12), e8540.

Small, C.L., Shaler, C.R., McCormick, S., Jeyanathan, M., Damjanovic, D., Brown, E.G., Arck, P., Jordana, M., Kaushic, C., Ashkar, A.A. and Xing, Z. (2010) Influenza infection leads to increased susceptibility to subsequent bacterial superinfection by impairing NK cell responses in the lung. *Journal of Immunology* 184(4), 2048–2056.

Whitney, C.G., Farley, M.M., Hadler, J., Harrison, L.H., Bennett, N.M., Lynfield, R., Reingold, A., Cieslak, P.R., Pilishvili, T., Jackson, D., Facklam, R.R., Jorgensen, J.H., Schuchat, A. and Active Bacterial Core Surveillance of the Emerging Infections Program Network (2003) Decline in invasive pneumococcal disease after the introduction of protein–polysaccharide conjugate vaccine. *New England Journal of Medicine* 348(18), 1737–1746.

15 Pandemic Vaccines

PETER CARRASCO[1] AND GEERT LEROUX-ROELS[2]

[1]*Former Policy Adviser – Vaccines and Immunization, World Health Organization, Geneva, Switzerland, Retired;* [2]*Ghent University and Hospital, Ghent, Belgium*

- What is the relationship between seasonal and pandemic influenza vaccines?
- What were the biggest successes related to the manufacture and use of pandemic vaccine in 2009/10?
- What were the biggest challenges related to the manufacture and use of pandemic vaccine in 2009/10?

15.1 Introduction

Since the last edition of this book, the world has confronted, managed and mitigated the first influenza pandemic of the 21st century. The global response during 2009 and 2010 included the production and distribution of over 900 million doses of pandemic influenza vaccines, in contrast to the previous pandemic in 1968, when vaccines were little used and hardly available outside the USA. Thus the science and practice of vaccination against pandemic influenza is no longer theoretical.

As a public health tool, influenza vaccines can be formulated in three ways to provide protection against influenza morbidity and mortality:

- seasonal influenza – against the annual circulating influenza strains;
- 'pre-pandemic' – against a novel strain of influenza virus that poses a pandemic threat, e.g. avian influenza A(H5N1); and
- pandemic influenza – against a novel virus that has recently been identified in various regions of the world and declared to be pandemic by the World Health Organization (WHO).

In most countries, seasonal influenza vaccination efforts are focused primarily on persons at risk of influenza complications, though some, notably the USA, have gradually moved towards universal vaccination.

An influenza pandemic is considered a global public health emergency. Because the virus is novel, a new vaccine must be manufactured to protect humans against the disease; by definition seasonal vaccines will be of no benefit. The stockpiling of a pre-pandemic influenza vaccine, based on the potential of the selected influenza virus to cause the next pandemic, is risky in public health policy terms. Between 2007 and 2009 some countries stockpiled an A(H5N1) 'pre-pandemic' vaccine. This decision was based on the fact that this was a novel virus associated with high mortality and almost all persons were deemed susceptible. Countries that stockpiled this vaccine (e.g. the UK and Finland among others) were undoubtedly effecting good 'insurance' against an avian influenza A(H5N1) pandemic. It is clear that this strategy did not pay off in relation to the emergence of an A(H1N1) pandemic virus in 2009; but if an A(H5N1) pandemic began 'tomorrow', these countries would likely have a 'head start'.

At the start of a pandemic, pandemic virus-specific vaccine supplies will be limited or non-existent. Vaccine cannot be stockpiled in advance of a pandemic because the emergence of a pandemic virus is unpredictable, and production can only start once the virus has been isolated. Furthermore, it is unknown if one or two doses of vaccine will be required to adequately protect people from the disease caused by a future pandemic virus. For example, in 2009, scientists determined that only one dose of the pandemic A(H1N1)pdm09 vaccine was required to provide protection; however, studies carried out with a pre-pandemic vaccine for A(H5N1) influenza showed that two doses would be required to confer adequate protection.

15.2 Seasonal Influenza Vaccines: the Essential Backdrop to Pandemic Vaccines

The first seasonal influenza vaccines were approved for use in humans in the USA in 1945. The ability to grow large quantities of influenza virus in embryonated hens' eggs and the development of chemical inactivation procedures enabled large-scale production of influenza vaccines. Antigenic variability of the influenza virus (Chapter 3) poses a major challenge for vaccine production. To address this, the WHO Global Influenza Surveillance Network (GISN) gathers twice annually to review the composition of the seasonal influenza vaccine for the northern and southern hemispheres. Based on the latest surveillance data collected by the GISN, the influenza vaccine strains for the subsequent season are selected. As vaccine strain selection takes place 9 to 12 months prior to the start of the influenza season (to allow time for manufacturing), drifted variants can emerge in the meantime. This can result in a mismatch that renders the vaccine less effective. During the 31-year period from the 1980/81 season to the 2011/12 season, the vaccine composition has changed 11 times for the A(H1N1) component, 19 times for the A(H3N2) component and 15 times for the influenza B component.

Most of the current seasonal influenza vaccines are trivalent inactivated vaccines (TIV) containing 15 µg of haemagglutinin protein (HA) from each of three circulating influenza strains (currently A(H1N1), A(H3N2) and B). The seed strains of the influenza B component are usually prepared from field isolates that grow well in embryonated hens' eggs. As most wild-type influenza A viruses do not grow well in hens' eggs, the influenza A reference viruses are not immediately suitable for vaccine production. Instead 'high-growth' reassortant viruses are developed as vaccine seed strains by laboratories at the New York Medical College, the UK's National Institute for Biological Standards and Control (NIBSC) and the vaccine manufacturer CSL in Australia, by 'mating' the wild-type virus with a laboratory variant that grows well in eggs. The candidate seed strains are then sent to the vaccine manufacturers to start production.

Most vaccines manufactured since the 1970s are split and subunit preparations (Table 15.1). Despite their increased reactogenicity, especially in children, whole virus vaccines are still used for seasonal influenza vaccination in some countries and have also been applied in the context of the A(H1N1)-pdm09 pandemic. In the USA and Europe, an intra-nasally administered live-attenuated influenza vaccine (LAIV) is licensed for use in healthy individuals aged between 2 and 49 years.

Despite the lengthy production process, which can take up to 8 months (Fig. 15.1), to date, eggs continue to be the primary platform for vaccine production. Some vaccine manufacturers are beginning to apply cell culture techniques as an alternative method to produce influenza vaccines. This approach has several advantages such as:

- no dependency on egg supply and scheduling of egg production;
- enables use of the natural virus instead of reassortants;
- lower susceptibility to microbial contamination than egg-based production;
- reduction of vaccine production time by about 10 weeks;
- no concerns about allergy to eggs;
- preservation of the antibody-combining site on the HA.

The first seasonal influenza vaccine produced in mammalian cells (Madin–Darby canine kidney or MDCK cells) was registered in 2007. Other cell lines that are in use or under development are Vero cells and PER.C6® cells. Influenza vaccination aims primarily at inducing HA-specific antibodies, the sole mechanism providing immediate and sterilizing immunity in the case of influenza virus challenge. Based on a study performed in 1972 in which healthy volunteers were challenged with influenza virus, a surrogate marker of protection has been defined that is still in use to the present day. In this study a haemagglutination inhibition (HI) titre of 1/36 corresponded with a 50% reduction of infection rate. The licensure criteria set by most regulatory bodies are all derived from this basic standard.

In general, countries with recommendations for seasonal influenza vaccination target populations at increased risk for complications of influenza infections: essentially, young children (aged ≥6 months to 59 months), adults aged ≥65 years, pregnant women and people suffering from chronic pulmonary, cardiovascular, renal, hepatic, neurologic, haematologic or metabolic disorders. The Western European countries, the USA, Japan, Korea and Australia purchase the majority of the seasonal

Table 15.1. Vaccine types.

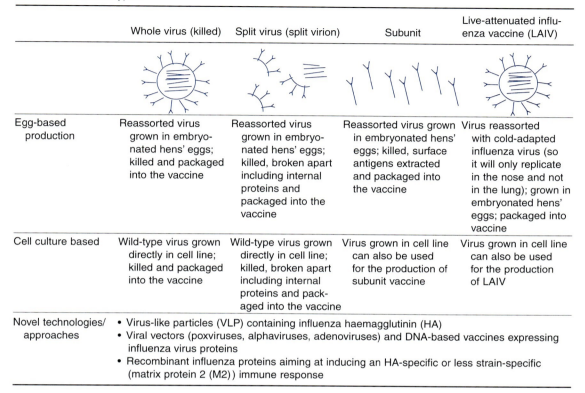

	Whole virus (killed)	Split virus (split virion)	Subunit	Live-attenuated influenza vaccine (LAIV)
Egg-based production	Reassorted virus grown in embryonated hens' eggs; killed and packaged into the vaccine	Reassorted virus grown in embryonated hens' eggs; killed, broken apart including internal proteins and packaged into the vaccine	Reassorted virus grown in embryonated hens' eggs; killed, surface antigens extracted and packaged into the vaccine	Virus reassorted with cold-adapted influenza virus (so it will only replicate in the nose and not in the lung); grown in embryonated hens' eggs; packaged into vaccine
Cell culture based	Wild-type virus grown directly in cell line; killed and packaged into the vaccine	Wild-type virus grown directly in cell line; killed, broken apart including internal proteins and packaged into the vaccine	Virus grown in cell line can also be used for the production of subunit vaccine	Virus grown in cell line can also be used for the production of LAIV
Novel technologies/ approaches	• Virus-like particles (VLP) containing influenza haemagglutinin (HA) • Viral vectors (poxviruses, alphaviruses, adenoviruses) and DNA-based vaccines expressing influenza virus proteins • Recombinant influenza proteins aiming at inducing an HA-specific or less strain-specific (matrix protein 2 (M2)) immune response			

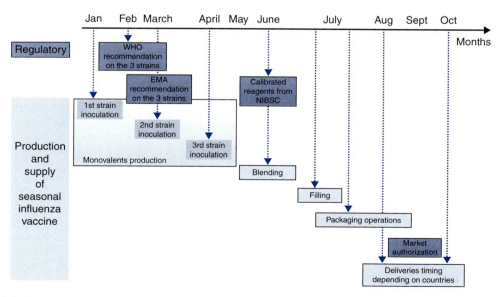

Fig. 15.1. The seasonal influenza vaccine approval and production process in the EU. EMA, European Medicines Agency.

vaccines produced. In the last decade many countries in Latin America and the Caribbean have also included seasonal influenza vaccine in their immunization schedules.

Despite strong recommendations from governments, sometimes with direct funding, influenza vaccine uptake remains stubbornly low. A survey in 11 European countries during two consecutive seasons revealed that vaccination coverage levels in the general population ranged from 10% (Poland) to 29% (UK) during season 2007/08. The coverage in the elderly target group ranged from 14% in Poland to 70% in the UK, and of chronically ill people from 11% (Poland) to 56% (UK). This survey and many other reports have shown that vaccination levels among healthcare workers are generally low. Sustained recommendation and use of seasonal influenza vaccination remains important, not only to prevent influenza infections and severe secondary complications, but also to create a state of willingness in the general public to accept pandemic vaccine when it is deployed.

15.3 Managing Challenges in the Development of a Pandemic Influenza Vaccine

To mitigate a severe pandemic, sufficient doses of pandemic vaccine are needed to vaccinate the global population and these vaccines need to be available 'in time' and convey protection against the influenza strain that causes the pandemic. These requirements represent enormous challenges for pandemic vaccine development and production.

The pandemic threat posed by influenza A(H5N1) since 2003 and the call by WHO to prepare for a pandemic have given influenza vaccine development an enormous stimulus over recent years that has led to significant progress in a field that had hitherto hardly evolved in several decades. Global manufacturing capacity has increased substantially, from 350 million doses in 2003 to almost 900 million doses of TIV by 2008, and numerous safe and immunogenic A(H5N1) 'mock-up' vaccines have been developed with fast-track licensure procedures put in place. These developments certainly contributed to a more rapid deployment of vaccines than would otherwise have been possible during the 2009 pandemic.

Prior to the 2009 pandemic most developed nations prepared for a pandemic using severe 1918-like scenarios; this was not unreasonable given the rapid spread of the A(H5N1) avian influenza virus in poultry and the occurrence of very severe human cases with high lethality. We now know that there are at least two scenarios that need to be planned for regarding use of a future pandemic influenza vaccine: a *mild to moderate* scenario such as the one that commenced in 2009, in which demand for a pandemic vaccine may be limited to those people deemed at highest risk of morbidity and mortality; and a *severe scenario* leading to policies of near-universal vaccination and demand that will far outstrip supply. Protecting against a severe global influenza pandemic will call for vaccination of more than 7 billion people, who may require a total of more than 14 billion doses (if two doses are required for protection). On the eve of the 2009 influenza pandemic, WHO estimated that the total installed production capacity for producing an influenza vaccine was 900 million doses. However, a survey sent to 36 potential influenza vaccine manufacturers by WHO revealed that up 3 billion doses of a monovalent A(H1N1)pdm09 could possibly be made available in a period of 12 months, or a weekly production of 95 million doses under optimal conditions and using 'dose-sparing' technology (Section 15.4).

Given current influenza vaccine production technology and the global distribution of manufacturing facilities, it will take several months to produce the first doses of a pandemic vaccine and make them widely available (Fig. 15.1), as was the case in the 2009 pandemic. The rapid spread of the A(H1N1)pdm09 virus made the production and implementation of a vaccine a global priority. The time schedule for vaccine production was extremely tight: on 29 April 2009, 2 weeks after the identification of the new virus, the A/California/7/2009(H1N1) strain was selected as an international reference strain and by the end of May the reassortant viruses to be used for vaccine preparation were shipped to the manufacturers. One month later the first seed lots were ready and over the 2009 northern hemisphere summer months, manufacturing, licensure and clinical evaluation took place. Large-scale vaccination could start by the end of September 2009 in some countries (e.g. China) and in October in many others. In first-affected countries such as Mexico, the USA, Canada and the UK, vaccine arrived long after the first pandemic wave had peaked. However, almost all countries that depended on donations of the 2009 pandemic vaccine received their first vaccine donations only after January 2010 (Chapter 25), in effect making it a post-pandemic or late-pandemic vaccine in many places. A total of 26 manufacturers, including new manufacturers in China, India, Thailand and South America, prepared split-virion, subunit, whole-virion and live-attenuated influenza vaccines, egg-grown or cell-derived.

It is now clear that many countries with emerging economies that do not currently produce their own influenza vaccine are unlikely to secure supplies of a pandemic influenza vaccine when needed. Indeed, this was one of the major lessons identified in the aftermath of the 2009 pandemic. Additional production facilities, new production methods and possibly new vaccine formulations are still needed to produce at least 7 billion doses of vaccine within a period of 6 to 12 months, especially if the next pandemic influenza virus has high lethality. Production capacity is especially lacking in some world regions, notably sub-Saharan Africa, Eastern Europe and Central Asia. Increasing the production capacities for the manufacturing of a pandemic influenza vaccine in these areas of the world is made more difficult because of lack of demand for seasonal influenza vaccines. Indeed, many countries in the world do not have a policy in place recommending the use of seasonal influenza vaccine. Furthermore, there are many other urgent health priorities requiring the allocation of scarce resources that impact policy and funding decisions regarding the use of seasonal influenza vaccine.

15.4 Pandemic Vaccine Production and Technology Constraints

An analysis by WHO indicates that, unless there are innovations in production methods, a minimum delay of 3 to 4 months can be expected between the development of the vaccine reference seed strain and production of the first doses of a pandemic vaccine. Approximately 90% of current influenza vaccine is realized via egg-based production processes. The constraints to producing sufficient doses of a pandemic vaccine using egg-based technology in the shortest timeframe possible lie in:

- the time required to produce a vaccine reference seed strain;

- having a sufficiently large supply of embryonated eggs;
- availability and access to novel adjuvants that reduce the amount of antigen required in a dose of vaccine, thereby permitting more doses to be produced (the antigen- or dose-sparing approach); and
- having sufficient installed manufacturing capacity that is distributed uniformly throughout the world to permit all nations to have access to the pandemic vaccine in the shortest possible timeframe.

The possible use of LAIV can lead to more doses being produced; up to 15–30 fold higher when compared to that of an 'inactivated' or 'killed vaccine' and within less time. However, only Russia, the USA and India currently manufacture LAIV. In addition, the administration of LAIV requires a special syringe to be filled for nasal administration. Therefore, in a pandemic influenza situation where the production of LAIV has increased over time, the lead time required to manufacture the nasal syringe may be a rate-limiting step.

An adjuvant is a substance or mixture of substances that is added to an antigen and increases the immune response following vaccination and permits the reduction of the amount of antigen from $15\,\mu g$ to as little $3.8\,\mu g$, thereby allowing more doses to be produced – the 'dose-sparing' approach referred to previously. Until quite recently aluminium salts (hydroxide, phosphate) were the only adjuvants licensed for human use; however although widely used these only modestly improve the immunogenicity of inactivated influenza vaccines, if at all.

MF59 was licensed in 1997 as the first oil-in-water (O/W) emulsion adjuvant included in a seasonal influenza vaccine. It has been shown to increase the immune response in the elderly and other at-risk populations. More recently, MF59 and the other proprietary O/W emulsions AS03 and AF03 have been developed and successfully evaluated as adjuvants for pandemic influenza vaccines. O/W emulsions have been shown to trigger the release of cytokines and chemokines, thereby inducing local inflammation and enhancing the immune response to the vaccine antigen; in addition the breadth of the immune response is also enhanced leading to broader (but not unlimited) cross-protection against different but related influenza strains.

Focus Box 15.1. Industrial perspectives from the 2009 pandemic.

Stephen D. Gardner, Bernadette Hendrickx and the Influenza Working Group of the European Vaccine Manufacturers (EVM)

In April 2009, signs of an influenza pandemic due to the emergence of a novel A(H1N1) strain took many by surprise. Not because a pandemic was unexpected, but because it was a different virus to that which many had anticipated would emerge as the next global influenza crisis (i.e. avian influenza A(H5N1)). The critical need for a quick and effective response to this emerging health threat prompted an unprecedented collaboration between international organizations, national governments, health authorities, scientists and influenza vaccine manufacturers. For the first time in history vaccine was made available shortly after the emergence of a pandemic. Indeed, within 3 months of the pandemic declaration by WHO in mid-June 2009, several manufacturers had completed vaccine development and production scale-up and obtained regulatory approval, allowing the initiation of vaccination programmes. This effective response was possible thanks to a decade of joint preparedness efforts conducted since 2001 involving the research-based vaccine industry to collectively address scientific, technical, regulatory, policy and advocacy issues, thus assisting public bodies in their preparation against pandemic influenza.

The 2009 pandemic clearly demonstrated that a pandemic is not only a public health threat, but also a major 'political' event in its broad socio-economic and communication dimensions. The performance of all stakeholders has to be assessed in an objective and balanced way, identifying which aspects were successful and which others require improvement. Many lessons have to be learnt in order to improve our global preparedness for further health threats.

From the vaccine industry perspective, the following elements of the response were positive and can be built upon as part of ongoing pandemic preparedness:

- **A high level of preparedness**: throughout the interpandemic period, vaccine manufacturers developed prototype ('mock-up') pandemic vaccines and modified facilities in readiness for their manufacture. Anticipating the need for a rapid regulatory response, authorities established 'fast track' processes to achieve this objective. As a result, it took only 3 months from the formal declaration of the pandemic to the first approval of A(H1N1)-pdm09 pandemic vaccines, an unprecedented timeline for the development of a new vaccine.

- **Global communication and cooperation between the industry and its partners**: the well-orchestrated scientific communication, virus-sharing programme and processes to share technical information proved essential for the rapid development, testing and production of a targeted influenza pandemic vaccine. As the pandemic progressed, this process was extended to include the sharing of clinical testing data to help authorities develop recommendations on vaccine use.

- **Resolution of technical issues:** WHO laboratories and manufacturers worked to improve low-yielding vaccine virus strains. The use of reagents for standardizing vaccines was possible due to the close cooperation of teams in Essential Regulatory Laboratories (ERLs) in the USA, the UK and Australia; and scientists agreed on alternative vaccine standardization methods for use early in the production process, to facilitate the fast release of clinical lots.

- **The establishment of vaccine monitoring systems** was critical to ensure robust surveillance during wide-scale vaccine use. These included continued regulatory assessment, ongoing clinical testing in thousands of adults, children and other special populations, as well as wide-scale surveillance allowing authorities to rapidly assess the safety of the vaccines.

Although the planning put in place prior to the A(H1N1)pdm09 pandemic greatly strengthened the response to the newly emerged threat, improvements in a number of areas could enhance future responses:

- **The decision-making process to declare the pandemic and to start producing vaccines** was critical, especially as the production of seasonal influenza vaccine for the northern hemisphere was still ongoing. Whilst recognizing the need to start pandemic vaccine production, health officials and WHO also considered that this should not interfere with the ongoing production of seasonal vaccines, which, in many cases, was well advanced. This led to both delays in start time and initially reduced pandemic production capacity for several manufacturers.

- **Technical issues** arose in a number of areas including:
  - the time to prepare suitable virus strains for vaccine production, which took 2 months from the isolation of A(H1N1)pdm09;
  - reagent production for vaccine standardization – in 2009, reference antigens were not available

Continued

until 13 July in Australia, 27 July in the UK, 11 August in the USA and 11 September in Japan;
- logistics planning including provision for the rapid coordination of importation licences for a broad range of products;
- lack of clarity regarding bio-containment requirements for working seed production and vaccine production;
- a simplification of the labelling processes, without jeopardizing the information needed by healthcare professionals and patients.

● *Enhancing regulatory processes*: despite having fast-track approval processes, the coordination of regulatory requirements and mutual recognition of approvals from other jurisdictions, the avoidance of duplication and reduction of bureaucracy could further streamline these processes, thereby accelerating vaccine supply.

● *Negotiating supply agreements in advance:* at the start of the A(H1N1)pdm09 pandemic many countries did not have vaccine supply agreements in place. This resulted in large numbers of complex concurrent negotiations between multiple governments and manufacturers, at a time when time pressures were already intense. The establishment of agreements in advance of a pandemic would allow both parties to plan for key contractual elements, including supply requirements, logistics and liability issues.

● *Enhancing communications with healthcare workers and the public:* throughout the pandemic, vaccine uptake remained low in many countries, though high in some others. Beyond the unexpectedly low clinical severity of the disease, the differences seem to have been due to the extent to which governments engaged healthcare professionals, media and the public in the pandemic planning processes and in communication of the need for pandemic vaccination.

15.5 Regulatory Hurdles

Another major lesson learned from the production of the 2009 influenza pandemic vaccine is that any candidate pandemic vaccine must be shown to be safe and effective. Because of the concern that the avian influenza virus A(H5N1) had the potential to cause the next influenza pandemic, major manufacturers of influenza vaccine (in the industrialized countries) had worked with their regulatory bodies and developed pathways for 'fast tracking' the approval and licensure of a 'mock-up' pandemic vaccine. This was possible because these manufacturers developed a potential pandemic influenza vaccine based on the production methods for producing their seasonal influenza vaccine. Since their seasonal influenza vaccine production processes have been reviewed and manufacturers have worked to maintained their certification as 'GMP compliant' (all facilities that produce a vaccine must meet the standards set out in Good Manufacturing Practice (GMP)), the argument was that the only change in the production methods used in producing a pandemic influenza vaccine would be substitution of the vaccine virus strain, followed by a very limited clinical trial taking around 30 days to complete. This agreement between the major manufacturers and their regulatory bodies facilitated the development of a specific registration process called the 'mock-up dossier'. The purpose of the 'mock-up dossier' is to expedite the licensure of a true pandemic vaccine by presenting data in advance on the effectiveness, safety and other information gathered from clinical trials on the candidate pre-pandemic vaccine. This process will greatly shorten the time from many months to less than 2 weeks for a regulatory body to license a pandemic vaccine in an emergency.

15.6 Research and Development: the Way Forward Towards Improving Influenza Vaccine Production Capacity

Besides the approach of switching from egg-based to cell-derived production processes mentioned earlier, there are new vaccine platforms that hold promise for improving the rapid production of a pandemic vaccine. One such approach that appears to be very promising in terms of producing a pandemic vaccine very quickly and in required quantities is the use of the baculovirus expression vector system. The HA gene of the influenza virus of interest is isolated and introduced into a baculovirus expression vector. Baculovirus is a virus that infects the armyworm caterpillar (*Spodoptera frugiperda*). The baculovirus vector is then introduced into cultured insect cells that will produce large amounts of HA. Alternative ways to present influenza antigens (HA and/or other) to the immune system consist of cloning these proteins into viral vectors (vaccinia viruses, adenoviruses). Upon injection in a muscle, the recombinant viruses express influenza antigen(s) and trigger cellular and humoral immune responses. Influenza-specific immune responses can also be elicited by intramuscular injection of DNA sequences comprising one (HA) or more (neuraminidase, nucleoprotein, M2) influenza gene segments.

Another approach to resolving the shortage of a pandemic influenza vaccine is to develop a vaccine targeting a particular protein of the influenza virus that, unlike the HA antigen, is conserved (i.e. does not or barely mutates) across all influenza A viruses. Such a conserved protein is matrix protein 2 or M2. Early research provided proof of concept that this approach induces a broad protective immune response against three of the then 16 subtypes of influenza HA (a seventeenth HA was identified in early 2012). The challenge is to show that this approach will provide a robust immune response and protection against all influenza A subtypes for a number of years.

Until a 'universal' influenza vaccine is made available, research opportunities should be encouraged and funded, including the establishment of multi-usage production facilities that could be used to produce both influenza and other vaccines (e.g. cell culture-based influenza vaccine and rotavirus vaccine, or egg-derived influenza and yellow fever vaccines). One effort in this direction is the WHO's Global Action Plan (GAP) to establish influenza production facilities in countries with emerging economies for increasing the supply of influenza vaccine. Under the GAP, WHO is facilitating technology transfer to six developing country vaccine manufacturers for establishing influenza vaccine production.

However, one important lesson that cannot be underscored enough is: if the world continues to rely on egg-based *inactivated* pandemic influenza vaccine production, with a global population of 7 billion, there will not be sufficient influenza vaccine in the required quantities and in the required timeframe to effectively use the pandemic vaccine to mitigate the impact of the influenza pandemic upon societies in a severe pandemic scenario. This will be the case even if additional egg-based production facilities are established in the next few years.

15.7 Managing Use of the A(H1N1) pdm09 Pandemic Vaccine

One of the many lessons identified from the A(H1N1)pdm09 influenza pandemic is that government authorities will need to decide on the effective allocation of the pandemic influenza vaccine as it becomes available. Under guidance from WHO and based on information collected in July 2009, countries were urged to prioritize or sequence which populations would be offered A(H1N1)pdm09 vaccination. All countries had to consider the goals of their mitigation efforts in using a pandemic influenza vaccine and which specific patient groups or populations would benefit the most from being vaccinated first. Considerations included reducing mortality and morbidity, limiting social disruption, ensuring maintenance of healthcare systems, ensuring the integrity of critical national infrastructures and limiting economic losses.

When the epidemiological data from countries emerged during the first few months of the 2009 pandemic, WHO recommended the following sequencing of populations that should be offered a dose of the A(H1N1)pdm09 pandemic influenza vaccine as it became available (in order of priority):

- healthcare workers;
- pregnant women;
- individuals aged >6 months with one of several underlying chronic medical conditions;
- healthy young adults between 15 and 49 years of age;
- healthy adults between 49 and 65 years of age;
- healthy adults above the age of 65 years.

Whilst helpful, this order of priority should not be regarded as 'cast in stone' for the future; a different future pandemic virus with a different epidemiological profile might necessitate the re-ordering of priority groups.

The safety of the A(H1N1)pdm09 pandemic vaccines has been thoroughly assessed during numerous clinical trials in various age cohorts. The safety of the O/W adjuvants MF59 and AS03 had previously been extensively documented with data from clinical trials with A(H5N1) and seasonal influenza vaccines (MF59 only). Adjuvanted vaccines are known to cause more reactions at the injection site (pain, swelling and redness) and systemic adverse events (such as fever, headache, fatigue and myalgia) as compared to non-adjuvanted vaccines. Most of these events are mild to moderate in intensity and resolve within 2 to 3 days. This decrease in tolerability is regarded as clinically acceptable in view of the increased risk of serious illness associated with pandemic influenza and the substantial benefit of an effective vaccine. The overall safety of pandemic A(H1N1)pdm09 vaccines in the general population, including use in vulnerable groups such as pregnant women or young children, has since been confirmed during the mass immunization campaigns that took place in the autumn of 2009. Despite increased alertness for the occurrence of Guillain–Barré syndrome during the recent mass vaccination campaign, only a small number of cases have been reported which turned out to be lower than the expected number of background cases.

Reports of cases of narcolepsy in Finland, Ireland and Sweden that were temporally associated with the use of the AS03-adjuvanted A(H1N1)pdm09 vaccine have prompted the European Medicines Agency (EMA) via its Committee for Medicinal Products for Human Use (CHMP) to review all available data on this suspected link. The CHMP has required that the manufacturer conducts preclinical/clinical studies to elucidate the potential link between vaccination and narcolepsy.

Notwithstanding the known increases in reactogenicity associated with adjuvanted pandemic vaccines, and the recent concerns over a potential association between AS03 and rare cases of narcolepsy, the overall risk–benefit profile for the 2009 pandemic vaccines strongly favours their use. Studies conducted in several European countries (Scotland, Germany and in seven countries (France, Hungary, Ireland, Italy, Romania, Portugal and Spain) via the I-move network) reported overall vaccine effectiveness data of monovalent pandemic vaccines of approximately 70% against laboratory-confirmed cases of influenza.

15.8 Procurement of Pandemic Influenza Vaccines

After declaration by WHO that the world was facing its first influenza pandemic since 1968, countries had four means available through which to purchase the A(H1N1)pdm09 pandemic influenza vaccine:

- use any pre-existing advance purchase arrangements already in place with manufacturers;
- place *de novo* contracts;
- use regional bulk purchasing mechanisms to place orders for the A(H1N1)pdm09 pandemic vaccine; or
- make a request to WHO and donor governments for donations of vaccine and syringes or funds for the purchase of the same.

Because of the potential threat that the avian influenza virus A(H5N1) posed to the world (and still does), many industrialized countries had established 'advance purchase agreements' with the major influenza vaccine manufacturers in the event that the aforementioned avian virus acquired the potential to cause a pandemic. Under these agreements the vaccine manufacturer agrees to provide all the doses contracted and, depending upon the terms stated in the agreement, within a stated timeframe. When it was evident that the A(H1N1)pdm09 virus met the conditions for causing an influenza pandemic, the manufacturers honoured the 'advance purchase agreements' they had in place with these countries and substituted the virus type for producing a pandemic influenza vaccine. WHO estimated that 16 countries (e.g. Austria, UK, Germany, Sweden, Switzerland) had such contracts in place with the industry and that these agreements totalled approximately 600 million doses in 2009. Under such arrangements the contracted influenza vaccine manufacturer is obligated to offer its first production lots to countries under pre-contract, before supplying new customers in the open market place – in effect this is a means by which high-income countries place themselves in priority positions 'at the front of the queue' for pandemic vaccine supplies.

Many middle-income countries with a higher gross domestic product (like Brazil, Argentina, Singapore, Malaysia, Macao and Tunisia) contacted the influenza vaccine manufacturers directly to negotiate the purchase of the required doses or issued tenders for manufacturers to bid against for the required doses.

Countries that belonged or had access to a regional vaccine bulk purchase mechanism were able to obtain their 2009 pandemic vaccine needs using this approach. The Pan American Health Organization (PAHO) has very successfully managed a Revolving Fund for the bulk purchase of vaccine for over 30 years for Member States that choose to procure their vaccine using this mechanism. Under this mechanism all orders for each vaccine and for each vial size are consolidated and WHO pre-qualified vaccine suppliers are invited to bid on the different tenders. Member States using this mechanism generally obtain very competitive prices. The PAHO Revolving Fund procured an estimated 30.5 million doses of the 2009 pandemic influenza vaccine.

WHO approached donor governments and influenza vaccine manufacturers for donations of the 2009 pandemic vaccine on behalf of 97 low-income countries. WHO had determined that if these countries could receive vaccine to cover up to 10% of their total population, they could vaccinate the high-risk populations and healthcare workers as recommended by WHO. WHO received pledges for 200 million doses including the donation of 70 million syringes from several manufacturers and donor governments. WHO donated approximately 77 million doses of the 2009 pandemic vaccine to 77 countries that confirmed their interest in receiving a donation and complied with the requirements stated by WHO for receiving it.

When the severity of the 2009 pandemic was determined to be mild to moderate, global demand for the vaccine waned considerably and there was an excess of unused vaccine on the market, which was offered to countries willing to pay for it. Indeed, some countries that found themselves with large quantities of unused pandemic influenza vaccine offered to sell this to others.

The major lesson learned from the efforts to purchase the 2009 pandemic influenza vaccine was that, apart from developed countries, most nations found it difficult to purchase the desired doses in sufficient quantities and in the timeframe required. This situation will be exacerbated if:

- the next influenza pandemic is severe and carries high lethality;
- more countries follow the example of establishing 'advance purchase agreements'; and
- if influenza vaccine production is not expanded to ensure that sufficient doses of a pandemic influenza vaccine can be supplied in the timeframe required to be effective as a tool in mitigating the effects of the pandemic.

15.9 Logistics of Vaccine Delivery

Underpinning any rapid response to a public health problem or civil emergency is the ability of governments to deploy personnel, equipment, supplies and other resources to address and mitigate effects. This surge capacity must exist and be built into a plan, have funds assigned to support the actions and be exercised well ahead of time. Responding to an influenza pandemic (or an outbreak of any other vaccine-preventable disease) requires rapidly moving vaccine supplies, consumables (e.g. needles, syringes, sharps bins, etc.) and personnel. Therefore, effective and efficient operations related to receiving, storing, packing/re-packing and distributing vaccines and consumables at each level is dependent upon:

- a pre-established schedule of shipments for each distribution point;
- an estimated minimum and maximum number of vaccine doses and consumable items to be shipped to each service/distribution point by route;
- lists of containers required, by size, for safely shipping the vaccines to each site;
- a pre-determined route schedule and the required types of transport, including estimated fuel requirements;
- lists of available transport and types required at each level;
- lists of the required human resources by skill types;
- lists of possible sites where additional vaccinators will be required, especially if the pandemic scenario is severe and many doses of vaccine will be distributed;
- having a supervisory schedule and transportation to support their movement;
- lists of important contact details by staff including civil and government authorities;
- lists of companies contracted to provide logistics services for receiving, packing and re-packing vaccine and ancillary items and their distribution.

The information gathered from the WHO workshops in July and November 2009 with all countries in the six WHO regions indicated that receiving, storing and distributing the A(H1N1)pdm09 vaccine would not be a major problem. Very few countries received all their vaccine requirements in one shipment. Therefore, as deliveries arrived, most countries distributed the vaccine and consumables to their health service providers or to the private logistics companies responsible for distribution. Apart from the industrialized countries in North America, Europe and Asia (with the exception of

Mexico and China), many countries have a long history of carrying out mass vaccination campaigns using their public health services to eradicate the wild poliovirus and to control the circulation of the measles virus. This experience was highly valuable in preparing countries to manage all aspects related to deployment and vaccination operations for the A(H1N1)pdm09 vaccine.

Countries that use private sector healthcare service providers to provide vaccination services to their clients generally outsourced the delivery of the A(H1N1)pdm09 vaccine via the same routes. However, regardless of the type of service providers, the logistics of delivery to healthcare facilities or service providers (especially at lower levels) was complicated by a lack of advance notification of firm delivery dates and quantities to be delivered, the number of people with medically confirmed high-risk conditions (including pregnant women) who were recommend for priority vaccination, and the packaging volumes and volume occupied per dose. Therefore, at different levels of the supply chain the exact quantities to be packed and re-packed, shipped and stored could not be determined with precision. This was especially true in low-income countries, but high-income countries such as Switzerland also experienced logistics difficulties.

Because the demand for the A(H1N1)pdm09 vaccine waned dramatically as the doses became available, many logistics systems were not tested to their limits. Data from all WHO regions confirm that there was a dramatic drop in the demand for the 2009 pandemic vaccine after it became available in January 2010. Without doubt the abrupt waning in demand made it easier for supply and logistics managers and their systems to receive, store, pack and re-pack, and distribute the vaccine. Whether this capacity would have been efficient and effective in a severe influenza pandemic can only be guessed at.

However, there are indications that, without external support, resource-poor countries would have been hard pressed to deliver the A(H1N1)-pdm09 vaccine to their healthcare facilities. In addition, at WHO review workshops held in 2011, some countries stated during the updating of their national deployment and vaccination plan for the next influenza pandemic that more funds should be budgeted for supporting logistics and vaccination operations. In workshops conducted by WHO between July and November 2009, it was evident that many existing pandemic influenza preparedness plans did not elaborate sufficiently on the use and deployment of a pandemic influenza vaccine.

15.10 Public Acceptance of Pandemic Influenza Vaccine

Public demand for the A(H1N1)pdm09 pandemic influenza vaccine waned dramatically in almost all countries within 6 to 7 months of the declaration of the pandemic. The reports prepared by the different WHO regions all attest to a lack of demand by the public in seeking the vaccination. In the WHO Eastern Mediterranean Region (EMRO) 19 countries received approximately 24 million doses of vaccine; however the utilization rate was 14%. The utilization rate for countries in the Western Pacific Region of WHO indicate that of the 25 countries that submitted data, 12 reported utilization rates above 80% or better. The PAHO region reported coverage rates for their targeted populations based on doses administered (199 million doses) ranging from 1% to 100%; however, only nine of 29 countries (31%) reported obtaining coverage above 80% for their targeted population. For the WHO African Region (AFRO) a similar picture emerges, with nine of 34 countries reporting utilization rates above 80% against dose distributed, but many countries reporting below 30%.

Communicating public messages on the benefits and purpose of pandemic vaccination is critical and cannot be overstated. The success or failure of national vaccination campaigns using the A(H1N1)pdm09 vaccine were largely influenced by the manner in which these campaigns were presented in the media (especially newspapers, television and social media). Where community-based groups were involved in planning the public communications activities, vaccine uptake on the part of the targeted groups was better. The results of a WHO survey undertaken in 84 countries (of whom 55 received WHO donated vaccine) revealed that public acceptance for the A(H1N1)pdm09 vaccine was somewhat ambivalent, and waned because of concerns about vaccine safety and whether the vaccine was really needed given the mild to moderate nature of the 2009 pandemic. In all WHO regions, public enthusiasm for the vaccine was dampened because of rumours of adverse events that quickly surfaced via the Internet and other forms of electronic media. Contributing to the dramatic drop in demand for the A(H1N1)pdm09 vaccine was the late arrival of vaccines in almost all countries where the number of cases of pandemic influenza was declining in the face of disease that was considered mild to moderate by most of the public. In countries where seasonal influenza vaccination was not well engrained, reaching populations not normally targeted by the national immunization programme also proved difficult. The communication lessons identified from the 2009 pandemic are discussed in Chapter 20.

15.11 Planning for the Next Influenza Pandemic

The principal obstacle likely to be encountered in a future pandemic will probably be the lack of vaccine, especially if the virus has high lethality and public concern is high. The lack of a deployment and vaccination plan will be the second obstacle that a country could face when using a pandemic vaccine. The third obstacle will be the lack of awareness and provision of trustworthy information on the benefits and the safety of the pandemic influenza vaccine. Until a new 'universal' vaccine and/or influenza vaccine production technology changes, no country will have all the vaccine it requires at the time it requires it. Countries must therefore plan for and rehearse over a range of severity scenarios (at least two) detailing which groups of patients or sectors of the populations will be offered vaccine. In all cases we reiterate that the use of a pandemic vaccine is about saving lives, including vaccinating essential personnel, such as healthcare workers, who will provide life-saving interventions to those who become critically ill during a pandemic. The vaccine industry is a critical partner and must be fully engaged in international planning efforts. The scientific community, political leaders and all public health officials now know that it was simply luck that the 2009 pandemic virus had low lethality. Today we do not know what severity of disease the next influenza pandemic may cause, but the ultimate purpose of using a pandemic influenza vaccine will remain to reduce public health impact.

- Increasing the use of seasonal influenza vaccines will be decisive in manufacturing a pandemic influenza vaccine when one is needed. The manufacturing capacity and global demand for seasonal vaccines provide the infrastructure and a platform for switching rapidly to pandemic production. Public acceptance of and familiarity with seasonal vaccination is important in terms of subsequent acceptance of pandemic vaccination.
- At the beginning of the 2009 pandemic, global pandemic vaccine production capacity stood at no less than 900 million doses per annum and possibly as much as 3 billion doses. From a standing start in late April 2009, most manufacturers had begun releasing pandemic vaccine in large quantities within 5–6 months. This was neither slower nor faster than anticipated, but emphasizes the need for new rapid manufacturing technologies and 'universal' influenza vaccines that can be stockpiled or given in advance.
- The biggest challenges related to pandemic vaccine in 2009/10 related to four main areas: a discordance between the appearance of the main pandemic wave and vaccine availability in many countries; global equity of supply; public acceptance of pandemic vaccine, often related to communication issues; and the logistics of vaccine delivery to front-line vaccinators.

Further Reading

Abelin, A. Colegate, T., Gardener, S, Hehme, N. and Palache, A. (2011) Lessons from pandemic influenza A(H1N1): the research-based vaccine industry's perspective. *Vaccine* 29, 1135–1138.

Blank, P.R., Schwenkglenks, M. and Szucs, T.D. (2009) Vaccination coverage rates in eleven European countries during two consecutive influenza seasons. *Journal of Infection* 58, 446–458.

Cox, M.M. and Karl Anderson, D. (2007) Production of a novel influenza vaccine using insect cells: protection against drifted strains. *Influenza and Other Respiratory Viruses* 1(1), 35–40.

Hickling, J. and D'Hondt, E. (2006) A review of production technologies for influenza virus vaccine and their suitability for deployment in developing countries for influenza pandemic preparedness. Available at: www.who.int/entity/vaccine_research/diseases/influenza/Flu_vacc_manuf_tech_report.pdf (accessed 1 April 2012).

Kieny, M.P. (2009) WHO supports fair access to influenza A(H1N1) vaccine. *Bulletin of the World Health Organization* 87(9), 653–654.

Lambert, L.C. and Fauci, A.S. (2010) Influenza vaccines for the future. *New England Journal of Medicine* 363(21), 2036–2044.

Leroux-Roels, I. and Leroux-Roels, G. (2009) Current status and progress of prepandemic and pandemic influenza vaccine development. *Expert Review of Vaccines* 8(4), 401–423.

Stephenson, I., Nicholson, K.G., Wood, J.M., Zambon, M.C. and Katz, J.M. (2004) Confronting the avian influenza threat: vaccine development for a potential pandemic. *Lancet Infectious Diseases* 4(8), 499–450.

Valenciano, M., Kissling, E., Cohen, J.M., Oroszi, B., Barret, A.S., Rizzo, C., Nunes, B., Pitigoi, D., Larrauri Cámara, A., Mosnier, A., Horvath, J.K., O'Donnell, J., Bella, A., Guiomar, R., Lupulescu, E., Savulescu, C., Ciancio, B.C., Kramarz, P. and Moren, A. (2011) Estimates of pandemic influenza vaccine effectiveness in Europe, 2009–2010: results of Influenza Monitoring Vaccine Effectiveness in Europe (I-MOVE) multicentre case–control study. *PLoS Medicine* 8(1), e1000388.

World Health Organization (2006) Global pandemic influenza action plan to increase vaccine supply. Available at: www.who.int/influenza/resources/action_plan_vaccine_supply/en/ (accessed 1 April 2012).

World Health Organization (2011) Second WHO Consultation on Global Action Plan for Influenza Vaccines. Available at: www.who.int/influenza_vaccines_plan/news/gap2_july11/en/ (accessed 1 April 2012).

16 National and International Public Health Measures

ANGUS NICOLL AND VICENTE LOPEZ CHAVARRIAS

European Centre for Disease Prevention and Control (ECDC), Stockholm, Sweden

- What is meant by the term public health measures?
- From the available data and analyses, what could be the value of public health measures in terms of health outcomes?
- Can the same measure be applied in all circumstances?
- What suggested measures are likely to be the most helpful and which the least?

16.1 Introduction

In the context of seasonal and pandemic influenza, public health measures can be defined as 'group actions taken that are intended to reduce human-to-human transmission of influenza and by that means mitigate the adverse effects of an epidemic or pandemic'. Some actions are individual actions designed to give personal protection (e.g. hand washing, mask wearing) that when taken en masse result in overall reductions in transmission and so have a public health benefit.

The most effective countermeasure will be a population-wide specific pandemic vaccine. However, this is not likely to be developed, produced and deployed in any quantity until at least 6 months after the pandemic begins. Additionally, it is likely that many parts of the world, particularly resource-poor countries, will have poor access to antiviral drugs and vaccines. Thus, non-pharmaceutical measures, the focus of this chapter, will potentially be of importance in many settings as the only interventions available. Antiviral drugs and vaccines, which can also have a role in reducing human-to-human transmission of influenza at a population level, are discussed in Chapters 14 and 15, and are not covered in detail in this chapter.

16.2 Rationale and Objectives

The application of public health measures is aimed at reducing the number of people who are infected,

need medical care and die during an influenza pandemic, or at least reducing the rate of transmission. By lowering the peak of a pandemic curve and reducing the numbers affected (Fig. 16.1) the measures can theoretically also mitigate the secondary consequences of pandemics that are most likely to result when many people fall sick at the same time. These include pressures on healthcare services (especially demand for higher levels of hospital care which are usually in short supply) and the impact of mass absenteeism on key functions (e.g. delivering healthcare, food supplies, fuel distribution, utilities, etc.). They may potentially even push back the epidemic curve of a pandemic to a point where influenza transmission declines naturally in the summer months, or when a pandemic vaccine starts to become more widely available, allowing local or national authorities to 'buy' time to prepare and implement other responses. This chapter focuses on measures that would be taken during the time when a pandemic is spreading widely both in a country and across international borders. It does not address the somewhat different circumstances of the first emergence of a putative pandemic strain as described in the World Health Organization (WHO) Rapid Containment Strategy (see Further Reading) nor the complex planning and policy issues that arise over how to sustain key services in a pandemic (Chapter 10).

A range of interventions has been suggested as public health measures (Table 16.1). Some are simple actions to be taken by large numbers of individuals (e.g. regular hand washing and early

Primary objective
- Reduce transmission and thus the number of infections, illnesses and deaths

Secondary objectives
- Delay and flatten outbreak peak
- Reduce peak burden on healthcare system
- Buy some time for preparation, and development of pandemic vaccines

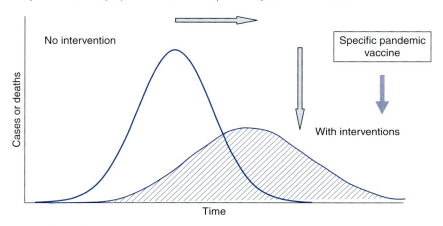

Fig. 16.1. Objectives of applying public health measures in a pandemic.

self-isolation), whilst others require considerable detailed preparation by communities (e.g. closing schools). For many years non-pharmaceutical public health measures were the only options. Nevertheless, their use varied between countries during the three pandemics of the 20th century with the greatest uptake in North America, while their use in the 2009 pandemic was generally not justified because of the largely benign nature of the disease at a population level. This chapter aims to summarize what can be conveyed about their likely effectiveness, costs (direct and indirect), acceptability, public expectations and other practical considerations.

It is thought that combinations of different types of measures will be more effective than single measures, so called 'defence in depth' or 'layered interventions'. This is probably the case but it should be remembered that no measures are cost-free and that attractive as combining measures may be to increase protection, this will inevitably also increase their overall cost and inconvenience. A few of the measures are relatively straightforward to implement (e.g. hand washing) while others are costly and potentially highly disruptive (e.g. school and border closures). In addition, modelling data suggest that some public health measures would only be impactful if applied and withdrawn at specific

times (e.g. school closures), whereas others (e.g. hand hygiene) are less time-sensitive.

16.3 Effectiveness and Secondary Effects

The effectiveness of most measures cannot be readily predicted and a number of them are controversial. Effectiveness varies according to the characteristics of the pandemic. For example, the 1957 and 2009 pandemics, when transmission was especially concentrated in children, were especially sensitive to mass school closure where practised, while that was probably not the case for the 1968 pandemic, when transmission occurred across all age groups. In addition, public compliance may be highly variable between countries and within countries over time. For example, it is known that 'fatigue' ensues when populations are asked to practise hand hygiene for a prolonged period (weeks instead of days) and compliance therefore declines over time. Hence, it is not possible to have rigid plans for every pandemic or for all countries and settings. However, there should be default plans (i.e. plans that will be implemented in the absence of other information) which should be applied with considerable flexibility within a risk-based approach, and command and control structures that allow rapid changes to be made.

Table 16.1. Potential public health measures for reducing influenza transmission (listed in no particular order of preference or hierarchy or effectiveness).

Travel measures – restrictions on international travel	• Travel advice • Entry screening • Border closures or severe travel restrictions
Personal protective measures	• Regular hand washing • Good respiratory hygiene (use and disposal of tissues) • General mask wearing outside the home • Mask wearing in high-risk situations • Mask wearing by people with respiratory infections • Early self-isolation of ill people • Quarantine measures
Social distancing measures[a]	• Internal travel restrictions • Reactive school closures • Proactive school closures • Reactive workplace closures • Home working and reducing meetings • Cancelling public gatherings, international events, etc.
Antivirals[b] – early treatment	• All those with symptoms • Health and social care and/or 'essential' workers
Antivirals – prophylaxis following a case	• Family • Family and other social contacts • Family and geographical contacts
Antivirals – continuous prophylaxis	• Health and social care and/or 'essential' workers
Vaccines[c] – human 'pre-pandemic' vaccines	• Whole population • Health and social care and/or 'essential' workers • Children first
Vaccines – pandemic-specific vaccines	• Pandemic-specific vaccines

[a]Most authorities recommend only considering and implementing each 'social distancing' measure following consideration of the individual merit of each one. [b]Antivirals are dealt with in detail in Chapter 14. [c]Vaccines are dealt with in detail in Chapter 15.

There are more gaps than knowledge concerning the effectiveness and unwanted secondary effects of most measures, and many will require careful consideration. The more drastic societal measures that have been suggested (e.g. proactive school closures and travel restrictions) have significant costs and consequences that will themselves vary according to setting. Limited experience of these disruptive measures shows that they are difficult to sustain, especially where they are not well practised. Hence, for ordinary seasonal influenza or a more benign pandemic like that of 2009, their application (especially their early application) can be more damaging than just allowing the infection to run its course whilst treating those with more severe illness.

16.4 Implementation

Early assessment of the strategic parameters of an evolving pandemic is crucial in deciding what public health measures should be applied and when. Some, like the easier personal measures, should be applied under all circumstances. There is benefit in countries rehearsing their policy options for these measures guided by the recommendations of the WHO and guidance issued by bodies like the European Centre for Disease Prevention and Control (ECDC), as well as national plans where these are available. Because of the diversity of countries, a 'one size fits all' approach will not be appropriate. However, common discussions on the measures will be helpful and make for more efficient implementation. Some countries have already undertaken considerable amounts of relevant scientific work, some of which this chapter draws upon.

Even within a comprehensive book such as this, it is not possible to go through the relevant parameters individually for each measure; instead, each aspect is summarized in Table 16.2.

A. Nicoll and V. Lopez Chavarrias

Table 16.2. Characteristics of potential non-pharmaceutical interventions to reduce transmission during WHO Pandemic Phases 5–6 and severe epidemics of seasonal influenza. (Reproduced with kind permission of the European Centre for Disease Prevention and Control (ECDC).)

Intervention	Quality of evidence[a]	Effectiveness (benefits)	Direct costs	Indirect costs and risks[b]	Acceptability	Practicalities and other issues
International travel (border closures, entry restrictions, travel advice)						
1. Travel advice	B	Minimal	Minimal	Massive	Good	International travel will anyway probably decline considerably, perhaps massively
2. Entry screening	B, Bm	Minimal	Moderate	Moderate	May be expected by resident population	Severe disruption at entry points. Many staff needed to screen travellers and implement follow-up action
3. Border closures or severe travel restrictions	B, Bm	Minimal unless almost complete	Massive	Massive	Variable, but may be expected by some in the resident populations	International travel will probably decline anyway
Personal protective measures						
4. Regular hand washing	B	Probably reduces transmission	Minimal	Nil	Good, but compliance is unknown	Moderate[c], but requires targeted communication and facilities to be made available to maximize compliance
5. Good respiratory hygiene (use and disposal of tissues)	B	Unknown but presumed	Minimal	Minimal	Good, but compliance is unknown	Minimal, but requires targeted communication to maximize compliance
6. General mask wearing outside the home	C, Cm	Unknown	Massive	Minimal	Unknown, but little culture of mask wearing in many countries	Massive – difficulties of training, supply and types of masks, disposal and waste. May be perverse effects from misuse and re-use of masks
7. Mask wearing in high-risk public settings (non-health)[d]	C	Unknown	Moderate	Minimal	Unknown but makes sense	Moderate – difficulties of training, defining high-risk situations, supply and types of mask
8. Mask wearing by people with respiratory infections	C	Unknown but presumed	Moderate	Minimal	Unknown but makes sense. Extends current hospital advice into home and public settings	Difficulties of defining those who should comply, and supply and types of mask. Also compliance for those with restricted breathing due to respiratory infection May permit those ill and infectious to still circulate and infect others
9. Early self-isolation of ill people[e]	C	Unknown but presumed	Moderate	Moderate[f], will increase risk to carers and they will be off work	Already standard advice in many countries	Need to train and equip home carers who will be at risk. Issue of compensation for lost wages and agreement of employers
10. Quarantine measures[g]	C	Unknown	Massive	Massive due to lost productivity	Unclear	Very hard to make work equitably and issue of compensation for lost wages

Continued

Table 16.2. Continued.

Intervention	Quality of evidence[a]	Effectiveness (benefits)	Direct costs	Indirect costs and risks[b]	Acceptability	Practicalities and other issues
Social distancing measures						
11. Internal travel restrictions	Cm, C	Minor delaying effect suggested	Moderate	Massive, including social and economic disruption[h]	Unknown	Key functions threatened. Issue of liability and legal basis[i]
12. Reactive school closures	Bm, C	May have greater effect than other social distancing	Moderate	Large because of children needing to be cared for at home[j]	Unknown, does not happen often in most countries	Children out of school need to be kept away from other children (if not, epidemiological rationale is weakened). Issue of liability and legal basis[j,k]. Difficulties of timing, sustainability and re-opening
13. Proactive school closures	Bm, C	May have greater effect than other social distancing and be better than reactive	Moderate	As above[k]	As above	As above but more difficulties of timing (may close too early), sustainability and re-opening[j,l]
14. Reactive workplace closures	Cm	Unknown[h]	Massive	Massive	Unknown compensation issue crucial	Issue of liability, compensation and legal basis, also sustainability and re-opening. Not possible for key functions[l]
15. Home working and reducing meetings	Cm, C	Unknown	Moderate	Moderate	Likely to be acceptable	Less possible for key functions[m]
16. Cancelling public gatherings, international events, etc.	C	Unknown	Massive[h,i]	Massive[h,i]	Probably depends on compensation issue and if insurance applies! May be expected by the public	Issue of liability and legal backing. Difficulty of definitions about what is a public gathering, international meeting and when to lift bans[l]

[a]Evidence of effectiveness: grades A, B and C represent strongly, reasonably and poorly evidence-based recommendations, respectively. Grade A: systematic reviews where there are diverse primary studies to draw from (not primarily modelling), well-designed epidemiological studies or especially experimental studies (randomized controlled trials). Grade B: represents evidence based on well-designed epidemiological studies, substantial observational studies or experimental studies with five to 50 subjects, or experimental studies with other limitations (like not having influenza as an end point). The code Bm indicates modelling work, with emphasis placed on studies which have available good-quality primary data. Hence quality can be both Bm and C. Grade C: represents evidence based on case reports, small poorly controlled observational studies, poorly substantiated larger studies, application of knowledge of mode of transmission, infectiousness period, etc. Cm refers to modelling with few or poor-quality primary data. [b]Sometimes called second-order and third-order effects – e.g. closing borders resulting in disruption of trade and movement of essential supplies and workers. [c]Need to make frequent hand washing far more available and possible in daily settings, e.g. in public places, fast food outlets, etc. [d]People having face-to-face contact with many members of the public, in crowded travel settings. [e]Usually at home of a person who is starting to feel unwell and feverish. [f]Person requires care at home and they and their carers are lost from work. [g]Isolation at home for some days of well people considered to have been exposed to infection. [h]An advantage of this and some other interventions is that they will bring forward in a planned way what will probably happen anyway with time. [i]Issue of who provides compensation if there is economic loss because of public (government) action. [j]Child requires care at home and their carers are lost from work and may or may not lose income. [k]Interventions targeted at children often assume they play an especially significant role in transmission which may not be the case in every pandemic. [l]There is a complex process of distinguishing what are and are not *key functions* which is important but beyond the scope of this document. [m]The evidence from trials is that with seasonal influenza early treatment reduces duration of illness and transmission. Estimates of the effect on hospitalization and mortality are observational, limited and far weaker.

A. Nicoll and V. Lopez Chavarrias

16.5   Specific Measures

Scientific evidence and experience

The scientific evidence on the effectiveness of the measures generally contains more gaps than certainties. To an extent, this reflects significant large gaps in knowledge about the basic characteristics of influenza transmission (Chapter 8). There have been examinations of existing data and historical information on measures that were applied or happened spontaneously in the three pandemics of the 20th century and the 2009 pandemic. These have revealed important and interesting observations. But these kinds of data can only generate hypotheses and suggestions, as the evidence base is limited and primarily comprises anecdotal observations from seasonal influenza outbreaks, other respiratory infections (notably the outbreaks of severe acute respiratory syndrome (SARS) in 2003) and previous pandemics including 2009. There have been few field studies and hardly any trials of public health measures during a pandemic, or even during seasonal epidemics, to evaluate their likely effectiveness and possible adverse secondary effects (for further details see Chapter 8). Although randomized controlled trials or randomized placebo controlled trials (for pharmaceutical measures) might be desirable, many public health interventions simply cannot be trialled effectively because to do so would cause widespread disruption. In addition, the conditions of a pandemic (novel virus and widespread population concern) cannot be adequately simulated in community trial settings. In the light of this, mathematical models have sometimes been used along with analyses of observational data to project the possible impact of the interventions. Modelling is essential to investigate possible mechanisms and suggest which measures are more or less likely to work (Chapter 13).

Diversity in characteristics and severity between pandemics

Pandemics are not homogeneous (Chapter 5). In particular, they differ in terms of:

- their severity;
- the groups experiencing the most transmission and those most affected by disease;
- the influenza A subtype.

The severity of a pandemic will determine which public health measures can be justified. Measures like extensive proactive school closures might be considered for a severe pandemic like that of 1918, could be excessive and ineffective in a 1968-like scenario, and are generally considered to have been of very limited benefit in Europe and North America during the 2009 pandemic. Similarly, if transmission is focused in one age band (as it was the younger age groups in 1957 and 2009) it may be worthwhile prioritizing measures that protect and reduce transmission in those age groups.

Individual pandemics may change in severity over time, as was the case in 1918 (the second wave), in 1968 (the winter wave in 1969/70 in some European countries) and in 2009 (the second winter wave in New Zealand in 2010 and the winter wave of 2010/11 in a few European countries). Whatever severity is found in the early stages of a pandemic, it is important to measure the epidemiological parameters at intervals, and in different settings, and use these data to assess which measures could and should be usefully applied or stopped as the pandemic progresses.

Diversity within the pandemic

Influenza never affects all localities in the same way at the same time. In the 2009 pandemic in Europe, mainly the UK and Spain were affected in the spring of 2009. Transmission then slowed down in the summer as schools closed, before picking up again in the autumn when the rest of mainland Europe experienced its first significant activity. In countries with appropriate command and control structures, it may be possible to move some resources to relieve the most badly affected areas; however, it can be a challenge for communicators to explain why certain measures are being enacted in one place but not in another. With measures involving limited resources (antivirals, masks, etc.), care will be needed to ensure that supplies are not expended in the areas first affected while leaving other populations with none when they are affected later.

Diversity within and between countries

It is self-evident that countries' demographies are highly diverse, with varying population densities and social and legal frameworks; but this diversity sometimes also exists within countries. Hence, a 'one size fits all' approach will not apply to some public health measures. Taking into account proactive early school closures, for instance, these may make particular sense in schools serving dispersed rural areas, where such institutions function as important foci where young people from scattered communities can meet together. However, they may make less sense (and actually be counter-productive) in dense urban areas, where many parents may have to take time off work to care for children and where it might be difficult to stop children mixing out of school anyway. Such considerations may rationalize implementation, but equally increase the challenges of communicating with the public with one single message.

Isolated communities

Few places are sufficiently isolated to miss a pandemic altogether. Although this was seen in a few places in the 1918 pandemic, these places were exceptional and relatively self-sufficient. The world has become far more inter-connected since the early 1900s and it is unlikely that more than a tiny percentage of citizens in Westernized countries live in communities that could practise self-isolation in this way. However even in the absence of a policy of deliberate self-isolation, the timing of influenza may be delayed in some world regions. For example, in the 2009 pandemic the major surge in disease activity in West Africa was actually seen in 2010, the reasons for which are not fully clear (Chapter 25).

Secondary effects

This concept, essentially looking at what are the costs, risks and consequences of applying the measures themselves, is of paramount importance. The complexity underlying seemingly simple solutions to the pandemic threat, such as 'close the borders' or 'close the schools', can be summarized in a famous saying attributed to the humorist H.L. Mencken: 'for every complex, difficult problem there is frequently a simple and attractive solution – that doesn't work'.

Public health measures, especially social distancing measures, can have major unintended effects. Although they might reduce influenza transmission, they might also be judged negative or unacceptable, certainly if there has not been any planning to overcome these secondary effects. For example, considering internal travel restrictions, these might slow down or reduce transmission, but if they also result in interruption of food or fuel supplies in highly inter-dependent societies, they would not be regarded as a success. Equally, if schools are closed it has to be determined who will look after and educate the children who are not at school. Would, perhaps, important staff like healthcare workers, have to take time off to look after their children? In the 2009 pandemic, when default plans for school closures were enacted in some parts of France and the USA, local authorities felt this was disproportionate to the threat and, after discussion, these policies were reversed. In contrast in parts of China, Japan and Eastern Europe, where these closures are considered the norm, they were enacted relatively smoothly. Public health measures also have the potential to raise significant ethical issues relating to autonomy and curtailment of freedom (Chapter 19).

Timing of introduction and sustainability

If public health measures are to be applied, it is agreed that they generally need to be undertaken early on if they are to be most effective. Overall, there is a suggestion from 1918 that public health measures instigated early tended to delay the peak in mortality by up to 2 weeks and reduce excess mortality. For example, it is suggested that proactive school closures (as the pandemic approaches) will be more effective in reducing transmission than reactive closures (waiting until cases occur in the school).

However, some of the measures are difficult to sustain because of their secondary effects. If they are introduced too early the measures may break down as people grow frustrated with apparently pointless inhibitions to their daily lives, generally meaning that compliance wanes and transmission re-starts. Again, there is some historical evidence of this happening in the USA in the 1918 pandemic, when a number of the larger cities attempted social distancing measures.

Along with planning for decisions about the timing of initiation of public health measures, there must be planning for how and when measures will eventually be lifted. These must make epidemiological sense (e.g. after schools are re-opened there can be 'rebound' increases in transmission among schoolchildren) and sense to the general public (e.g. borders closed one week, but open the next).

A. Nicoll and V. Lopez Chavarrias

Focus Box 16.1. Modelling case study: travel restrictions.

Dr Peter G Grove, Senior Principal Analyst, Health Protection Analytical Team, Department of Health, London, UK

When dealing with any pandemic, a natural response of an individual or community is to try to separate or cut oneself off from the source of infection. Clearly, cutting a community off completely from the world would indeed prevent infection reaching that community. However, in the modern world, few countries are self-sufficient, particularly in terms of food and medical supplies. Only in a few special cases, therefore, could a 100% travel ban be imposed and held in place until the population had been vaccinated. Given this, would temporary or less complete restrictions help?

The limited usefulness of temporary restrictions of any kind is an immediate consequence of the epidemiological theory underlying any kind of model. As long as a large fraction of the community is susceptible (that is, neither having gained immunity by exposure to the virus nor by vaccination) an epidemic will occur as soon as the first cases of the pandemic strain – perhaps having become a form of 'seasonal' influenza elsewhere – enter the country. The policy only makes sense if one can sustain the restrictions long enough for a pandemic-specific vaccine to become available in large quantities. Unless a pre-pandemic vaccine was developed for the right virus this would be at least 6 months after the beginning of the pandemic.

What about reducing the flow of people into a country or other community? Will this provide a significant delay in the arrival of the pandemic? The problem here is that influenza typically affects ten times as many people every 7 to 14 days. Thus the reduction of initial cases entering the community by 90% would be expected to produce at best a 2-week delay in the epidemic in the community. Similarly a 99% reduction produces on a 3–4 week delay, 99.9% perhaps a couple of months.

These expectations have been supported by the findings from a number of explicit models of international travel (e.g. Cooper *et al.*), which also show more subtle effects; such as with a cooperative policy where travel *out* of each community is reduced after the first few observed cases in that community, then the delay of the pandemic in other communities is twice that of a similar universal *entry* restriction imposed unilaterally by those communities.

The same argument backed up by explicit modelling also indicates that, given the period of approximately one day between infection and symptoms, neither exit or entry screening is likely to be effective, producing only a few days' delay in the community's epidemic at most. The delay is even less if there is significant pre-symptomatic and asymptomatic transmission from individuals.

Similar arguments apply to travel within a geographically extended community such as a country. Only very significant reductions (i.e. considerably more than half) in travel could be expected to make any significant difference to the spread of the national epidemic. Even then, the effect would be to decouple the timing of 'local epidemics' in different parts of the country. Each local epidemic would put similar strain on the local health responders, whether or not they were synchronized with other parts of the country.

In summary, formal travel restrictions and screening of those entering from affected countries are generally considered ineffective and not cost-effective.

Complete protection or mitigation?

Many of the measures discussed in this chapter are not expected (or even intended) to give complete protection. They will mitigate or reduce the risk, but not eliminate it; they are a public health approach to reduce the overall impact on the population. This is especially important with the measures that have significant secondary effects, where complete implementation may be unacceptable. That is why some governments intend to apply a number of measures in combination. However, given the nature of infection and pandemics, there are some measures for which only almost complete implementation would be effective, notably those intended to totally block the entry of the virus to a population (e.g. border closures) (Chapter 13). In these cases, the intervention may have greater negative consequences than the disease itself.

Layered containment measures – 'defence in depth'

Current thinking is that the impact of any single public health measure will be limited, because they are hard to enact and do not work perfectly, and some may fail entirely. By applying a number of

Focus Box 16.2. Modelling case study: social distance measures and other non-pharmaceutical interventions.

Dr Peter G. Grove, Senior Principal Analyst, Health Protection Analytical Team, Department of Health, London, UK

As stressed in Chapter 13, modelling is based on data. Its main task is to make obvious information that is not obvious in simply looking at the data used to construct the model. If there are no data, modelling can be of only limited value. Unfortunately, for many socially based interventions there are very few data and therefore little assistance is available from modelling. A typical example is the value of the public use of face masks. There is currently no useful information on the effectiveness of face masks in reducing the transmission of influenza in the general community, and hence no data to put in a model. All that modelling can do here is say, 'we could buy so many face masks which we have no information will save a single life or we could use the same resources for an intervention which will avoid *N* deaths'.

Some information can be inferred on the possible effectiveness of social distancing interventions by seeing if it is possible, for instance, to model the epidemic profies during the 1918 pandemic in a number of American cities that adopted different social distancing measures. Such an investigation was carried out by Bootsma and Ferguson. They showed that it was indeed possible to fit models of interventions to the observed epidemic profiles for major cities, the most convincing evidence for the effectiveness of interventions being a second rise in the number of cases as interventions were relaxed. However, it is not clear if this provides useful information for policy development. While a failure to explain the variation in terms of the interventions applied would be of interest, it is likely, given that we do not know how effective the interventions were, that some combination of assumptions about the interventions applied will in many cases be consistent with the observed data. The question is whether these assumptions are plausible. But this cannot easily be answered by fitting models to data.

The authors recommend caution in extrapolating from 1918 to the current day. Household sizes were much larger and many urban workers lived in large, crowded boarding houses, within which transmission was probably intense. Far more people interacted within large extended families, children spent far fewer years in full-time education, and there were different travel patterns. Overall infectious disease mortality was much higher than it is today. Even taking the results at face value, the authors point out that to save substantial numbers of lives the measures would need to be kept in place until there was enough vaccine to immunize the population. There would be huge social and economic consequences of imposing such measures during the many months that they might be required for optimal effect.

The social measures that do have the most supporting information are school closures, particularly for attending pupils. Even here the effectiveness of closing schools depends critically on how children are assumed to mix with other children and adults, as well as on the profile of any existing immunity. A wide range of impacts has been claimed in the literature. The UK government's scientific advisory group for pandemic influenza considers the most credible results come from studies based on school holidays in the UK and France. These indicate that the school closures are most effective at reducing illness in schoolchildren, although there may be substantial effects in the general population. In a pandemic similar to those recorded in the 20th century, the total effect on the number of clinical cases in the entire population would be expected to be in the range of 10–20%, although the reduction in peak incidence could be higher, up to 50% (spreading the pressure on health services over a longer period but at a more manageable level). Although of limited value themselves, school closures are a very effective adjunct to a household post-exposure prophylactic approach using antivirals (Chapter 14). When estimating the effect of school closures it is important to take into account that children would not stop mixing if schools are closed, so this would reduce the effectiveness of the policy.

On the other hand, if there were significant background immunity amongst adults there may be a more considerable impact on the pandemic. For example, in the UK in the 2009 pandemic the combination of school holidays and general summer holidays suppressed the epidemic over the summer months. However, to be used successfully as a suppression strategy, closures would need to be maintained until a pandemic-specific vaccine was available. Indeed, if ill-timed, the closing of schools might make the epidemic worse by precipitating spread at the point of re-opening.

Closing schools, in countries like the UK, has the potential to create large amounts of absenteeism from work as working parents would have to stay at home to look after their children. The UK government's scientific advisory group estimated that such absenteeism could be as high as 17–20% of the workforce, similar to that expected directly from illness at the peak of the epidemic.

A. Nicoll and V. Lopez Chavarrias

measures simultaneously there will be a cumulative effect on transmission. Some public health experts have argued that, given the relatively low infectivity of influenza, it may be possible to prevent transmission chains building up or to interrupt transmission altogether; however, that assumes a cumulative effect of the measures which is currently a theoretical concept. There is some encouragement for this view from the experience when SARS cases were occurring in Hong Kong in 2003. Multiple measures were enacted by the authorities (including closing schools, forbidding public events) or just happened because they made sense to the citizens (such as staying home and wearing masks when people went out). This is not thought to be what ultimately controlled SARS (a different disease with different transmission parameters), but there was a contemporaneous significant impact on influenza incidence, as reflected in laboratory reports. Additionally, there are also important considerations of cumulative costs and secondary effects with multiple measures, i.e. not only the benefits will increase but so also would the adverse effects.

The necessity of inter-sectoral planning and preparation

Inter-sectoral planning and preparation are critical for many of the public health measures. If regular hand washing is important there need to be facilities in schools and public places to enable this. If it is thought that masks will be needed for some workers these will need to be ordered and stockpiled by employers. Actions involving schools will need preparation, not just by educational authorities, private and public schools, but also by other sectors, industry and civil society. If parents have to seek other care for their children, that cannot be in groups, or the epidemiological rationale for the school closures will be undermined. If they have to take time off work, is it agreed that they will be paid?

Legal issues and liability

Enacting some of the public health measures requires legal powers, and this has to be planned for. There is also the complex area of who is liable for any financial loss that can be said to be due to the measures versus the pandemic. This is genuinely difficult. For example, if it is thought that an international or national meeting must be can-celled, should this be a decision by the authorities who may then be financially liable? Or is it better to wait until it is clear that many individuals are cancelling, in which case the organizers will have to cancel themselves? These considerations can prevent early action even when it is desirable.

General versus selective measures

General measures (such as everyone wearing masks, everyone taking antivirals, etc.) are simple and equitable by their very nature. However, they may not make sense to people who perceive obvious variation in risk, and therefore are less acceptable than selective measures for those at higher risk (e.g. people exposed to the general public wearing masks). Selective measures allow for more possibilities and for ensuring quality in the application of the measure, and can allow for more efficient use of limited supplies. However, the recurrent issues with selective measures are boundaries and 'policing', and deciding who should practise measures and who should not. Further issues would be preventing people feeling left out of benefiting from measures, or getting anxious or annoyed that some people seem to be breaking the rules.

Communications

The importance of communication for the public health measures cannot be overemphasized. All the measures require close cooperation by the public, professionals and decision makers. Communication materials explaining them will need to be prepared ahead of time, pre-tested and probably re-written. Equally there will need to be surge capacity in communication specialists for the pandemic as there is for other key staff (Chapters 10 and 20).

Special groups and special considerations

There will be a number of groups who will find it especially difficult to comply with some measures: the elderly (especially those living alone); children; homeless people or those living in poverty or institutions such as prisons; people travelling but 'caught' in another country; people with physical or learning difficulties; or those with special communication needs (e.g. hearing difficulties, visually impaired, not speaking the national languages). In some cases, numbers will be substantial and planning will need to take this into account.

Work quarantine

This is where quarantine is observed or special measures are taken by health or social care workers who have been exposed and who work in settings where influenza is especially liable to transmit, or where there are people at higher risk from infection, for example people working in care homes or nurses in high-risk settings (such as neonatal care nurseries or intensive care units). This practice was quite common during the SARS crisis but has far less relevance during a pandemic where, in contrast, the threat of infection will be prevalent throughout society and not just in the healthcare environment.

Interoperability

This multifaceted term has a number of meanings, both positive and negative (Table 16.3). For example, neighbouring states or regions need to consider the impact on their neighbours of enacting public health measures, e.g. closing borders if that stops the movement of essential workers. Because of modern communications there can also be indirect effects through the media; for instance if one state is seen enacting measures such as border screening entrants or mask wearing, whereas neighbouring states do not.

As can be seen, the public health measures (including the mass application of individual measures) do not offer a panacea for a pandemic. However, in many countries, especially in resource-poor settings, they will be the most readily available tools to hand for authorities to use, in addition to healthcare (Chapter 25). Some can always be recommended (hand washing) while others will almost always be unwise to enact (border closures). However, between those extremes, the deployment of public health measures requires planning, practice, flexibility and an evidence-based approach. But above all their use has to be guided by the application of public health principles and skills.

Table 16.3. National and international interoperability and pandemic planning.

Negative	Positive
• A country does something that impacts negatively and directly on your state, e.g. closing borders if that stops daily commuting for work	• Some countries perform work from which all (or its neighbours) benefit. Actions that can be undertaken most efficiently in a few Member States (MSs) rather than all MSs but of benefit to all, e.g. monitoring for the development of antiviral resistance
• A country does something that causes questions in another state – especially if its done without warning, e.g. starting to publicly screen people coming off flights or enacting 'containment'	• A group of countries share thinking and analyses on particular policy areas so that conclusions emerge from a common understanding of what is known and not known, e.g. whether and when to close schools proactively
	• Countries share experience and development while recognizing the diversity across a global region (one size will not fit all) – the MS to MS approach: measures enacted in one state that will potentially cause some confusion in other states are discussed, e.g. mask wearing
	• A country talks specifically with its immediate neighbours in relation to all the above
	• A country warns all others as to what it plans to do in a pandemic
	• International bodies like ECDC and WHO develop common mechanisms and tools for preparing and dealing with pandemics, e.g. the ECDC/WHO Pandemic Preparedness Assessment Tool

A. Nicoll and V. Lopez Chavarrias

- Public health measures can be defined as group actions taken that are intended to reduce human-to-human transmission of influenza and mitigate the adverse effects of a pandemic. Some actions are really individual actions designed to give personal protection (e.g. hand washing, mask wearing) or even treatment (e.g. taking of antiviral drugs and use of vaccines) but when taken en masse can result in overall reductions in transmission, and so have a public health benefit.
- Many of the measures would have some impact in terms of reducing transmission although they are less than might be at first imagined, because even if influenza is stopped by one route or in one setting, it may well encroach through another. The greatest impact may, therefore, be through using multiple measures 'in layers' or 'defence in depth'. Then the effects may be additive, but so will be the costs and disruption.
- The same measures should not necessarily be applied in all circumstances. Each pandemic studied so far has had some distinct features implying different responses. Nevertheless, there need to be default sets of recommended public health measures. Also, because of different circumstances in different countries, the measures will not be implementable equally or have the same effect in every country.
- It is difficult to determine which of the suggested measures is likely to be most helpful and which the least, as this depends on the circumstances and the pandemic. Furthermore, there are some suggested measures for which the evidence of effectiveness is simply unknown. However, there are some that we know will not be effective in a pandemic or they are simply impractical – such as trying to screen people at borders (does not work), sealing borders (usually impractical), and mass case finding, contact tracing and PEP (exhausting and largely ineffective).

Further Reading

Bish, A. and Michie, S. (2010) Demographic and attitudinal determinants of protective behaviours during a pandemic: a review. *British Journal of Health Psychology* 15(Pt 4), 797–824.

Bootsma, M.C. and Ferguson, N.M. (2007) The effect of public health measures on the 1918 influenza pandemic in U.S. cities. *Proceedings of the National Academy of Sciences USA* 104(18), 7588–7593.

Cauchemez S., Ferguson N.M., Wachtel C., Tegnell A., Saour G., Duncan B. and Nicoll A. (2009) Closure of schools during an influenza pandemic. *Lancet Infectious Diseases* 9(8), 473–481.

Cooper B.S., Pitman R.J., Edmunds W.J. and Gay N.J. (2006) Delaying the international spread of pandemic influenza. *PLoS Medicine* 3(6), e212.

ECDC (2009) Technical Report. Guide to public health measures to reduce the impact of influenza pandemics in Europe: 'The ECDC Menu'. Available at: http://ecdc.europa.eu/en/publications/Publications/0906_TER_Public_Health_Measures_for_Influenza_Pandemics.pdf (accessed 1 April 2012).

Halloran, M.E., Ferguson, N.M., Eubank, S., Longini, I.M. Jr, Cummings, D.A., Lewis, B., Xu, S., Fraser, C., Vullikanti, A., Germann, T.C., Wagener, D., Beckman, R., Kadau, K., Barrett, C., Macken, C.A., Burke, D.S. and Cooley P. (2008) Modeling targeted layered containment of an influenza pandemic in the United States. *Proceedings of the National Academy of Sciences USA* 105(12), 4639–4644.

Inglesby, T.V., Nuzzo, J.B., O'Toole, T. and Henderson, D.A. (2006) Disease mitigation measures in the control of pandemic influenza. *Biosecurity and Bioterrorism: Biodefense Strategy, Practice and Science* 4(4), 1–10.

Nicoll, A. and Coulombier, D. (2009) Europe's initial experience with pandemic 2009 – mitigation and delaying policies and practices. *Eurosurveillance* 14(29), pii.19279.

World Health Organization (2007) WHO Interim Protocol: Rapid operations to contain the initial emergence of pandemic influenza. Available at: http://www.who.int/influenza/resources/documents/draftprotocol/en/ (accessed 1 April 2012).

World Health Organization (2009) Pandemic influenza prevention and mitigation in low resource communities. Available at: http://www.who.int/csr/resources/publications/swineflu/low_resource_measures/en/index.html (accessed 1 April 2012).

17 Port Health and International Health Regulations

David Hagen

Health Protection Agency (South-East), Horsham, UK

- How rapidly can pandemic influenza spread between countries?
- What are the International Health Regulations (IHR)?
- Could the spread of disease be interrupted by travel-related countermeasures?
- What does WHO advise as effective measures that can be undertaken at ports?

17.1 Introduction

Based on previous pandemics, including the recent one in 2009, the next pandemic will begin in one discrete location, from which it will spread nationally and internationally. Prior to the 2009 pandemic, many experts predicted that the next pandemic epicentre would be in South-east Asia. This was based on the behaviour of the 1957 and 1968 pandemics, the emergence of influenza A(H5N1) and the opportunities in this region for interspecies transmission of influenza viruses. The 2009 pandemic, however, apparently originated in Central America, demonstrating the continuing uncertainty and unpredictability of pandemic influenza. Based on the 2009 experience, it is also clear that, in the current era of globalization, dissemination from the epicentre to neighbouring countries is extremely rapid: many of the first cases of influenza A(H1N1)pdm09 in 2009 in Europe were reported in travellers returning from Mexico or the USA within a few days of the outbreak being announced; in addition travel-associated cases emerged rapidly in New Zealand.

It is intuitive and instinctive to consider whether the spread of disease worldwide could be interrupted or delayed through travel-related countermeasures such as border controls, screening and forced reductions in international travel (Chapter 16). Whilst it is clear that these measures are highly unlikely to succeed, alone or in combination, even the idea of successful travel-related countermeasures inevitably draws attention to international ports and how port health functions should be handled during a pandemic. Although there is an inevitable focus on how port health issues will be used to handle the first few cases of pandemic influenza introduced into a country from outside its borders, the more relevant reality is that once pandemic influenza is established within a country's borders (i.e. is transmitting in the resident community) then control measures at ports will definitely have no further effect on the course of the pandemic within the country. For example, once pandemic influenza has entered a community, coming into contact with someone with symptoms on board an aircraft will have no greater relevance than coming into contact with someone with symptoms on a local bus.

Nevertheless port health issues will continue to present throughout a pandemic. Although international travel is expected to decline sharply during a severe pandemic period as people spontaneously change their behaviour and contact patterns, it will not cease completely; there is a natural instinct to 'return home' during a crisis and some international business travel will continue. Thus, passengers with influenza symptoms are still likely to present at ports (arriving and departing) and will need to be dealt with appropriately. It is also possible that 'health tourism' may encourage citizens from one country to attempt to cross into another because pandemic treatments (e.g. the availability of hospital care, antiviral drugs and vaccines) may be more readily available or cheaper elsewhere.

17.2 International Health Regulations (2005)

To understand the foundation upon which a response to a case of pandemic influenza at a port is to be planned, we must first examine the International Health Regulations (IHR). Via these regulations it has been stated that 'the global community has a new legal framework to better manage its collective defences to detect disease events and to respond to public health risks and emergencies that can have devastating impacts on human health and economics'. The World Health Organization (WHO) issued its first set of regulations intended to prevent the spread of diseases in 1951. They concentrated on only six 'quarantinable' diseases: cholera, plague, relapsing fever, smallpox, typhus and yellow fever, and were called the International Sanitary Regulations. These were renamed the International Health Regulations in 1969, and other public health issues have since appeared as international concerns and been incorporated into the framework. Three fundamental principles (below) have subsequently been included in the latest version of the IHR, which came into force in June 2007 and provides an international agreement that is legally binding on 194 countries (States Parties), including all WHO Member States:

1. Replacing the list of specific diseases with more generic illness.
2. Including chemical, biological and radiological agents as well as infectious agents.
3. Making some incidents notifiable within 24 hours to the WHO if they fulfil the criteria to constitute a Public Health Emergency of International Concern (PHEIC). The decision to report and responsibility for reporting PHEICs rests firmly with the individual state and these are reported through a National Focal Point to the WHO.

In addition, the emphasis for member states has changed from control at borders to containment at source for international threats. This is consistent with the stated intention of the IHR: 'to prevent, protect against, control and provide a public health response to the international spread of disease in ways that are commensurate with and restricted to public health risks, and which avoid unnecessary interference with international traffic and trade.'

Below is a summary of the member states' key obligations:

1. **Reporting PHEICs** – as noted above, which requires notification to WHO for all cases of: (i) certain specified diseases; and (ii) all events involving at least two of the following four criteria regardless of the particular disease or risk: (a) serious public health impact, (b) unusual or unexpected nature, (c) risk of international spread, and (d) risk of interference with international trade.
2. **Public health capacity** – to develop national *core capacities* for detection, assessment, control and reporting of public health events notable here; at certain international ports, airports and ground crossings.
3. **Travellers** – to provide proper treatment of international travellers, including some human rights and other protection such as personal health data and prior informed consent for examination and procedures.
4. **Measures** – authorizations and limits on health/sanitary measures applied to international travellers, conveyances (e.g. aircraft, ships), cargo and goods.
5. **Certificate/document requirements** – on sanitary requirements for international air, sea and ground traffic.

It must be borne in mind that member states' fundamental obligations to develop and/or maintain key public health capacities for surveillance and response apply, regardless of whether or not a PHEIC has been notified. It was envisaged that PHEICs would be relatively rare events, and this has subsequently been demonstrated.

17.3 WHO Review of the Implementation of the IHR in May 2011

In January 2010 the WHO Executive Board accepted the Director-General's proposal, which included a request to review the experience gained in the global response to the influenza A(H1N1)-pdm09 pandemic. The three key objectives were:

1. To assess the functioning of the IHR (2005).
2. To review the role of WHO in pandemic preparedness and response.
3. To identify lessons for the future.

The independent Review Committee consisted of 25 members from 24 countries and the proceedings included four plenary sessions plus deliberative sessions where information was sought not only from WHO's Secretariat, but also evidence was received from experts around the world, which included testimonies and written submissions.

The final report has three main components: the first section, entitled 'Preparation for a Global Public-Health Emergency', provides the background for the committee's assessments; the second section, entitled 'Pandemic Influenza A(H1N1) 2009', is a chronology of events; and the third section assesses the functioning of the IHR and the WHO's role in the 'Management of the Global Response'.

Three overarching conclusions were reached by the Review Committee and are summarized below:

1. 'The IHR helped make the world better prepared to cope with public health emergencies, however in terms of borders they note that core national and local capacities called for in the IHR are not yet fully operational and are not now on a path to timely implementation worldwide.'
2. 'WHO performed well in many ways during the pandemic, confronted systemic difficulties and demonstrated some shortcomings. The committee found no evidence of malfeasance.'
3. 'The world is ill-prepared to respond to a severe influenza pandemic or to any similarly global, sustained and threatening public health emergency....'

Within these conclusions are many recommendations that are applicable throughout this textbook's topic areas, but we will examine more closely those related to response at borders.

Recommendation #1 notes that the implementation of *core capacities* required by the IHR needs accelerating. As noted earlier, there are various obligations of member states which the report notes will not be completed by 2012. This applies to the states' infrastructure such as public sector organizations' processes and laboratory capacities for the most part, but includes the capacity to respond at ports of entry for international travellers, conveyances, cargo and goods.

Recommendation #3 notes a requirement to reinforce evidence-based decisions on international travel and trade. Specifically it is critical of those states that attempted to apply more stringent health measures at ports, which would have significantly interfered with international traffic. It goes on to note in IHR Article 43 that there is a requirement that States Parties shall inform WHO of their actions if this interference means 'refusal of entry or departure of international travellers, baggage, cargo, containers, conveyances, goods and the like, or their delay, for more than 24 hours'. It goes on to state that the WHO should 'energetically seek to obtain the public-health rationale and relevant

scientific information...and where appropriate request reconsideration'.

Recommendation #4 briefly notes that the necessary authority and resources for all National IHR Focal Points be made available. This includes procedures and training for their implementation.

Further findings of the Review Committee included:

- #78 – the Committee noted that 'the temporary recommendation issued on 27 April 2009 that remained unchanged until the end of the PHEIC, was not to close borders and not to restrict international travel'. WHO surveyed States Parties, airports, airlines and shipping operators and noted that most provided information in the form of posters or leaflets to incoming travellers. The report continues that 'During the early stages of the pandemic, 34 of 56 (61%) responding countries "screened" incoming passengers for disease. In most of the countries, screening was combined with isolation of suspected or confirmed cases and quarantine of their asymptomatic close contacts for 3–10 days (median eight days)' although usually this was at home.
- #79 – the Committee noted that 'two of the surveyed countries reported denying entry to people from affected countries. Six out of the 56 surveyed countries (11%) reported restricting the entry of animals or goods from affected countries'.
- #80 – the Committee noted that 'five out of 56 surveyed countries reported having denied free *pratique* to at least one mode of transport, mostly owing to the presence of ill people on board'. This reflects 'the experiences of a few ship operators and airlines that were refused permission to embark or disembark passengers or crew because of illness or having visited affected countries'.
- #81 – the Committee noted 'half of the surveyed countries recommended that their citizens avoid travelling to affected countries during the early stages of the event; the median duration of travel advisories was 5 weeks. There were also instances of flights to affected countries being cancelled', although this was often due to lack of sufficient passengers.
- #82 – on a positive note, the Committee pointed out the results of the survey that suggest that 'measures introduced at borders changed during the first four months of the pandemic, showing that countries adapted to changing epidemiology and recommendations'. Early strategies shifted from a broad precautionary approach to more focused

response measures implemented at points of entry. It was noted that 'control measures later shifted to communities as more information about the virus became available, perceptions of risk changed, and community transmission [within the member states' own country] became more prevalent'.

Evidence to the Review Committee from IATA (below), whose members comprise all major passenger and cargo airlines, indicated that countries' varying approaches to border control were confusing for airlines. Not all countries advertised their measures and pilots did not know what to expect upon landing. This had a cascade effect, delaying aircraft turnaround times. The Committee again pointedly noted that such measures should be based on evidence.

17.4   International Organizations

There are three primary organizations that advise the international air travel industry on public health and other issues, and hence on response to an influenza pandemic. These are the:

- International Civil Aviation Organization (ICAO), which represents its contracting countries and whose responsibilities are at country level;
- Airports Council International (ACI), which represents its individual airports; and
- International Air Transport Association (IATA), which is a trade association representing the airline industry worldwide.

Each has developed contingency plans and guidelines for its respective areas of responsibility, most of which are available on the Internet and are well worth examining.

17.5   Cooperative Arrangements for the Prevention of Spread of Communicable Disease through Air Travel (CAPSCA)

This project commenced in 2006 in order to provide guidance for all public-health-related events. The project is managed by ICAO, in close collaboration with the WHO and additional partners including the ACI and IATA, and is directed towards devising and amending ICAO Annexes and facilitating their implementation. These Annexes provide guidance on specific areas such as operations, air traffic services, aerodromes and procedures for air navigation services. It was first established in the Asia Pacific region following the severe acute respiratory syndrome

(SARS) epidemic, and took the form of providing workshops, seminars and training to address two main points: strengthening preparedness planning for public health emergencies affecting the aviation sector; and improving cross-sectoral communications and collaboration. Their latest initiative is the expansion of the project to the European Region, and two meetings have taken place at the time of writing: the first in September 2011 and the second in July 2012. Support from the European States was achieved and work continues to ensure a consistent approach to public health emergency planning in the aviation sector.

17.6   Misconceptions of Risk

There is a mistaken belief amongst the travelling public, often reinforced by public health officials, that if one person has boarded an aircraft with symptoms of an infectious disease then all remaining passengers are at high risk of acquiring that infection. Widespread influenza transmission has indeed been documented on board an airliner in Alaska; however, that aircraft was grounded, the ventilation was switched off and passengers were free to walk about. An analysis of data obtained from two long-haul flights entering Australia in May 2009 revealed that sitting in the same row or within two rows of those who were symptomatic with A(H1N1)pdm09 before the flight carried a 4% increased risk of developing A(H1N1) pdm09, rising to 8% if seated within two seats of a case. However, similar data from a flight entering the UK from Mexico in 2009 suggest that the risk of secondary infection, even with several potentially infectious persons on board, is still small (under 5%) but not limited to those within two rows.

17.7   SARS Provides Lessons

Those planning for a public health response to an influenza pandemic often look at the international response to the SARS outbreak in 2003 for lessons.

SARS demonstrated just how rapidly the international spread of disease can occur in the modern age of air travel. From first appearing in the Guangdong province of southern China in November 2002, it only took 4 months to spread to 26 countries causing nearly 800 deaths and over 8000 cases of infection. Transmission was facilitated by a Chinese doctor who had treated patients with the 'unknown' respiratory illness, before himself flying to Hong Kong and infecting others, as well as failures in isolation and infection control measures in healthcare facilities as far afield as Toronto in Canada.

SARS is a milestone with regard to air travel due to several factors:

- It was a newly emerging global threat first recognized only recently.
- It spread rapidly to more than two dozen countries in North America, South America, Europe and Asia before the outbreak was contained.
- It was spread readily by close contact.
- It was more amenable than influenza to proactive efforts due to the fact that peak infectivity occurred well after symptom onset and the incubation period was relatively long (3–10 days) compared with influenza (1–3 days).
- General infection control precautions are the suggested actions (see Chapter 8).

Much publicity was given to exit screening in affected countries, both by medical questionnaire and thermal imaging, but these proved disruptive, ineffective and costly – requiring individual and public health action for febrile people.

According to flight schedule provider OAG, the number of scheduled flights worldwide fell by 3% (equivalent to 2.5 million seats) in mid-June 2003 compared to the same period in 2002. Flights to and from China showed a 45% drop in passenger numbers, and the outbreak is estimated to have cost the world's airlines and travel-related industries approximately US$40 billion. Furthermore, the public's perception of risk of in-flight transmission of disease was influenced, despite the lack of evidence for this.

In addition, the previously mentioned WHO Review Committee noted three generic lessons to be learnt from SARS:

1. The importance of early detection and for transparent reporting of unusual disease events, notably communicating information to policy makers, politicians, public health professionals and the public.
2. The importance of zoonoses as a source of infections in humans, whereby infection can occur following contact with infected animals, animal products or contaminated environments; as well as human-to-human transmission.
3. The important role of national veterinary services (both in SARS and avian influenza) in planning and responding to a pandemic with collaboration between animal health and public health authorities.

17.8 Travel Restrictions

Widely accepted modelling suggests that a 90% restriction on European air travel would delay the peak of the pandemic by less than 2 weeks (Chapter 13). Restrictions on travel from specific locations, for instance South-east Asia, would also be ineffective given the indirect flows of people from Asia to the rest of the world as well as flows of people who would rapidly become infected in outbreaks in other countries. Although there was a study in 2006 indicating that restricting air travel to the USA might have some domestic effect, most planners still accept the findings of a WHO technical consultation which was held in Geneva in 2004, attended by more than 100 experts from 33 countries, which stated that:

> … providing information to domestic and international travellers (risks to avoid, symptoms to look for, when to seek care) is a better use of health resources than formal screening. Entry screening of travellers at international borders will incur considerable expense with a disproportionately small impact on international spread, although exit screening should be considered in some situations.

However, there will be intense political pressure to strengthen port health vigilance and implement restrictions in the early stages of the next pandemic, which was borne out by experience in 2009.

17.9 The Layered Approach

Both North America and the UK have adopted what is termed a *layered approach* to port health, whereby several levels of response overlap and complement each other. This approach is necessary in an influenza pandemic as it is likely that: (i) the causes of influenza-like illness in passengers will be varied; (ii) asymptomatic infected individuals will not be detected by screening; and (iii) some travellers who are asymptomatically incubating the illness at the start of a long-haul flight may develop symptoms en route. The layered approach divides the actions into those at pre-embarkation, en route and upon arrival at the destination airport.

17.10 Pre-embarkation

Pre-embarkation measures would be applied throughout the pandemic, but as with most measures outlined here the real value is in the early pandemic period before cases are found within a country. These measures may include:

D. Hagen

- medical assessment of fitness to fly;
- screening by check-in or gate staff supported by airline contracted ground-based medical support (routine at present);
- self-administered medical questionnaire with assessment;
- questioning of passengers by trained staff; and
- thermal imaging.

Early on, identification of cases will be a high priority given the enormous implications of a confirmed case and will be facilitated by rapid or near patient tests when they become available. The real value in identifying cases before or once the virus is isolated in the country is to offer prophylaxis to those caring for the traveller and 'contacts' of the case, as well as for surveillance purposes. This would be of little value once outbreaks begin to occur within the destination country.

17.11   Generic Communicable Disease Control Applied to Pandemic Influenza

En route generic measures include enforcing existing IATA guidelines on dealing with suspected communicable diseases. These facilitate appropriate action in recognizing and dealing with any passenger fulfilling the criteria stated. Implementing these guidelines should give cabin crew the confidence to avoid overreaction, such as the removal of a 16-year-old girl from a flight from Hawaii to New York due to an acute episode of coughing in March 2007.

IATA guidelines indicate that cabin crew obtain contact details from all travellers seated in the same row, two rows in front and two rows behind the sick traveller utilizing passenger locator cards (PLCs). PLCs were developed by the WHO to obtain public health contact tracing information and have been adapted for use by airlines and public health authorities internationally. Obtaining passenger data through airline manifest information continues to be problematic due to the nature of the details held by airlines, which are for financial purposes, and also because of confidentiality issues. In addition to the above measures, in July 2007 ICAO introduced a system to provide earlier warning of public health events which would increase the window for mounting a public health response by reporting suspected cases of communicable disease via air traffic control services. This was subsequently refined in further communications to industry.

Despite evidence from the SARS response showing lack of effectiveness, arrival measures may include consideration of thermal imaging as a screening method, utilizing newer generation equipment and/or having public health staff perform assessments on self-administered questionnaires completed upon landing or en route. Current generic arrival measures rely on *isolation*, which is the separation and restriction of movement of ill and potentially infectious individuals. *Quarantine* is the separation and restriction of movement of persons who, while not yet ill, have been potentially exposed to a communicable disease. It would require a large investment in resources to staff, accommodate and supply basic day-to-day needs in a secure area. This would require each country to pass legislation to ensure compliance and enforcement; and would also require a policy in place for removal of quarantine through near patient or rapid testing or evidence-based clinical assessment. Neither isolation nor quarantine measures at ports would have any impact on population spread once cases of pandemic influenza had already been reported within a country.

17.12   Management of Pandemic Influenza at Ports

Management of pandemic flu at ports of entry and exit to a country will require the cooperation of a myriad of organizations involved in the travel industry, as well as close liaison between public health and healthcare service providers. The greatest call on resources will occur early in the pandemic when there will be political pressure to be seen to be protecting the country from disease, despite the lack of evidence to support control measures.

Symptomatic individuals may need to be sent to hospitals or assessment centres for further investigation, and where possible these should be located near the airport. Early in the pandemic antivirals for cases and contacts may be available at ports, but this facility would be quickly overwhelmed. Quarantine would require pre-arrangement of facilities which could provide all accommodation requirements as well as security to prevent escape and entry, as well as a pre-determined end point to its application.

Any arrangements made at ports will require mechanisms to minimize direct contact with passengers and crew who may be subject to public health intervention, yet still satisfy security and immigration requirements. Table 17.1 summarizes the range of possible port health actions during a

Table 17.1. Potential measures at ports at different stages of an influenza pandemic.

Measures	Pandemic declared	Virus isolated in country	Outbreaks within country	Widespread activity in country	Declining numbers	Comments
Information to travellers						
Details about the outbreaks	+	+	+	+	+	Full information on outbreaks must be shared
Advice – e.g. avoid non-essential travel	+	+	+	+	+	Country should issue advice early in pandemic
Repatriation (citizens and dead bodies)	–	?	?	–	–	Each country will have its own policy, but practicalities are immense
Border closures	–	–	–	–	–	No evidence to support effectiveness
Port closures	–	–	–	–	–	Impractical
Pre-embarkation measures						
Medically fit to fly	+	+	+	+	+	Current practice
Screening at check-in	+	+	+	+	+	Current practice
Self-administered questionnaire	+	+	–	–	–	Only useful in early part of response
Questioning by trained staff	+	+	–	–	–	Supports self-administered questionnaire
Thermal imaging	?	?	–	–	–	No evidence to support effectiveness
En route measures						
IATA guidelines – generic						
ID sick passengers	+	+	+	+	+	Current practice
Infection control measures	+	+	+	+	+	Current practice
Consult ground-based support	+	+	+	+	+	Current practice
Advise port health	+	+	+	+	+	Current practice
Passenger locator cards	+	+	–	–	–	May be impractical later
Arrival measures						
Thermal imaging	?	?	–	–	–	No evidence to support effectiveness
Self-administered questionnaire	+	+	–	–	–	Only useful in early part of response
Assessment by medical staff	+	+	–	–	–	Supports self-administered questionnaire
Isolation	+	+	+	+	+	Current practice, but unlikely to prevent population spread once cases are occurring within country
Quarantine	?	?	–	–	–	No evidence of effectiveness and impractical

+, Consider as potentially beneficial; –, not useful at this stage of the pandemic; ?, currently not supported.

D. Hagen

pandemic, and the stages at which these might be most relevant to consider.

17.13 Disruption to the Global Economy

Despite the relatively mild nature (for the majority of people) of the A(H1N1)pdm09 pandemic, in 2011 the Organisation for Economic Co-operation and Development (OECD) noted in its report *Future Global Shocks* that a new pandemic remains amongst the top five major potential causes for disruption. The other four being a cyber attack disrupting critical infrastructure, a financial crisis, socio-economic unrest and a

geomagnetic storm. It notes the increasing number of heavily populated megacities, notably in Asia, exacerbating this risk.

In the event of any future virulent influenza pandemic, or for that matter, any public health emergency on a global and sustained scale, there will clearly be massive disruption to the international travel sector. It may be that the degree of disruption is due more to the uncertainty of the potential impact of the virus at the early stages of a pandemic and the steps taken to reassure travellers and countries, rather than the properties of the virus; but the infrastructure is in place for a proportionate and evidence-based approach to both planning and response.

- Dissemination from the epicentre to neighbouring countries will be extremely rapid. Many of the first cases of influenza A(H1N1)pdm09 in Europe were reported in travellers returning from Mexico or the USA within a few days of the outbreak being announced and cases rapidly emerged in countries as far away as New Zealand.
- The International Health Regulations (IHR) were first issued by WHO in 1951 as the International Sanitary Regulations specifically to prevent the spread of six quarantinable diseases. In 1969 they were renamed the IHR and were updated to reflect further public health issues. The current IHR (2005) are legally binding on 194 countries who have agreed to their adoption.
- Travel-related countermeasures such as border controls, screening and forced reductions in international travel are highly unlikely to interrupt or delay the spread of a pandemic, alone or in combination. A 90% delay on European air travel could delay the peak of the pandemic by less than 2 weeks. Restrictions on travel from specific locations would also be ineffective due to indirect passenger flows.
- Provision of information to travellers (e.g. risks to avoid, symptoms to look for, when to seek care) is a better use of health resources than formal screening. Entry screening of travellers at international borders will incur considerable expense with a disproportionately small impact on international spread, although exit screening should be considered in some situations.

Further Reading

Airports Council International (2009) Airport Preparedness Guidelines for Outbreaks of Communicable Disease. Available at: http://www.airports.org/aci/aci/file/ACI_Priorities/Health/Airport%20preparedness%20 guidelines.pdf (accessed 9 April 2012).

Anonymous (2010) Public health measures taken at international borders during early stages of pandemic influenza A(H1N1)2009: preliminary results. *Weekly Epidemiological Record* 85(21), 186–195.

Foxwell, A.R., Roberts, L., Lokuge, K. and Kelly, P.M. (2011) Transmission of influenza on international flights, May 2009. *Emerging Infectious Diseases* 17(7), 1188–1194.

International Air Transport Association (2011) Suspected communicable disease: general guidelines for cabin crew. Available at: http://www.iata.org/whatwedo/safety_

security/safety/health/Documents/health-guidelines-cabin-crew-2011.pdf (accessed 9 April 2012).

International Air Transport Association (2012) Business continuity plan: specific issues for public health emergencies. Guidelines for air carriers. Available at: http://www.iata.org/whatwedo/safety_security/safety/health/Documents/public-health-emergency-bcp.pdf (accessed 9 April 2012).

International Civil Aviation Organization (no date) Guidelines for States Concerning the Management of Communicable Disease Posing a Serious Public Health Risk. Available at: http://legacy.icao.int/icao/en/med/AvInfluenza_guidelines.pdf (accessed 9 April 2012).

Leder, K. and Newman, D. (2005) Review: Respiratory infections during air travel. *Internal Medicine Journal* 35, 50–55.

Moser, M.R., Bender, T.R., Margolis, H.S., Noble, G.R., Kendal, A.P. and Ritter, D.G. (1979) An outbreak of influenza aboard a commercial airliner. *American Journal of Epidemiology* 110, 1–6.

World Health Organization (no date) Public health passenger locator card. Available at: http://www.who.int/ihr/ports_airports/locator_card/en/ (accessed 9 April 2012).

World Health Organization (2004) WHO Consultation on priority public health interventions before and during an influenza pandemic, Geneva 16–18 March 2004. Available at: www.afro.who.int/index.php?option=com_docman&task=doc_download&gid=5116 (accessed 9 April 2012).

World Health Organization (2005) The International Health Regulations. Available at: http://www.who.int/ihr/en/ (accessed 9 April 2012).

World Health Organization (2011) External review of pandemic response. Available at: http://www.who.int/ihr/review_committee/en/index.html (accessed 9 April 2012).

World Health Organization (2011) Implementation of the International Health Regulations (2005) Report of the Review Committee on the Functioning of the International Health Regulations (2005) in relation to Pandemic (H1N1) 2009. Available at: http://apps.who.int/gb/ebwha/pdf_files/WHA64/A64_10-en.pdf (accessed 9 April 2012).

18 Socio-economic Impact

Patricia R. Blank[1,2] and Thomas D. Szucs[2]

[1]University of Zurich, Zurich, Switzerland;
[2]University of Basel, Basel, Switzerland

- What are the potential socio-economic impacts of an influenza pandemic?
- How might pandemic influenza mortality and morbidity differ to patterns seen with seasonal influenza?
- How big could the financial impact of a pandemic be and where could it be felt?
- What aspects of business might be impacted by a pandemic?

18.1   Introduction

This chapter explores some of the possible effects of a future pandemic on societal functioning. Much will depend on the virulence and rapidity of spread of the emergent virus and the response taken by governments and the public. Previous pandemics have been highly variable in impact and unfortunately, only limited data are available on which to make predictions due to the fact that these are relatively infrequent events. Given improved healthcare provision, extensive, international cooperation and the recent experiences from 2009, it is almost certainly true that preparation to face a pandemic is better than it has ever been. However key changes to global society such as increased global mobility, urbanization, social inequalities and population growth will further facilitate rapid spread of a future pandemic. The uncertainties surrounding the possible impact of future influenza pandemics make planning and preparedness a difficult endeavour. While there is the potential to be accused of scare mongering on the one hand, when a serious outbreak does occur, questions will inevitably be asked as to why not more action was taken before the event. The former Secretary of US Health and Human Services, Michael O. Leavitt, famously remarked: 'Everything you say in advance of a pandemic is alarmist; anything you do after it starts is inadequate'.

18.2   Social Impact

Mortality

While it is anticipated that future pandemic mortality could be orders of magnitude greater, history is not very consistent on this fact. The 1918 pandemic produced a high global mortality, 20–40 million people worldwide are thought to have died with some estimates placing this figure nearer 100 million. The events later in the century had a much smaller mortality impact, thought to be in the region of 1 million excess deaths, not vastly different from the annual death toll attributed to seasonal influenza. Finally, the recent A(H1N1)pdm09 pandemic in 2009 was extremely mild in terms of total mortality, but less so in terms of premature deaths (years of life lost).

The variability in mortality experienced between pandemics makes it very difficult to predict with any precision what will be experienced in the next one. Nevertheless, governments around the world have planned for a pandemic that could realize deaths in the upper range of that experienced in 1918. For example, prior to the 2009 pandemic, the UK government planned for a 'reasonable worst case scenario' of a 50% clinical attack rate and a case fatality rate of up to 2.5%. Accordingly, 50,000 to 750,000 additional deaths would be expected. In 2008, the World Bank estimated that more than 74 million people could be killed during an influenza pandemic, but some researchers even suggest higher figures of up to 250 million deaths worldwide. The World Health Organization (WHO) suggests that 25% of the global population might be rapidly affected during a future pandemic. What is known from the last century is that the spike in deaths caused major problems with dealing with the dead, particularly so in 1918. The numbers of deceased overwhelmed undertakers and burial authorities.

Conventional seasonal influenza tends to afflict the very young, old and those with weak immune systems or certain chronic diseases. The same was experienced with the two milder pandemics of 1957 and 1968. However, the 1918 pandemic behaved differently; while the first wave conformed to this pattern, the second saw large numbers of working-age adults (aged 20–45 years) killed with relative sparing of the very young and old. The reasons for this are not fully understood. According to the European Centre for Disease Prevention and Control (ECDC), around 3000 laboratory-confirmed deaths were attributable to the mild A(H1N1)pdm09 pandemic in Europe in 2009/10. However, the pattern of death differed considerably from the previous influenza seasons. Indeed, 80% of fatal cases occurred in people under 65 years of age. Although the majority of deaths were reported in people with one or more chronic underlying conditions, there were increased numbers of deaths among children and around 30% of all reported influenza deaths occurred in previously healthy people. The US Centers of Disease Control and Prevention (CDC) reported about 12,000 deaths in the USA due to A(H1N1)pdm09 in 2009.

Morbidity

With up to 50% of the population being affected by symptomatic influenza over the course of an influenza pandemic, it is clear that the potential for disruption due to the ill health will be substantial. While it is expected that most illness will be self-limiting and relatively minor, there will be a minority who become more severely ill. The less badly affected are nevertheless predicted to be absent from work for approximately 5–10 days due to the illness itself (Chapter 1).

US estimates have indicated that approximately one-sixth of the population will seek 'outpatient' care. Of all influenza cases, about 0.7–3% will require hospital care, with up to 0.5% needing intensive care. Other estimates suggest that of those

who become infected with symptoms, up to 25% will need medical help, with between 0.6% and 4% needing hospital treatment and up to 1% requiring intensive care. During the A(H1N1)-pdm09 pandemic period, approximately 60 million Americans were infected and 274,000 hospitalizations (41,914 laboratory-confirmed, influenza-associated hospitalizations) were reported by the CDC, with indications of an increase in the hospitalization rates among younger age groups compared to previous winter influenza seasons.

18.3 Economic and Socio-economic Burden

Macro-economic business impact

The financial costs of an influenza pandemic could be enormous. Modelling studies have suggested that this could be in the region of several trillion US dollars. The costs will be felt across society, from increased healthcare provision requirements, through lost productivity of industry, to early deaths and short- and long-term disability of victims. However, it is not only these expenditures immediately associated with a pandemic that should be borne in mind. The financial outlay made in preparation for a pandemic is ongoing and substantial. This poses significant dilemmas for planners in terms of the opportunity costs of making these investments. In resource-poor settings where healthcare provision or public health infrastructure for current health problems is currently lacking (e.g. childhood vaccination programmes), allocation of resources to pandemic preparedness may raise important bioethical dilemmas (Chapter 25). Post-pandemic recovery costs can also be considerable.

According to the World Bank, the labour supply shock of the first year of a pandemic can account for 1.3% of the global gross domestic product (GDP). If preventive means are taken into account, the costs can increase to about 2% of the GDP leading to total decline in GDP of 3% per year, with an even higher estimate for a severe scenario (4.8% of world GDP or US$3 trillion (€2.28 trillion)).

A recent study determined the potential macro-economic impact of behavioural responses, school closures and vaccination in the UK in terms of GDP by accounting for different economic sectors and equivalent variation. The proposed cost of illness was estimated at 0.5–1% (£8.4–16.8 billion or

€9.8–19.7 billion) or 3.3–4.3% of the UK GDP (£55.5–72.3 billion or €64.9–84.6 billion), depending on a low or high fatality scenario, respectively. Closing schools, changed behaviours or absence from workplaces would increase the economic toll without substantial health gain. On the other hand, it is estimated that vaccination would be cost saving over a broad range of disease scenarios. Similar results have been derived from modelling in France, Belgium and the Netherlands, which assessed the cost implications of implementing policies of school closure, vaccination, antiviral drugs and prophylactic absence from work. Loss of between 0.5% and 2% of GDP in those European countries was calculated, mainly driven by school closure and precautionary absenteeism.

Industrial impact

Modelling has suggested that a severe influenza pandemic could cause industrial output to decline to a level consistent with the recessions that have occurred since the end of World War II. Some sectors of the economy are likely to face bigger declines than others. In particular, mass transport, restaurants, large social gatherings and hotels will probably be affected most. Life and health insurance businesses would also suffer appreciably due to the morbidity and mortality of influenza cases.

The demand for services such as tourism, retail trade, transport or entertainment will likely be reduced by individuals' precautionary behaviours during a severe pandemic. Likewise, productivity may be affected by the decline in labour supply due to influenza morbidity and mortality. The financial consequences of an influenza pandemic are expected to vary by country, region and industry type. Those more dependent on tourism, travel and entertainment are likely to be hit hardest with GDP reductions of up to 8%, whereas those with more diverse economies will probably fare better with GDP decreases of up to 5%. European research suggests that, during an influenza pandemic, labour-intensive segments such as insurance, health and social services, and education would suffer most, whereas agriculture would be the least affected sector in terms of loss in GDP.

The industrial burden during the 2009 pandemic was mainly concentrated on the transportation sector. Not only did air travel from and to Mexico decrease considerably, but the entire Mexican tourism revenue also decreased by about 43%, resulting in an enlarged financial gap. The World Bank estimated a loss in the Mexican GDP of up to 2.2%, given the disruption in the commerce, restaurant, hotel and transportation sectors. A similar picture was seen during the severe acute respiratory syndrome (SARS) outbreak in 2003, where significant correlations were found for SARS cases or deaths and the volume of public transportation, tourism, household consumption and GDP reduction in Beijing. The World Bank estimates that the SARS outbreak led to an overall decline of 0.5% in the GDP of the East Asian economy, with a steeper decline of 2% in the second quarter of 2003 when publicity about the disease was at its peak.

Governments around the world work on the presumption of maintaining business and services towards as normal a state of affairs as possible because to advise otherwise would risk causing even greater harm. The virulence of the outbreak will determine whether this is achievable. If mild it may not be difficult to persuade people to continue to work, but if severe many may consider the risks as too great for them. Management of the perceived risks will be important as people are not always good at determining the degree of threat they face, which can lead to inappropriate responses. Businesses should make preparations for an influenza pandemic to enable them to maintain their services and protect their staff during the crisis. However, it is a fallacy to consider that even the best plans will be 100% effective (Chapter 9).

While many businesses will be negatively impacted during a pandemic, others may see a surge in demand. As people choose to stay away from crowded areas, there may be an increase in online purchasing, especially for groceries. There will inevitably be elevated demand for over-the-counter healthcare products and environmental cleaning/disinfectant products among the general public, and companies will need to ensure they can manufacture and supply enough to meet the need.

The direct costs of a pandemic are only a small proportion of the economic impact. In a small country like Switzerland, the total direct costs are estimated to reach CHF2.4–5.0 million (€2.0–4.6 million) during a pandemic situation. It is expected that by trying to avoid infection, the resultant behaviour changes will cause 60% of the predicted economic losses. Nevertheless, according to a recent Cochrane review there is little evidence that social distancing or screening at entry ports would be an effective measure to delay the spread of respiratory viruses. The experience with SARS provides some useful parallels; the number of deaths was relatively small and yet the losses due to people trying to avoid infection were substantial. The World Bank estimates that the financial losses that will occur due to deaths and infection are, respectively, only 20 and 40% of the cost of anticipated behavioural changes.

Absenteeism

Work absence during an influenza pandemic is likely to be determined by the severity of the outbreak, the degree of concern generated and the subsequent public response. It will be affected to varying degrees throughout the pandemic. By definition, if the attack rate is in the range 25–50%, then over the course of the pandemic it is likely that 25–50% of staff will not attend work for a period of time. More problematic to predict are the possible levels of absence at the peak of a pandemic wave. Estimates vary from 10 to 30% of the working population or between a doubling and a two-thirds increase in absence levels in the private and public sector, respectively. This will vary by industry type, with health and social care likely to have a greater problem than for example goods distribution because of the larger potential for exposure to the infection. Some of the non-attendance will be due to caring responsibilities (either through sickness or school closure), transport disruptions and also possible work avoidance due to fear of catching the virus either at work or on the way to work. Equally troublesome is presenteeism and associated externalities, i.e. when infected, virus-shedding individuals attend their working sites.

Modelling from Canada indicates that seasonal influenza absenteeism normally ranges from 5 to 20%, with higher rates associated with multiple circulating strains. The absenteeism due to influenza was estimated at 12 and 13% per year for seasonal and A(H1N1)pdm09 pandemic waves, respectively. However, employees took on average more hours off during the pandemic (25 h versus 14 h, respectively).

Estimating the potential impact a pandemic might have on the economy of a country is fraught with the same problems that all aspects of pandemic planning face – the large number of unknowns. The UK government has calculated that the potential financial impact to that country due to illness-related absence from work could reduce the year's GDP by between £3 and 7 billion (€3.5 and 8.2 billion). The excess deaths caused by a severe pandemic could result in a further reduction of between £1 and 7 billion (€1.2 and 8.2 billion) in the pandemic year. The variance comes from the uncertainty around the case fatality rate and whether earnings or gross output are calculated. In the longer term, further calculations can be made around the financial impact of the premature deaths due to a pandemic, taking into account assumptions about the age ranges of those affected by the pandemic and future economic trends. The potential reduction in future lifetime earnings could range from £21 to 26 billion (€25–30 billion) at a low case fatality rate and from £145 to 172 billion (€170–201 billion) at a high case fatality rate.

Travel

During the A(H1N1)pdm09 pandemic, countries tried to slow the international spread of the virus by travel limitations as well as traveller screening on airport entry. As a result, the international air traffic from and to Mexico decreased by 40%. Similar impacts were experienced during the SARS outbreak of 2003, where international travel to the affected areas declined markedly. The WHO advised against non-essential travel to those areas and people also voluntarily reduced their flying. However, modelling has suggested that restricting compulsorily travel would not significantly delay the spread of the disease internationally (Chapters 13 and 16).

Pharmaceuticals and vaccines

Several specific examples of where supplies may come under particular pressure are influenza vaccines, antiviral drugs and antibiotics. Routine seasonal influenza vaccine manufacturing facilities will have to be diverted to the production of pandemic-specific vaccines. Seasonal vaccine manufacturing has little in the way of spare capacity after meeting the annual demand for seasonal vaccine. Only a proportion of the countries around the world have annual influenza vaccination programme. While the existing manufacturers can switch their facilities to produce a pandemic-specific vaccine, the capacity would not be sufficient to meet the needs of the entire global population by some considerable degree. Therefore there will be delays and shortages in the supply of the vaccine (Chapter 15).

Vaccination can be argued as the most cost-effective mean of avoiding influenza. The costs and health outcomes of vaccination versus no-vaccination can be assessed by computer simulation model. During the A(H1N1)pdm09 outbreak, research determined the health economic impact of using vaccines in a target population of 6 months and above from a US social perspective. Vaccination prior to the outbreak was cost saving for the population below 64 years of age. Depending on age and risk status, an incremental cost-effectiveness ratio of US$8000–52,000 (€6300–41,200) per quality-adjusted life year (QALY) gained was achieved. Hence, A(H1N1)pdm09 vaccination for children and working adults was a cost-effective mean of disease prevention. The delay in vaccine availability seemed to have a considerable influence on the cost-effectiveness ratio. However, a vaccine can only be effective if a high vaccine take-up rate can be achieved. Swiss research suggests that by achieving 60% vaccination coverage among all age groups, net savings would be highest from a social perspective during a pandemic situation. In addition, other externalities such as herd immunity, providing protection against influenza among unvaccinated persons, should be considered. In a cluster-randomized trial, it has been shown that selective vaccination of children and adolescents can interrupt 61% of influenza transmissions if vaccine take-up rates of about 80% are reached.

Likewise, influenza antiviral drugs and antibiotics to treat secondary bacterial respiratory infections will be in high demand. The antiviral drugs do not have much routine demand outside the seasonal influenza period (except in Japan), therefore manufacturing capacity is restricted under normal commercial rules. Stockpiling of antiviral drugs by national governments can partially alleviate this problem. While in normal times antibiotics are in fairly constant demand (some seasonal winter increase) and manufacturing capacity covers that 'steady state' requirement, this is not likely to be the case during a pandemic. Some countries have considered antibiotic stockpiling as part of their pandemic preparedness arrangements (Chapter 14).

Consumables

As the pandemic threat starts to increase, there is likely to be a surge in demand for certain types of supply, in particular personal protective equipment, healthcare equipment and some pharmaceuticals. Most countries import at least some of these items and therefore have little direct control over the maintenance of supply. Prices are likely to rise under these circumstances. Those countries with the deepest pockets will be best able to access these scarce resources, leaving poorer areas more vulnerable to being unable to fulfil their needs. Some regions will experience the onset of the pandemic earlier than others and therefore may be better placed to get in supplies early, while those affected later may have more difficulties.

Food, utilities and other essential supplies are all vital to maintain the population. Any significant disruption to such systems would be rapidly felt. Contrast this with more rural, self-sustaining communities already used to having to fend for themselves who will perhaps be in a better position to cope. Authorities in the former therefore need to emphasize the maintenance of 'business as much as usual' as is possible during the pandemic.

18.4   Wider Social Impact

What will be the impact of an influenza pandemic on normal social functioning? The experience of previous disasters can give an indication. The pandemic of 1918 saw considerable difficulties, but press reports at the time indicate that in the large part people continued about their normal daily lives as best they could. The population as a whole continued to go to work and school; banks and businesses continued to operate. In short, there was no meltdown of society. Some specific issues related to social epidemiological influences of influenza outbreaks are described in the following paragraphs.

Schools and education

Children are efficient spreaders of influenza in that they excrete the virus in higher concentrations and for longer than adults. Compliance with hygiene measures can be more difficult to maintain and the close proximity in the school setting assists greater efficiency of transmission. For these reasons the scientific advice is that in the event of a severe pandemic, school closures could be considered, to protect children and also to reduce transmission in the wider community. Modelling has suggested that this intervention would help to flatten the peak of an outbreak and therefore reduce the acute demand for healthcare (Chapter 16).

During the 1918 influenza epidemic, school closure could be linked to a significant reduction in disease mortality. In the recent A(H1N1)pdm09 pandemic, a reduction in cases could be achieved by school closures. However, school closure in response to the pandemic also resulted in parental workplace absenteeism, wage loss and the need to pay for alternative childcare. US research showed that during school closures in 2009, 30% of students visited at least one locality outside their homes. If both parents were employed, an ill child was less likely to leave home and instead someone took time off work. As a result, at least one adult missed some work in 17% of the households affected. Interestingly, if the household was composed of other children, an adult was less prone to take time off work. Modelling suggests that closing schools during the A(H1N1)pdm09 outbreak would have taken a substantial economic toll on society and outweighed the savings of preventing influenza cases. From an individual perspective, the economic burden seemed to be tolerable.

Health and social care capacity

During an influenza pandemic the services likely to come under the most pressure are health and social services, and initial planning for pandemic influenza quite rightly concentrates heavily on the response of the healthcare services to ensure patients can be cared for.

Healthcare services are likely to be affected at an early stage in the outbreak and remain under sustained pressure until the end of the outbreak and into the recovery period. Dependent on the severity of the outbreak, demand for health and social care support is likely to rise steeply at the same time as organizations are facing rises in staff absenteeism due to sickness or caring responsibilities. It is probable that at some point during the local epidemic wave of a severe pandemic the capacity of these services to respond will be exceeded. Difficult decisions will have to then be taken regarding the allocation of these scarce health and social care assets.

Delays in access to treatment can not only result in poorer outcomes but also result in delays of recognition and control of the pandemic itself. Indeed, experts have argued that one reason for the high mortality associated with the A(H1N1)pdm09 virus in Mexico was due to delays in accessing healthcare, partly due to cost barriers. In contrast, the emergency departments of New York City experienced heavy surge.

Primary and secondary healthcare and social support agencies will have to act at an early stage to prioritize which services to maintain and which to scale back or curtail completely. The implication is that, particularly at the peak of the pandemic, it is possible that only the most urgent and ill cases will be prioritized to access secondary-level healthcare especially intensive care/therapy (where available). Authorities will need to help the remainder of the population to support themselves through the crisis or through access to basic healthcare. Natural and voluntary community support networks will be particularly important for helping the vulnerable through the episode.

Personal protective equipment

The WHO together with individual states' advisory and regulatory bodies has issued guidance on the use of personal protective equipment by certain key staff in a pandemic. Much of this is based on sound reasoning rather than hard evidence. Some evidence on physical interventions to interrupt the spread of respiratory viruses is given by a recent meta-analysis from the Cochrane Collaboration. Evidence from randomized controlled and observational studies suggest that low-cost interventions such as hand washing, especially among children, or using surgical masks seemed to be effective in reducing the spread of the disease. However, long-term implementation of some preventive means might be difficult to realize (Chapter 16).

Given that potentially at-risk workers will need to use the equipment for the duration of each wave, which may be as long as 15 weeks, compliance with use and availability of supplies may become a problem. Moreover, differences in approaches adopted between and within countries has the potential to cause confusion and divisiveness within the population at large and in specific occupational groups.

Existing poor health and socio-economic status

The impact of an influenza pandemic on countries already ravaged by war, poverty and/or other major infectious disease problems (e.g. HIV) is likely to be greater than on those not compromised by such difficulties. War, poverty and political breakdown will make it much more difficult for those countries affected to prepare in advance for a major infectious disease outbreak.

Changes in societal cohesion may have also had effects on the population's reaction. Cultural differences may also be of relevance in between-country responses. A new influenza pandemic is therefore likely to have different social manifestations across the globe.

18.5 Summary

An influenza pandemic is complex and difficult to plan for because the range of possible impacts is so vast. It may be that the next one will be minor and have only marginal effects (as in 2009), or it could be severe with extensive consequences to the social and economic fabric of the world. What is clear is that by careful and effective planning these effects can be mitigated, at least in part.

During past influenza pandemics, reductions of nearly 5% in global GDP were assimilated through a combination of direct economic losses and the consequences of altered patterns of human behaviour. Workplace absenteeism – due to direct sickness, indirect absence to care for relatives and friends and inability to attend work if schools are closed – is an additional driver of the economic and social burden. It seems to be crucial that school closures and other means to mitigate a pandemic need to be carefully planned. Vaccination remains a cost-effective measure to reduce the clinical and economic toll of an influenza outbreak.

However, achieving this without engendering excessive concern, while maintaining sufficient engagement to obtain the resources needed, is complex and will require continued effort by relevant stakeholders if attention is not to be diverted by other competing priorities. Ultimately, an influenza pandemic cannot be tidily packaged as a purely health problem, solvable by a health service-driven solution. Instead, although health remains at the heart of the problem, pandemic influenza is a whole-of-society phenomenon because diverse sectors will be affected over an extended period of time. This, in turn, demands a whole-of-society response.

- Socio-economic impacts include population mortality and morbidity; impacts on specific businesses such as pharmaceuticals, health and social care; impacts on wider business e.g. through staff absenteeism, disruption to supplies or markets; and wider societal impacts such as to schools and education.
- Seasonal influenza typically afflicts the very young, old and those with a weak immune systems or chronic disease. However the 1918 pandemic saw the greatest impact in working-age adults, while 80% of fatal cases in the 2009 pandemic were in people under 65 years of age.
- Modelling indicates that the global financial costs of a pandemic could be up to several trillion US dollars. These costs could be felt across societies through increased healthcare requirements, loss of productivity and early deaths, as well as through pandemic preparations (e.g. allocation of resources to pandemic preparedness over other health problems). Workplace absenteeism will be dictated by the severity of the pandemic, but will be at least as bad as the clinical attack rate.
- A severe influenza pandemic could cause industrial output to decline to a level consistent with the recessions that have occurred since the end of World War II. Some sectors of the economy are likely to face bigger declines than others. In particular tourism, entertainment, mass transport, restaurants, large social gatherings and hotels. The insurance business would also suffer appreciably due to the morbidity and mortality of influenza cases. Conversely, other businesses may see a surge in demand: there may be an increase in online purchasing (especially for groceries) and there will inevitably be elevated demand for over-the-counter healthcare products and environmental cleaning/disinfectant products.

Further Reading

Bajardi P., Poletto C., Ramasco J.J., Tizzoni M., Colizza V. and Vespignani A. (2011) Human mobility networks, travel restrictions, and the global spread of 2009 H1N1 pandemic. *PloS One* 6(1), e16591.

Brown S.T., Tai J.H., Bailey R.R., Cooley P.C., Wheaton W.D., Potter M.A., Voorhees R.E., LeJeune M., Grefenstette J.J., Burke D.S., McGlone S.M. and Lee B.Y. (2011) Would school closure for the 2009 H1N1 influenza epidemic have been worth the cost?: a computational simulation of Pennsylvania. *BMC Public Health* 11, 353.

Chen, W.C., Huang, A.S., Chuang J.H., Chiu C.C. and Kuo H.S. (2011) Social and economic impact of school closure resulting from pandemic influenza A/H1N1. *Journal of Infection* 62(3), 200–203.

Esposito, S., Molteni, C.G., Daleno, C., Tagliabue, C., Picciolli, I., Scala, A., Pelucchi, C., Fossali, E. and Principi, N. (2011) Impact of pandemic A/H1N1/2009 influenza on children and their families: comparison with seasonal A/H1N1 and A/H3N2 influenza viruses. *Journal of Infection* 63(4), 300–307.

Jefferson, T., Del Mar, C.B., Dooley, L., Ferroni, E., Al-Ansary, L.A., Bawazeer, G.A., van Driel, M.L., Nair, S., Jones, M.A., Thorning, S. and Conly, J.M. (2011) Physical interventions to interrupt or reduce the spread of respiratory viruses. *Cochrane Database of Systematic Reviews* 6(7), CD006207.

Keogh-Brown, M.R., Smith, R.D., Edmunds, J.W. and Beutels, P. (2010) The macroeconomic impact of pandemic influenza: estimates from models of the United Kingdom, France, Belgium and The Netherlands. *European Journal of Health Economics: HEPAC: Health Economics in Prevention and Care* 11(6), 543–554.

Keogh-Brown, M.R., Wren-Lewis, S. Edmunds, J.W., Beutels, P. and Smith, R.D. (2010) The possible macroeconomic impact on the UK of an influenza pandemic. *Health Economics* 19(11), 1345–1360.

Mota, N.V., Lobo, R.D., Toscano C.M., Pedroso de Lima, A.C., Souza Dias, M.B., Komagata, H. and Levin, A.S. (2011) Cost-effectiveness of sick leave policies for health care workers with influenza-like illness, Brazil, 2009. *Emerging Infectious Diseases* 17(8), 1421–1429.

Prosser, L.A., Lavelle, T.A., Fiore, A.E., Bridges, C.B., Reed, C., Jain, S., Dunham, K.M. and Meltzer, M.I. (2011) Cost-effectiveness of 2009 pandemic influenza A(H1N1) vaccination in the United States. *PloS One* 6(7), e22308.

Smith, R.D., Keogh-Brown, M.R., Barnett, T. and Tait, J. (2009) The economy-wide impact of pandemic influenza on the UK: a computable general equilibrium modelling experiment. *British Medical Journal* 339, b4571.

19 Ethical Issues Related to Pandemic Preparedness and Response

Elaine M. Gadd

Queen Mary University of London, London, UK

- How should ethical issues be dealt with in preparing for, and responding to, pandemic influenza?
- Do health professionals have an unlimited obligation to care for patients regardless of the risk to themselves?
- In what circumstances can countries impose mandatory measures to control people's behaviour?
- How can prioritization decisions be addressed in an ethical way?

19.1 Introduction

Ethics concerns how it is right to behave. As decisions concerning pandemic preparedness and response potentially impact on individuals, they always have an ethical dimension. The ethical issues involved may be complex and difficult. Such issues would be hard to resolve under the pressure of responding to an influenza pandemic, and should therefore be addressed in advance as far as possible. Similarly, as an ethical justification is required to treat people in similar circumstances differently, advance consideration of ethical issues makes it more likely that, at least at national level (given how widely the circumstances of different countries vary), people will be treated consistently. Consideration of ethical issues should therefore be an integral part of pandemic planning, rather than a separate or side issue.

In complex situations, particularly where resources are limited, there is seldom a single 'right' answer or an ethically perfect solution. However, there may be several ethically appropriate or ethically acceptable solutions between which a decision maker can choose. The challenge is to ensure that ethically inappropriate solutions are not adopted. The ethical issues raised by an influenza pandemic range from wide questions of global justice to medical treatment of individuals. This chapter outlines issues from a health perspective and some of the approaches that countries and international organizations, such as the World Health Organization (WHO), have taken (and are continuing to take) to address them.

19.2 Ethics as an Integral Part of Pandemic Preparedness and Response

As every aspect of pandemic preparedness and response has an ethical dimension, this chapter is not a full account of all the ethical issues that need consideration. Other health issues include those concerning management of people detained by the State, whether in prison or on mental health grounds (given that infection rates may be higher in closed institutions), and finding an appropriate balance between requirements for medical safeguards in death and cremation certification and the needs of the living for doctors. As ethics concerns how we should behave to others, ethical issues are not confined to the health sector but also include issues such as the availability of food and fuel or access to services such as banking or the courts.

Advance preparation is central to an effective pandemic response. This raises ethical issues, as countries vary greatly in the resources they can devote to preparation, both in terms of planning and materially (e.g. developing a stockpile of antiviral medication). Some developing countries, for example, faced with overwhelming current healthcare needs that cannot be met, have to decide whether it is right to divert any of their limited resources to pandemic planning. In so doing, the potential harms to their population today caused by such diversion must be weighed against the potential future benefits to their population at some unknowable (as the onset of a pandemic cannot be predicted) future date.

19.3 Global Issues and the Role of the WHO

Pandemics respect neither national borders nor the legal status of individuals. For practical purposes, it is reasonable to assume that a pandemic will affect all nations at some point. The shared humanity of individuals globally gives rise to ethical concerns about the inequities between their situations and to an ethical duty to attempt to ameliorate such inequity. At global level, this is often expressed as the principle of solidarity. The ethical duty has been codified into a legal duty of international cooperation and assistance between States expressed in many international human rights instruments, such as the United Nations International Covenant on Economic, Social and Cultural Rights (1966). Article 12 of that Covenant particularly highlights that obligation in the context of the prevention, treatment and control of epidemic diseases. Assistance can take several forms including sharing of scientific and technological expertise as well as financial aid.

As well as their legal duties, some of which are embodied within WHO International Health Regulations (Chapter 17), all States have reasons of national interest to cooperate. Effective global surveillance offers the opportunity to attempt to control the pandemic at source, and even if this is unsuccessful, provides all States with the maximum possible degree of warning of an imminent pandemic. Achieving such a level of surveillance means that assistance needs to be provided to some States that would not otherwise be able to achieve this goal. Furthermore, timely and effective sharing of scientific information, for example through the sharing of virus and other specimens, has the potential to enhance preparedness and response at global level.

The WHO is the United Nations body responsible for health and has therefore been responsible for coordinating global pandemic preparedness work. Under its aegis, after 4 years' negotiation, a global framework for pandemic influenza preparedness was agreed in 2011 that covers global sharing of influenza viruses and access to vaccines and other benefits for developing countries. This includes measures to strengthen surveillance and laboratories in developing countries.

WHO also recognized the importance of ethical issues in preparedness planning and has produced a series of discussion papers on key issues. These were subject to consultation with WHO's 193 Member States, after which guidance was produced in 2008 on ethical considerations in developing a public health response to pandemic influenza. The relatively mild nature of the 2009 pandemic meant that the ethical challenges were not as severe as they might have been. However, this may not be the case in a future pandemic and the guidance on ethical issues produced by WHO and by national bodies (see below) is of continuing value.

National self-protection is a State's first obligation, and during a pandemic (particularly if it is severe) there may be limits to the international assistance that States can offer. It is ethically important that what is available is used to best effect, and which again requires advance discussion and planning, incorporating flexibility to respond according to the pandemic's actual characteristics.

The legal status of individuals is often relevant to access to national healthcare systems. The position of asylum seekers, refugees and displaced people during a pandemic therefore needs consideration. Many countries have reciprocal health agreements regarding the medical treatment of their citizens who become ill on the territory of the other country, but these are not universal. The treatment of citizens of States with whom no agreement exists therefore also needs thought, as does the practicality of healthcare staff enquiring about a person's legal status under the pressures of a pandemic.

'Health tourism' during a pandemic, in which people attempt to travel from a country thought to be ill-resourced or ill-prepared to another seen as being in a better situation, could present difficulties. Where countries share borders such travel may be relatively easy. The ethical dimensions of such a practice are quite complex, involving consideration of the position of others in both the original and receiving countries. It may be preferable to minimize the risks of the practice developing, both for ethical reasons and because of the potential disruption to pandemic response that might occur from such a practice if widespread. WHO has highlighted the need to try to avoid disparities of care across borders, and this is another reason for neighbouring countries to cooperate in pandemic planning.

E.M. Gadd

The pressures involved in planning for, and responding to, a pandemic mean that the need to plan for the recovery phase can be overlooked. International cooperation and assistance will again be important. While the full range of difficulties that countries may face in the recovery phase cannot be discussed here, the existing inequities between countries in terms of healthcare staff and services can be highlighted. Where few staff are available even in normal times, the loss of a critical number of these during a pandemic may produce an ongoing crisis in healthcare provision. The need for assistance both in terms of shoring up available provision and in training new staff may be profound.

19.4 Voluntary and Mandatory Non-medical Measures

Given the different resources available to them, countries will vary in the extent to which they can use medical measures such as antiviral medication or hospital care to respond to a pandemic. The use of some non-medical measures, such as border controls and entry or exit screening (even if largely ineffective – see Chapter 13), also has resource consequences. However, measures such as isolation or quarantine may be relevant to a wide range of countries, although the potential to enforce such measures will vary widely.

The rights to associate freely with others and not to be deprived of liberty without just cause are recognized in international human rights instruments at both the global and regional level (e.g. in the European Convention for the Protection of Human Rights and Fundamental Freedoms (ECHR)). These support the ethical principle of self-determination, or autonomy. However, the international legal instruments do recognize that these rights can legitimately be limited in certain circumstances, including the need to protect public health.

However, not all restrictions are legitimate. The Siracusa Principles, as noted in WHO's guidance on ethical considerations referred to above, are widely accepted as a standard for assessment of the legitimacy of a restriction on human rights. These are that the restriction is: in accordance with law; based on a legitimate objective; the least restrictive and intrusive means available; and not arbitrary, unreasonable or discriminatory.

In practice this means that, first, there must be a reasonable belief that the proposed measure would be effective. Chapter 13 shows that modelling implies that even massive restrictions on air travel would be unlikely to have a significant effect on a pandemic's impact in the UK; thus, it would be unreasonable for the State to impose such a measure. It is ethically less problematic to encourage voluntary cooperation with a measure than to impose it, although if it cannot work in any circumstances there are no grounds for seeking voluntary cooperation. For a measure to be the least restrictive and intrusive means available, there must be reasonable grounds to believe that voluntary measures will not be effective and mandatory measures will.

If a voluntary measure would not be effective, the feasibility of enforcing a mandatory measure requires consideration. Could home isolation be enforced even in an influenza pandemic with a relatively low clinical attack rate of 25%, for example? How could it be monitored? Large-scale enforcement problems give rise to concerns about whether the measure can be effected in a non-arbitrary way. Furthermore, the potential benefits need to be proportionate to the burdens a mandatory measure places on individuals. By imposing and enforcing a measure for collective benefit, the State also has an ethical obligation to minimize the harm that it causes to the relevant individuals. So, for example, if a person were to be confined at home, the provision of food, medical care and other necessities of life to that person needs attention.

Measures chosen by individuals, such as not to attend a mass gathering or other place that is likely to be crowded in order to avoid infection, must be distinguished from measures imposed by the State. Imposed measures that limit the freedom of individuals require rigorous justification, balancing the potential collective benefits to society against the rights of individuals. This is a difficult test; it is much less ethically problematic to encourage people to cooperate voluntarily with measures that are likely to benefit society (such as isolation at home when ill with influenza) than to legally impose such measures.

Where voluntary measures are used, providing individuals with information explaining why the measure is being encouraged demonstrates respect for people and supports the right to self-determination. There may be situations where scientific evidence indicates that at population level a measure (such as avoiding mass gatherings) would make no, or minimal, difference to the pandemic's impact.

In such circumstances, it would be ethically appropriate to provide what information is available on the potential risks at individual level, and allow people to make their own choices on how to behave as a result.

Assessing the ethical dimensions of a potential measure requires clear thinking about the potential impact on all those who may be affected by it. School closures are a good example. Potential issues are harms through loss of educational opportunities and association with friends for the children, coupled with potential benefits in terms of reduced rates of infection for the children and (probably) in society more widely. But if schools are closed, childcare will be needed. This may present few problems in societies in which few women work outside the home, but for societies in which both parents often work the impact may be far greater.

In such societies, sectors employing a high proportion of working parents (particularly women), which may already be experiencing absenteeism through the direct health impact of a pandemic, may then be placed under an additional burden as parents face the conflict between their domestic and work responsibilities, which in turn may give rise to societal harms. Furthermore, the theoretical benefits of closing schools in terms of reduced transmission rates are predicated on decreased contact rates between the children. The 2009 pandemic illustrated the need to consider, particularly in relation to older children in urban areas, the extent to which such decreased contact rates would be achieved in practice.

The extensive potential impact of widespread school closures in some societies means that it is impossible to judge the best course of action until some information on the characteristics of the pandemic virus is available; what would be appropriate may differ depending on the clinical attack rate, mortality rate and differing vulnerabilities of subsections of the population associated with the virus. If school closures are a potential option in such countries, in order to minimize harms, society (and particularly sectors that may be disproportionately affected) needs to be aware of this well in advance so that individuals and organizations can incorporate it in their plans.

19.5 Health Professionals' Duty of Care

An influenza pandemic may place severe demands on healthcare services, and health professionals will be central to an effective response. But they will also face conflicting obligations, for example to family members, and particularly if the pandemic virus is associated with a high mortality rate, may be placed at higher risk as a result of their professional duties.

The extent of health professionals' duty of care has been debated. Sources of the duty include ethical and professional obligations as well as contractual and other legal duties. This section focuses on the situation in developed countries, rather than situations in which lack of health professionals is always a major problem.

Ethical obligations may arise from the specialized knowledge possessed by health professionals, particularly if their training has been funded by the State. Professionals may also feel an ethical obligation to work from solidarity with their colleagues, recognizing the burden that their absence places on others. Professional obligations, which themselves have an ethical base, derive from professional codes of conduct that require giving care, particularly in emergency situations. However, there is no universal agreement on the extent of the obligation, although there seems to be broad agreement (as expressed in WHO's guidance on ethical considerations referred to above) that the extent is not unlimited. In addition, in some cases caring for someone with an infectious disease might place a particular health professional at unusually high risk (for example due to a personal medical condition), and this also needs ethical consideration.

Historically, the professional response to serious infectious disease has been mixed. While there are examples of great heroism, there are also examples where doctors are reported to have fled the area. The experience of severe acute respiratory syndrome (SARS) provides an opportunity to examine this issue in a relatively modern context. However the situation was different in important ways from pandemic influenza: the cause of SARS was unknown for some time, and SARS in the developed world was largely confined to healthcare institutions. The risk of infection outside such institutions was negligible. In contrast, during an influenza pandemic, levels of infection in the community will be significant; a health professional may be exposed to infection travelling between work and home, while carrying out domestic tasks such as shopping or in the course of family life. Not working is therefore no guarantee of avoiding infection.

E.M. Gadd

During SARS, the majority of health professionals demonstrated high commitment to care (as a result of which some died), but this was not universal. The SARS experience suggests that keeping staff well informed of developments, the provision of personal protective equipment, and a non-punitive approach to those who felt unable to undertake direct care, may contribute to an effective response to pandemic influenza.

Attempts have been made to study health professionals' attitudes to working during an influenza pandemic. Studies of healthcare workers in Europe and the USA suggest that a significant number thought that they might not report for work, although clinical staff appeared significantly more likely to intend to work than non-clinical or support staff. Perception of the importance of one's role in responding to a pandemic appeared to be a significant factor. Fear of infection of oneself or family was raised as a reason for not working, but as noted above it may not be realistic to expect to avoid infection by avoiding work.

The need for information and for reciprocity – in terms of provision of protective equipment and expression of appreciation of the potential burdens staff may assume – has also been highlighted. In addition, staff may fear that the pressures of a pandemic may mean that they will be unable to deliver their normal standard of care, or that they may need to work in unfamiliar areas or take on new roles, and that this might have medico-legal consequences. Inappropriate care during a pandemic would always be regrettable, but (depending on the particular circumstances) it may not be appropriate to consider it ethically blameworthy. If health professionals deliver the best care they can during a pandemic, there is an ethical obligation to minimize the professional or employment consequences of so doing.

Involving health professionals – and indeed other staff – at an early stage in pandemic planning is important to gain commitment to cooperation in pandemic response. Such discussions should aim to clarify expectations concerning the duties of health professionals and to provide information, so far as it is known, about the potential risks of pandemic influenza and delivering care and about the measures available to support staff (including personal protective equipment, access to medicines or vaccines, etc.). Early discussions also provide the opportunity to address individual issues, such as personal health needs or childcare, which could

impact on the person's ability to deliver care. A person may be able to contribute to the pandemic response in other ways (e.g. staffing an advisory telephone help line). The ethical obligations of health professionals to patients are widely recognized; in pandemic preparedness and response it is also necessary for society, and in particular for those directing the preparedness and response phases, to remember the ethical obligations to those, including but not limited to health professionals, on whom the burden of response may fall particularly heavily.

19.6 Prioritization and Access to Healthcare

Questions of prioritization for access to healthcare are not new, although an influenza pandemic may present them in a more severe form. Many different approaches to healthcare prioritization and rationing have been proposed, but there is no general agreement on the best method – although it is clear that some approaches are less ethically acceptable than others. How a country approaches these issues during a pandemic will be dependent on the resources available to it, in terms of both the healthcare system and its staff and specific interventions such as antiviral medication and vaccines.

The potential impact of prioritization on individuals means that it is ethically highly desirable to involve society to the greatest extent possible in the process for deciding the approach and criteria to be used. Wide social understanding and acceptance of the chosen approach is also likely to facilitate the management of the pandemic.

In terms of general approach, when considering issues at a population level, the principle that one should do 'the greatest good for the greatest number' is often proposed. This principle of utility is not as straightforward as it seems, and has a practical impact on the choice of prioritization criteria. Ideas of what constitutes the 'greatest good' may vary – options include minimizing the clinical attack rate so that fewer people are affected; minimizing deaths; maximizing health benefits by saving most life-years (resulting in lowered priority for older people); and taking a wider view and aiming to minimize the impact of a pandemic on society (which leads to considerations of individuals' social roles and their impact on society). Some type of utility consideration will form part of any prioritization approach, but the form this takes may vary in different circumstances, such as the use of pre-pandemic vaccine or access to intensive care.

However, utility considerations fail to address significant ethical concerns. For example, if there are five items of a limited resource and many people who could benefit equally from it, the maximum number of people who can receive the resource is five. But most people would think there is an ethical difference between choosing the five by lottery or the person responsible for the resource choosing five friends over the other potential beneficiaries. This reflects an underlying concern with fairness, or equity, which concerns giving equal weight to equal claims.

In normal circumstances, equity considerations generally support giving priority to the worst off – in a casualty department, the sickest people are treated first, and those who will not be harmed by having to wait do so. Such considerations are also relevant in a pandemic; for example, one could consider prioritizing groups of people who may be at higher risk of death if infected to receive vaccine. However, considerations of equity may conflict with utility and a difficult balance may have to be found. For example, one very sick person with multiple underlying medical conditions might need to occupy a ventilator bed for several weeks to stand a chance of recovery. In that time, many other people who needed the ventilator for only a short period in order to make a full recovery could die.

These potential conflicts need to be widely debated in advance in order to reach agreement on the limitations to treatment that can be offered. Such limitations may vary depending on the pressures on the limited resource and other options available; it is ethically desirable that limitations are applied only to the extent necessary, so the application of a particular level of limitation needs to be reviewed regularly.

However, even with the strictest restrictions based on medical criteria in force, particularly in a severe pandemic, there may be more people with equal claims to, for example, an intensive-care bed than beds available. Very hard choices will need to be made – on equity grounds, these need to be made fairly but also in a way that is practical in the situation. 'First come, first served' approaches are difficult to operationalize fairly; how is 'first' assessed? The first person notified to the intensive-care consultant after the bed becomes available?

What if someone tried to call the consultant, who was otherwise occupied, and before the person called back another notification was made? A lottery between patients with an equal claim to the bed may be a more practical (and fair) answer, but implementation in practice would require careful thought.

The use of age in prioritization is very controversial. A much discussed equity-based argument is the 'fair innings' approach. This suggests that a young person may have a stronger claim to life-saving treatment than an older person who has already had a 'fair innings'. However, this makes age the defining characteristic of an individual and ignores other characteristics that might be ethically relevant. Furthermore, defining the cut-off for a 'fair innings' in the real world is always going to be highly problematic. Age may sometimes be relevant in prioritization: for example, if there is scientific evidence that statistically persons of a certain age are less likely to respond to certain forms of treatment, this may be relevant to considering potential benefits from treatment on utility grounds. However, this is not based on the concept of a 'fair innings', and needs to be tempered by individual consideration (some 70-year-olds are fitter than some 30-year olds), rather than blind application of population-level data.

Some criteria are never appropriate for use in prioritization, such as gender, religion, sexual orientation, political affiliation or socio-economic status. Unjustified discrimination is prohibited by legal human rights documents at global and regional level (such as the ECHR) and this applies in a pandemic as at other times.

During a pandemic, people will still have road accidents, heart attacks and strokes, develop cancers and give birth. Such people have ethical claims to care that need consideration in pandemic planning and in prioritization criteria for resources that both they and patients with influenza-related illness may need, such as intensive care. Similarly, the potential impact of decreasing preventive care such as childhood immunization during a pandemic needs thought, given that potentially severe childhood illnesses such as measles and whooping cough will remain risks.

As noted above, the needs of those who are 'worst off' require consideration on grounds of equity. In developed countries, many disabled, frail and otherwise vulnerable people are dependent on social care, often for many basic activities of daily

E.M. Gadd

living such as meals, dressing and bathing. Social care staff will be affected as others in society by a pandemic, and the impact of absenteeism on social services needs careful consideration.

The importance and effects of prioritization decisions are such that they need to be subject to the widest possible debate during the preparedness planning phase. Protocols need to be developed, made publicly available, and discussed, on issues such as limitations to care (for example in relation to intensive care). Information is also needed on how these will be reviewed (e.g. to take account of emerging information on the pandemic virus). All members of society should have the opportunity to contribute to the debate – not everyone uses or can access the Internet. Thus, making information available in community languages, large print and other formats, and accessible to groups such as the homeless or travellers, is important. The use of transparently developed, publicly available criteria will be important in assuring people that agreed principles are being applied fairly in individual cases during a pandemic, and this will assist in maintaining public trust in the pandemic's management. Nevertheless, clinicians may still be faced with very difficult decisions in individual cases. Arrangements to support them in taking those decisions and managing their emotional impact also require consideration in advance.

19.7 National Approaches to Ethical Issues

The importance of addressing the ethical dimension of managing an influenza pandemic has been recognized worldwide. This has been achieved in different ways, and informed by academic contributions. Of these, 'Stand on Guard for Thee', a report of the University of Toronto Joint Centre for Bioethics, is notable. This built on the work of the Centre after the Canadian SARS outbreak and proposed a series of ethical and procedural values to inform pandemic planning.

Some countries, such as France, New Zealand and Switzerland, have a national ethics committee that has examined pandemic influenza as well as other problems. The New Zealand National Ethics Advisory Committee's guidance sets out ethical values for a pandemic and also provides a range of hypothetical pandemic scenarios to illustrate the practical implementation of the values.

The UK does not have an overarching national ethics committee. In 2006, the Government set up

the Committee on Ethical Aspects of Pandemic Influenza (CEAPI) that produced an ethical framework for policy and planning, which was accepted by the Government as part of the pandemic response strategy. During the 2009 pandemic, CEAPI kept the handling of the ethical dimensions of the pandemic response in the UK under review. The Committee is also consulted on drafts of pandemic preparedness guidance on a range of issues.

Approaches based on setting out frameworks of principles or values recognize the impracticality of an ethics committee providing an answer to every ethical question that may arise in pandemic management. The values or principles may often be in tension, as noted with issues of equity and utility above, and how this tension is balanced will depend on the exact circumstances under consideration. Also, as scientific information changes (e.g. concerning the characteristics of a new pandemic virus), this may impact on ethical decisions, and plans need to be flexible enough to cope with this. Frameworks of values or principles can act as a decision support tool, by encouraging people to consider systematically the different ethical dimensions of a problem. Those involved in a pandemic's management are expected to be aware of the framework and to use it to inform their daily decision making where this is not covered by specific protocols (e.g. concerning limitations of care in certain circumstances).

As one might hope, there is considerable commonality between the approaches to setting out values or principles. For example, both the UK and New Zealand frameworks specify minimizing harm, and call for respect, fairness and reciprocity and (expressed in different words) working together, flexibility and procedural principles related to good decision making. The UK also has a principle of keeping things in proportion, and New Zealand a value of responsibleness, but it seems probable that if these slightly different frameworks were applied to the same situation the outcome would be very similar.

However, a framework is not a calculator – one cannot hypothetically feed an issue in at one end and expect a precise answer to simply emerge. Judgement is always required about the weight to be given to a particular principle in a specific situation; or with a broad principle such as minimizing harm, about which harms are particularly important. That is why the element of the framework dealing with good decision making is particularly important, as this aims to ensure that those difficult judgements are made in the most ethically appropriate manner.

Ultimately, all of those responsible for planning and responding to pandemic influenza need to be aware of the ethical dimensions of their work, and to ensure that ethical issues are appropriately addressed in the decisions they take. As this chapter has illustrated, the complexity of the issues is such that to ensure an ethically appropriate response to a pandemic, the benefits of thinking things through in advance cannot be overstated.

- All decisions that affect people have an ethical dimension, so ethical issues need to be integrated into the preparations for, and response to, pandemic influenza.
- Health professionals have a strong duty to care, but it is not unlimited. Willingness to care is enhanced by recognizing reciprocal obligations to health professionals (e.g. to consult them, provide protective equipment and keep them informed of developments).
- Mandatory measures can only be imposed if voluntary measures would be ineffective, and must meet certain legal criteria if they are to be legitimate.
- Criteria for prioritization decisions need to be subject to wide public discussion. Such criteria will involve a balance between ethical principles of utility and of fairness and must avoid unjustified discrimination.

Further Reading

Cabinet Office and Department of Health (2007) Responding to pandemic influenza: the ethical framework for policy and planning. Available at: http://www.dh.gov.uk/en/Publicationsandstatistics/Publications/PublicationsPolicyAndGuidance/DH_080751 (accessed 1 April 2012).

New Zealand National Ethics Advisory Committee (2007) Getting Through Together: ethical values for a pandemic. Available at: http://www.neac.health.govt.nz/moh.nsf/pagescm/1090/$File/getting-through-together-jul07.pdf (accessed 1 April 2012).

University of Toronto Joint Centre for Bioethics (2005) Stand on Guard for Thee. Ethical considerations in preparedness planning for pandemic influenza. A report of the University of Toronto Joint Centre for Bioethics Pandemic Influenza Working Group. Available at: http://www.jointcentreforbioethics.ca/publications/documents/stand_on_guard.pdf (accessed 1 April 2012).

World Health Organization (2007) Ethical considerations in developing a public health response to pandemic influenza. Available at: http://www.who.int/csr/resources/publications/WHO_CDS_EPR_GIP_2007_2c.pdf (accessed 1 April 2012).

World Health Organization (2008) Addressing ethical issues in pandemic influenza planning: discussion papers. Available at: http://www.who.int/csr/resources/publications/cds_flu_ethics_5web.pdf (accessed 1 April 2012).

E.M. Gadd

20 Pandemic Communication

Thomas Abraham[1] and Daniel Pople[2]

[1]The University of Hong Kong, Hong Kong;
[2]NHS London, London, UK

- Why is proactive communication important?
- What are the challenges of pandemic communication?
- What are the principles of pandemic communication?
- How important is social media in pandemic communication?

20.1 Introduction

Every public health measure taken during a pandemic relies for its success on communication between the authorities, the public and other stakeholders. Whether it is information about personal protection, school closures, vaccination or business continuity planning, communication is essential. Without effective communication it would be impossible for public health agencies and governments to respond to a pandemic. The World Health Organization (WHO) has noted 'Pro-active communication encourages the public to adopt protective behaviours, facilitates heightened disease surveillance, reduces confusion and allows for a better use of resources – all of which are necessary for an effective response'. It is often assumed that good communication is a matter of common sense, and does not require the kind of training or planning that other public health interventions require. But effective communication is rarely straightforward or spontaneous. It is the result of a well-thought-out, carefully planned, systematic process.

During a pandemic the authorities might well be required to take unpopular, and often controversial, decisions on quarantines, travel restrictions, access to scarce medical supplies and so on. It will be very difficult to get public acceptance of these decisions without effective communication. Many of the characteristic features of pandemic influenza (its unpredictability, its wave-like seasonality and the differing severity with which it affects different risk

groups) combine to make pandemic communication a challenge. The length of an influenza pandemic also poses challenges. Unlike other disease outbreaks, which are normally short-lived, an influenza pandemic is a fairly long-running event and can change in severity over its course. This can require rapidly updating advice to the public. At the same time, it is a challenge to hold public attention when a pandemic has been in progress for several months and complacency can set in. The length and variability of a pandemic can also lead to public distrust of the advice from health authorities.

To meet these challenges, communication planning is essential. One solid lesson learned from the experience of the 2009 pandemic is the value of advance planning and preparation. The preparation for a pandemic began in earnest from around 2005, when the A(H5N1) avian influenza virus became recognized as a pandemic threat. Pandemic communication plans were prepared in different countries and regions, shared with stakeholders and tested in planning exercises. So, when the pandemic emerged in April 2009, health agencies, governments, intergovernmental agencies and other responders were reasonably well prepared to communicate with the public and provide advice and information.

The 2009 pandemic also showed the importance of the WHO's Outbreak Communication guidelines as principles to guide communication. This chapter will provide basic advice on the planning process, explain the WHO Outbreak Communication guidelines, and provide some ideas on how to handle media relations and effective use of the Internet and social media tools.

20.2 Communication Planning

Without advance planning, effective communication during a pandemic or any other disease outbreak is extremely difficult. The huge demand for information from the media, the public and other stakeholders and partners is impossible to meet without preparation. The basis of preparation is a good communication plan. This chapter does not provide a ready-to-use communication plan because local conditions vary and there is no 'one size fits all' solution for communications planning. However, it sets out some preliminary steps to creating a good communication plan based on the WHO's planning guide for outbreak communication.

As a first step before beginning the planning process, it is useful to assess whether there are enough staff and other resources to meet the communication demands of a pandemic. A pandemic will make enormous demands on manpower. A huge volume of media queries will have to be answered, communication materials such as posters and leaflets have to be prepared and distributed and if necessary updated, communications with healthcare workers and other stakeholders will have to be managed and so on. If there are insufficient resources, then it is important to either plan to increase resources or to see whether partner organizations such as non-governmental organizations (NGOs) and international bodies have the capacity to fill any gaps.

A communication plan should broadly set out goals and objectives for different stages of a pandemic, and set out the mechanisms and procedures by which these objectives should be achieved. For planning purposes, the stages that a pandemic, or a disease outbreak, passes through can broadly be described as pre-outbreak or pre-pandemic (when preparation is made for a threat that has not yet appeared), first appearance of cases, acceleration, peak transmission, deceleration and post-outbreak or post-pandemic. Many countries have pandemic alert systems, corresponding to different stages of disease emergence and transmission. A communication plan should be tailored to these different levels of alert, setting out objectives appropriate for each level. The objectives themselves should be based on the public health assessment of what needs to be done to manage the disease at different stages. If for example during the early stages of a pandemic, promoting social distancing to reduce the speed of spread is decided as the main public health goal, then communication objectives should be to produce messages and materials to help achieve this.

Once goals have been set, the communication plan should then set out the people and processes though which these aims are to be achieved. It should assign responsibility for the following broad functions:

- **Communications leadership**: this includes overall responsibility for pandemic communication, setting out communication strategies, planning day-to-day communications, managing communication staff and representing the communications department in higher-level pandemic planning and response committees.
- **Spokesperson and media relations**: the news media is the major channel of information for the public during a pandemic, and providing information to the media is a key function.
- **Internal communications**: it is essential to communicate internally within an organization, so that staff are kept aware of latest developments, without having to learn about them from the media. Internal communications from top management can also be used to boost staff morale during the stresses and strains of dealing with a pandemic.
- **Message development, material production and distribution**: public health advice needs to be turned into messages and publicity material that the public can understand and act on. The needs of hard-to-reach groups and minorities have to be catered to as well.
- **Management of approvals and clearances for information release**: a system for the rapid release of information to the press and public is essential.
- **Listening to the public**: gathering feedback from the public and analysing public perceptions through mechanisms such as surveys and media monitoring are essential to ensure communications strategies are effective.
- **Website and social media management**: the Internet and websites are critical channels for communicating with the public.

- **Partner communication coordination**: coordination with other ministries and organizations involved in pandemic response is essential in order to avoid conflicting messages being sent to the public. Liaising and coordinating with partners and stakeholders is thus an essential communication responsibility.

In addition to this, it is useful that the plan establishes mechanisms and protocols in advance of a pandemic for carrying out functions such as:

- **Coordination**: identify partner agencies that will be involved in pandemic communication (e.g. state- and provincial-level organizations, different ministries, international agencies) and establish a coordination mechanism with them in advance.
- **Information release**: develop in advance a policy on information release that is agreed to by all key decision makers, and set out the procedures and clearances for information release.
- **Monitoring public perceptions and opinion**: during a pandemic, it is important to gauge public perceptions to understand public concerns, counter rumours and misconceptions, and tailor messages to meet public needs. It is therefore important to have in place mechanisms to gather public opinion and to feed these findings to policy makers.
- **Evaluation mechanisms**: it is important to be able to evaluate communications to ensure that messages are getting through to the public and being understood correctly. Typical evaluation mechanisms include quick surveys, which are easily done, but need to be planned for in advance.

As part of preparedness, it is worth considering creating basic public health messages and publicity material in advance of a pandemic and testing them with focus groups to ensure that they are clearly understood. These could be messages on hand and respiratory hygiene, cough etiquette, behaviours to be avoided and recommended behaviours.

20.3   Principles of Communicating During a Pandemic

The following section sets out some principles to guide communicating with the public during pandemics or other infectious disease outbreaks.

The main purpose of public communication is to ensure that the public is well informed about the disease, has access to the latest information, and is able to make informed decisions on how best to protect themselves. The WHO's Outbreak Communication guidelines list building trust between the public and authorities as a key to effective communication with the public. Building trust requires being open with information, so that the public knows that bad news is not being hidden, being as transparent as possible and explaining the reasons for various decisions and recommendations, and also listening to the public. The following paragraphs explain this in more detail.

Maintaining trust

A key challenge for health communicators is to maintain the trust of the public before, during and after an outbreak. Experience has shown that if the public ceases to have trust in health authorities it becomes extremely difficult to manage a disease outbreak. Absence of trust can flow from a variety of factors: lack of belief in the competence and knowledge of authorities, lack of belief in their fairness, lack of belief in their honesty and so on. Trust is built over time, but unfortunately it can disappear in a matter of days if the public perceives that the health authorities have not been open, or lack competence. The low uptake for pandemic vaccine in many countries during the 2009 pandemic was partly a consequence of low trust in authorities. Many of the attributes that lead to trust between an institution and the public, such as professional competence, are outside the scope of communication. But announcing disease outbreaks or bad news early, and being transparent with information, are two key strategies for building trust.

Early announcement

It is often tempting to delay the release of bad news such as the outbreak of a disease, rising numbers of cases and rising mortality during an outbreak. Public health managers worry that bad news could trigger panic. However, experience has shown that public anxiety and overreaction is more likely to happen when the authorities try to suppress news. In modern societies with a 24-hour news culture, it is virtually impossible to hide news, and if the authorities are not open, rumours will circulate instead. A classic example was during the early stages of the severe acute respiratory syndrome (SARS) outbreak in southern China in early 2003. The authorities, confronted with a rapidly spreading disease they could not identify and knew very little about, decided not to tell the people in order to avoid public panic. But the public soon found out as news leaked out from hospitals. Not knowing what to do, people flocked to shops to buy vinegar and face masks in the hope that this would protect them. Without proper information the people were unable to protect themselves effectively, or know what behaviours to avoid, leading to the spread of the disease across China and eventually globally. Suppressing information also leads to distrust of the health and government authorities. Therefore early announcement of significant news is an essential element of good communication during disease outbreaks. In the case of a pandemic, this would include early announcement of the first cases to enter a country, daily updates of figures, information on disease severity patterns, how well medical services are coping, and any other questions that might be on the public mind. Early announcement of information in the context of a fast-moving event like a pandemic brings with it the risk that information might turn out to be wrong and might need correction later. Therefore it is important in any public communication to acknowledge uncertainty, and prepare the public for changing information and circumstances.

Transparency

In addition to the early announcement of news, a general policy of transparency is a good tool to build trust. Transparency involves sharing with the public some of the dilemmas and challenges that the authorities are facing, and allowing the public to understand why certain decisions are being taken. This is especially so in the case of potentially controversial decisions such as quarantines, travel restrictions or vaccine availability. These are decisions which will not be universally welcomed, and it is helpful to the public to communicate the reasoning behind these decisions as fully as possible. In this way, even if people do not agree with a decision, they will be aware why it was taken. An example of how transparency could have avoided a controversy comes from the anthrax attacks in the USA in 2011, when letters containing *Bacillus anthracis* spores were sent to various high-profile recipients through the US postal service. Since the letters were passing through the postal service, it was decided to provide postal workers at risk with prophylactic antibiotics. However, this led to widespread dissatisfaction among the postal workers. This was because they had been recommended the drug doxycycline, while prominent people such as journalists and congressional staff who were targets of the letters had been recommended another drug, ciprofloxacin. The postal workers felt they were being treated as second class citizens by being given doxycycline. Doxycycline, rather than ciprofloxacin, had been recommended by the US Centers for Diseases Control (CDC) to reflect changing scientific knowledge. When the anthrax attacks first began, the CDC had recommended ciprofloxacin. Subsequently, CDC scientists found that doxycycline worked as well against the prevailing strain of anthrax. Therefore, CDC updated its recommendations to include doxycycline. However, as the reasons for this change were never communicated, this lack of transparency led to public dissatisfaction.

Similarly, in Germany during the 2009 pandemic there was public anger against the government when it was discovered that civil servants were being provided a vaccine without adjuvants, while the general public was being offered an adjuvanted vaccine. Both vaccines were licensed for use, and different groups had been given different vaccines depending on what was available from manufacturers. But this was not explained clearly enough, and the public was suspicious that it had been given a less safe, adjuvanted vaccine, while the government reserved the safer vaccine for itself.

Communicating in a transparent way is often difficult, and so it is important, as part of the planning process, to agree in advance with the leadership of an organization on transparency guidelines. These guidelines should include the timely release of information that allows the public to understand why certain decisions were taken.

Listening to and understanding the public

It is easy to think of pandemic communication as a one-way process where health officials provide advice that the public passively listens to and accepts. While this one-way model might have been accurate in previous pandemics, the public today has access to multiple sources of information, ranging from websites and blogs, to the news media and information from friends and family. People develop their own perceptions of a disease threat based on all these sources of information, as well as their own personal experience. This perception could be at variance with the risk assessments of public health authorities. Also, not all people accept biomedical explanations of disease, and communication based on scientific explanations of disease might not resonate with those who see disease through other frameworks. It is also possible that the issues that concern the public during a disease outbreak might not be the issues that health agencies are communicating about. An example of how important it is to listen to and understand audiences comes from an outbreak of Marburg which occurred in Uige province in the north of Angola in 2004/05. International teams from the WHO and different NGOs rushed to help contain the outbreaks. But they were met with hostility and suspicion. Villagers were alarmed to see foreigners dressed from head to toe in protective garb, their faces masked, descend on their villages and whisk away their sick family and friends. What was worse from the local point of view was that many of those who were taken to hospital died, since Marburg has a high mortality rate. The hospital thus came to be seen as a place where sick people were taken to be killed. Villagers were also prevented from burying their dead in the normal way, since traditional burial practices were a risk factor for the spread of Marburg. There had been no attempt to begin a dialogue with the villagers, understand their thoughts on the disease and then provide them with the help they needed. Not surprisingly distrust and anger at the foreign teams grew. It was only after medical anthropologists were brought in to understand the villagers' point of view that progress in controlling the outbreak was possible. While this may be an extreme case, the basic principle is relevant: it is essential to listen to and understand the public during an outbreak. Otherwise there is a danger that public health officials will talk past the public. It is the role of the communicator to be a bridge between the public and public health officials.

How is listening to be done? There are a variety of ways, depending on the context. As part of pre-pandemic communication planning, it might be worth considering KAP (Knowledge, Attitude and Practices) surveys among different risk groups. A KAP survey will provide information about how much people know about a disease, their beliefs about the disease, and their practices. Among other things, such a survey is useful in identifying knowledge gaps and differences in perceptions between public health agencies and the public.

Other methods of being in touch with audiences include setting up community advisory panels, which could help enlist the support of influential community members, give an insight into community perspectives and provide a way to reach groups who might otherwise be hard to reach, such as ethnic minorities. Town hall type meetings are another way of sharing information and understanding community perceptions.

Other methods of gauging public opinion and perceptions include media monitoring and the monitoring of blogs, websites and Twitter® feeds; the importance of exploiting social media data to assist in communication is being increasingly recognized. Once a pandemic starts, the kind of questions being received from the public on hotlines are also valuable sources of information on public concerns and perceptions. Communication messages and campaigns should be followed up with surveys to ensure that messages are getting through to people.

20.4 Media Relations

The news media is a major source of information for the public during a pandemic or any other disease outbreak, and it is essential to have a well-thought-out plan to provide clear information to the media, to respond promptly to media queries, and also to rebut rumours and inaccurate information that might be circulating in news reports. The demand for information from the media during a pandemic can be overwhelming. The number of daily phone calls from the media can increase several hundred fold, and it is vital to have a mechanism to bring in more people either from within the organization or from partner organizations to manage this demand.

Meeting the demands of the media requires several elements. These include:

- A system for the **timely release of information** such as the latest numbers of cases, hospitalizations and fatalities. It is important to have prior agreement within the organization, or organizations managing the pandemic response, on what kind of information will be released on a daily basis, and when it will be released. If information is released on a daily basis at a fixed time and in a fixed manner (i.e. through a press release, or press conference, at the same time every day), then this allows the media to plan accordingly, and will help to reduce the number of phone calls from the media asking when information is going to be released. Communications officers need to ensure that the managers responsible for pandemic response understand the importance of providing regularly updated information to the public.

- A system for **developing key messages** to be communicated to the public. While the media is primarily interested in the latest figures, it is important to use the media to convey key messages to the public. These messages will vary with changing circumstances. For example, if large numbers of people are rushing to hospital emergency rooms out of worry, it might be necessary to develop messages asking the public to only go to hospital if their symptoms are serious. It is important to have a process by which key messages are decided upon based on the needs of the day, and then turned into talking points for spokespersons to use.

- **Assigning a spokesperson** or spokespersons. A spokesperson, or spokespersons, who are trusted by the media, and are comfortable dealing with the media, is a key element to a media strategy. On big issues, it will often be the political leadership which will make announcements to the media. But the day-to-day media strategy requires competent spokespersons who are knowledgeable and able to communicate with the press. It is recommended that potential spokespersons be identified in advance and given training in dealing with the media, so that they are prepared to take on the responsibility at the time of a pandemic. If there is a lot of foreign media interest, it might be worth assigning a specific spokesperson with the requisite language skills to deal with the foreign media.

- **Media monitoring** is an essential part of media relations. It is important to monitor and analyse what the news media, both local and international, are reporting about the pandemic. If rumours and misinformation are circulating, it is important to rapidly intervene to set the record straight. Misinformation that is allowed to circulate for more than 24 h tends to be difficult to correct. The response to rumours and wrong information should be as rapid as possible. Media monitoring is also a good way to understand public concerns and public opinion, and is a useful input in forming communication strategy.

20.5 The Internet and New Media

The 2009 pandemic was the first influenza pandemic of the Internet age, and it became clear that the Internet as well as other social messaging sites such as Twitter® and Facebook® were powerful tools for health agencies to use, but also posed challenges.

On the positive side, websites and social messaging services are a quick and efficient method to provide up-to-date information for the public. Public health agencies around the world used their websites during the pandemic to post the latest information, as well as advice to the public. Many agencies also maintained Twitter® and Facebook® accounts to reach audiences.

At the same time, the Internet can also transmit rumours and misinformation at lightning speed, and health authorities need to know how to respond to this rapidly and effectively. During the 2009 pandemic, the Internet became an important channel for anti-vaccination messages and rumours about the safety and efficacy of pandemic vaccines. Anti-vaccine bloggers were able to get global audiences for their views through the Internet. The global nature of the Internet means that public health authorities are faced with the challenge of responding to rumours that might originate anywhere in the world.

The key issue for health agencies is to develop a strategy which will harness the benefits of communicating through the Internet, while at the same time responding rapidly to, and minimizing, the damage caused by misinformation. The following points should be considered while preparing to use the Internet and new media effectively:

- Monitor other websites, blogs and social media sites to understand what the public is saying about the pandemic. Be prepared to promptly counter wrong information and disinformation that might be circulating on the Internet. The longer misinformation circulates without being addressed, the harder it becomes to correct it.

- Ensure that your website is speedily updated as soon as new information is released. Ensure that your website is well designed and easy to navigate, so that users will be encouraged to use it and will be able to find information easily.
- Consider using social media such as Twitter® and Facebook®, if they are widely used by key audiences. Social media networks can also be used to counter rumours and misinformation.
- During the initial stages of a pandemic or any other health emergency, public demand for information could by overwhelming, so it is important to ensure that there is adequate server capacity to meet public demand.
- In addition to being a source of new information, a website should also be used to provide information about symptoms, recommended actions and other basic advice. If basic advice is available in an easily accessible form on a website, this can reduce the load on medical services.

20.6 Communicating with Healthcare Workers

Healthcare workers are a key audience during a pandemic, or any other major disease outbreak, and it is important to have procedures and channels of communication in place to rapidly provide updated advice and information, and also to collect information including epidemiological and clinical data. In countries where private and public health providers coexist, it is important to ensure that information gets through to doctors, nurses and other responders in both sectors. It is equally important to have mechanisms by which the views of front-line medical staff can be conveyed to pandemic managers and through which it can be established that messages are getting through and are understandable by end recipients. Particular problems arose during the 2009 pandemic in several Europe countries related to the ability of primary care staff to access Internet-based clinical guidance and its (over) complexity.

20.7 Summary

The key to being prepared to communicate efficiently during a pandemic is planning in advance. Pandemics by their very nature are unpredictable and so plans need to be flexible, and it may not be wise to plan in too much detail. However it is essential to have basic mechanisms and structures in place, and personnel who are identified and trained to perform key roles. It is important to plan for surges in information demand, and have enough manpower and infrastructure to meet this demand.

It is equally important to be aware of the principles on which communication should be based, particularly transparency and openness. Without these, it is difficult to maintain public trust. And once public trust in the ability of the authorities to manage the pandemic gets eroded, pandemic management becomes that much more difficult.

- The WHO states that proactive communication is important because it 'encourages the public to adopt protective behaviours, facilitates heightened disease surveillance, reduces confusion and allows for a better use of resources – all of which are necessary for an effective response'.
- A pandemic can be a long-running event and severity can change over its course. This can require rapid updating, as well as being a challenge to hold public attention when a pandemic has been in progress for several months and complacency may have set in. The length and variability of a pandemic (e.g. how different groups of the population are affected) can also lead to public distrust of health authority advice.
- The principles of pandemic communication are: maintaining trust, early announcement, transparency, and listening to and understanding the public.
- The 2009 pandemic was the first influenza pandemic of the Internet age. Websites and social messaging services (e.g. Twitter® and Facebook®) are a quick and efficient way to provide up-to-date information to the public. However, the Internet can also rapidly transmit rumours and misinformation and health authorities need to know how to respond to this. The global nature of the Internet means that public health authorities are faced with the challenge of responding to rumours that might originate anywhere in the world.

Focus Box 20.1. Case Study: Managing the communication response to pandemic influenza in a large conurbation – an example from London in 2009/10.

In the world of 24-hour news and social media, the challenge for communications professionals in a crisis is to cascade accurate information quickly enough to advise internal staff, the public and politicians and to inform balanced news coverage. What follows is a short overview of NHS London's communications activity during the 2009 pandemic.

Inform and reassure
In preparation for a pandemic, NHS London, as the capital's Strategic Health Authority (SHA) with responsibility for 70 National Health Service (NHS) organizations serving over 7 million people, developed a communications framework setting out the roles and responsibilities for communications professionals pre-, during and post-pandemic. This included three core objectives:

- provide accurate, timely and consistent information and advice to internal staff, the public, media and stakeholders, including government ministers and local councils;
- promote understanding of pandemic influenza and good hygiene amongst healthcare workers and the public to slow the spread of the virus and ease pressure on front-line healthcare services;
- explain how the NHS is responding to the pandemic.

Communicating to NHS healthcare workers was the first priority. Healthcare workers are the trusted ambassadors of the health service. As such, they needed to be kept informed and able to convey accurate and authoritative messages to their patients, family, friends and neighbours – and often to the media. NHS London's Pandemic Flu Team produced a daily 'noon brief' to all public health and emergency planners across the capital. This regular bulletin became the essential briefing for over 800 multi-agency partners involved in responding to the pandemic. At the same time, the SHA communications team regularly cascaded updated lines to take for hospital trusts and primary care services to use when briefing NHS staff face-to-face or in internal newsletters.

NHS London also adopted a 'command and control' protocol coordinating the responses to all pandemic media enquiries centrally. This 'do once' approach allowed front-line NHS communications staff within hospitals and primary care services to focus on managing the response of local health services, whilst the SHA acted as the one consistent voice of the NHS in London.

The biggest challenge was gathering information from many different organizations to keep up to date with changing messages. During the pandemic, the Department of Health, England (DH) determined the timing of health announcements and would cascade briefing material to all health organizations in England. SHAs would then gather information from the Health Protection Agency (HPA), local hospitals and GPs treating people with flu-like symptoms to inform the DH national understanding of the scale and response to the situation. The challenge was to interpret this information quickly to give prompt responses to the media and cascade consistent messages to NHS organizations and stakeholders. An example of this is the weekly reporting of deaths from pandemic influenza.

The DH, in conjunction with the HPA, held weekly press briefings to announce the number of cases and confirmed A(H1N1)pdm09-related deaths. However no regional breakdown of cases was available. This put local NHS organizations under increased media scrutiny. NHS London took the decision to confirm the number of confirmed deaths week-by-week along with the number of people in hospital intensive care units. No identifiable patient information was released. This reduced the pressure on NHS organizations and enabled the media to report the latest developments whilst allowing protection of patient confidentiality. In turn, this helped NHS London develop strong relationships with key journalists. More importantly, it contributed towards NHS London being viewed by the media and by other NHS organizations as a trusted, valuable and reliable source of information.

Promoting health messages
The NHS in London experienced significant pressures on services from the 'worried well' or people with mild influenza-like symptoms, particularly in accident and emergency (A&E) departments during the first wave. In response, NHS London with the DH launched a campaign to signpost patients to the most appropriate NHS service. The campaign aimed to remind the public of the many alternatives available for the treatment of mild symptoms, such as GPs, pharmacists and walk-in centres, and importantly encourage people not to call the emergency services or go to A&E unless it was a real emergency. This helped to reduce demand on front-line NHS services and enabled paramedic and A&E staff to care for the most critically ill.

Continued

T. Abraham and D. Pople

Focus Box 20.1. Continued.

Over a 3-week period at the height of the pandemic in the UK, a 40-second commercial was played in heavy rotation across London's radio stations. A half-page press advertisement was also printed in regional press and over 70 local newspapers. This work was supplemented by extensive internal communications and reinforcement through existing NHS websites. Primary Care Trusts were charged with targeting hard-to-reach black and minority ethnic groups. A proactive media campaign was also undertaken with interviews given to London's newspapers, television and radio stations to raise public awareness.

Over 800 people across London were interviewed to evaluate the effectiveness of the campaign. The results showed that one in five people had seen or heard the advertisement. Of these, 41% remembered the advice to stay at home or seek alternative treatment before going to A&E. The campaign materials were shared with NHS organizations across the country for local use.

Capacity and resilience

The pandemic remained a 'breaking news' story for almost 16 months. Managing the media's demands throughout this time was a significant challenge. Whilst adrenaline can get you through the early stages of a major incident, resilience is needed to sustain this response for as long as is required. Consequently, when media interest was it its highest, a rota for the NHS London communications team was agreed. This involved two members of the team dealing solely with swine flu media enquiries, while one team member provided additional support. This role was pivotal and involved gathering the latest information and updating lines to take to enable the media officers to respond to enquiries quickly and with authority. A further two members of staff would provide general administrative support. The team would then rotate to allow those dealing with a high volume of media enquiries to recharge and inject renewed energy into the team. Throughout, two senior directors would alternate to provide ongoing strategic oversight.

By rotating responsibilities, NHS London created a dedicated swine flu communications unit that had the knowledge and resilience to adapt to the changing demands of the situation whilst creating capacity to continue with business as usual. This enabled us to coordinate communications quickly and consistently. In doing so, NHS London became the 'go-to point' for NHS organizations on the ground and the DH, and a reliable source of information for the news media and other stakeholders.

Managing social media

Like pandemic influenza, misinformation can spread quickly from person to person and continent to continent through social media. Communicators have joined together to create an online forum, 'Social Media in the NHS', to put forward recommendations for best practice in the future. Using realistic scenarios from the 2009 pandemic, this forum discusses how social media can be used to reach at-risk groups, inform the news media and spread reliable information.

Further Reading

Pan American Health Organization/World Health Organization (2009) Creating a Communication Strategy for Pandemic Influenza. Available at: http://www.paho.org/English/AD/PAHO_CommStrategy_Eng.pdf (accessed 1 April 2012).

Social Media in the NHS, via the #nhssm hashtag. Blog: http://nhssm.org.uk. Twitter: @nhssm. Contact: @a_double_tt, Alexander Talbott, Communications Officer, NHS London.

World Health Organization (2008) WHO Outbreak Communication Planning Guide. Available at: http://www.who.int/ihr/elibrary/WHOOutbreakCommsPlanngGuide.pdf (accessed 1 April 2012).

US Centers for Diseases Control and Prevention (2007) Crisis and Emergency Risk Communication. Pandemic Influenza. Available at: http://emergency.cdc.gov/cerc/pdf/CERC-PandemicFlu-OCT07.pdf (accessed 1 April 2012).

21 Case Study 1: Mexico

Diana Vilar-Compte and Patricia Volkow

Instituto Nacional de Cancerología, México

21.1 Introduction

In 2003 the National Committee for Health Security in Mexico established an influenza preparedness and response plan as recommended by the World Health Organization (WHO). In 2004 antiviral drugs, antibiotics and medical supplies for an emergency were stockpiled.

21.2 The 2009 Pandemic

In early 2009, epidemiological surveillance systems identified clusters of influenza cases and public health reference laboratories observed an increased number of non-typeable influenza samples. By mid-March, morbidity reports showed an increased number of cases of acute respiratory disease, with high attack rates in some communities (La Gloria, Veracruz). At the same time, clinicians from referral centres (mainly Mexico City, San Luis Potosí and Oaxaca) were reporting an abnormally high number of patients with severe influenza-like illness (ILI) and rapidly evolving severe pneumonia. Most of these individuals were young and previously healthy.

On 17 April 2009, the national health authorities issued a country-wide influenza alert and commenced an active search for cases of severe pneumonia with ILI in Mexico City hospitals. Samples from non-typeable influenza A cases were sent to reference laboratories in Canada and the USA. On 23 April 2009, the existence of a novel influenza A(H1N1) virus of swine origin that had already been identified in samples from two children in San Diego, California was announced as the likely cause of the respiratory epidemic already underway. WHO later designated the virus A(H1N1)pdm09.

The response to the challenge was driven by the public health sector; in the face of a virus with pandemic potential, strong social distancing measures were specified, which included country-wide school closures. In Mexico City, the epicentre of

the epidemic, all non-essential activities were stopped. A mass media campaign was started on hand washing and respiratory etiquette.

Many emergency departments across the country experienced surge pressures and the number of people hospitalized with severe ILI and pneumonia increased over the following days, with almost half of those admitted requiring mechanical ventilation. Healthcare facilities reached capacity and areas outside the intensive care units were converted to allow for the care of patients requiring mechanical ventilation. Figure 21.1 illustrates the admissions of patients with ILI at a referral hospital for 2009–2011.

The Mexican health system faced enormous demands from patients. A total of 6129 cases of severe acute respiratory illness were hospitalized throughout the country from the first week of March to 7 July 2009. At the National Institute of Respiratory Diseases in Mexico City, which is a national referral centre and sentinel hospital for influenza, 1698 emergency room visits from 1 April 2009 to 15 May 2009 were registered compared to approximately 1418 over the same periods in 2007 and 2008 combined. Admissions for influenza-related pneumonia for that same period rose from 6% of all acute admissions in 2007 and 2008 to 29% in 2009, and the in-hospital mortality rate for all admitted patients increased from a 9% baseline to 13%. Both the nosocomial influenza rate and the nosocomial pneumonia rate also doubled during the outbreak compared with baseline. Referral hospitals were reorganized to increase surge capacity, deliver safe healthcare, and protect healthcare workers and visitors.

As initially recommended by the WHO, only laboratory-confirmed cases were registered. This generated confusion and even scepticism among some sectors of Mexican society as it became clear that many severe cases were not being registered through lack of confirmatory diagnosis, although

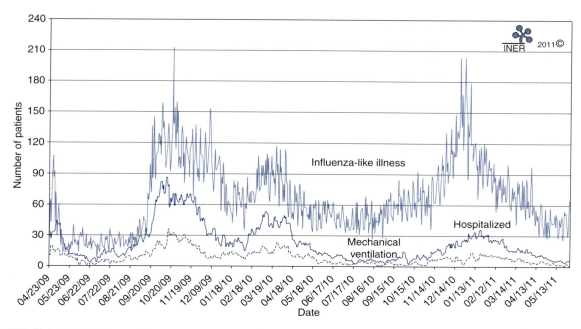

Fig. 21.1. Monthly aggregate of influenza-like illness in a referral hospital for respiratory diseases in Mexico City, Mexico (March 2009–May 2011). (Figure kindly provided by the Unidad de Vigilancia Epidemiológica Hospitalaria, Instituto Nacional de Enfermedades Respiratorias (UVEH-INER).)

still exerting overwhelming pressure on hospital bed capacity. The existing numbers of ventilators and monitors available for treating ill patients were insufficient in the country. The Ministry of Health conducted a rapid assessment of the number of ventilators available and capacity to handle critically ill patients (staff, electrical power and oxygen pressure under maximum usage). In response, the Government purchased 700 mechanical ventilators and monitors that were distributed among 100 hospitals.

As part of the influenza preparedness and response plans, Mexico had stockpiled oseltamivir active pharmaceutical ingredient (Chapter 14). Immediately after the announcement of the new virus, the powder was reconstituted into suspension to increase national availability, although distribution was hindered as this formulation required refrigeration. Oseltamivir was recommended for all ILI patients at the beginning of the outbreak, and was freely available for all patients who needed it.

As the epidemic evolved and knowledge about the virus and its behaviour increased, public health measures were relaxed and more focused information and prevention measures were implemented. As the country prepared to face a second wave, the

experience gained about hospital reorganization and the management of severe cases in the referral hospitals during the first wave was disseminated to other hospitals. The expertise gained by healthcare workers who had already cared for severely ill patients during the first wave was extremely valuable and helped to achieve better outcomes in the forthcoming months.

Twenty-eight million doses of monovalent pandemic A(H1N1)pdm09 vaccines were purchased; they arrived in the country gradually from November 2009 to January 2010. The target groups for vaccination were: pregnant women and women with children under 6 months of age, healthcare workers, infants aged 6 to 23 months, and people 25 months to 64 years with chronic conditions. Acceptance of the vaccine varied, but as observed in other countries (Chapter 15), was ultimately rather low among the population. By the end of January, 2010, vaccination was opened to all persons wishing to be immunized.

The influenza epidemic had a large and important impact in Mexican society. Economic activities were paralysed, with a decrease in contributory revenue towards major healthcare expenditure.

The cost of the epidemic up to June 2009 alone was estimated at US$5000 million, around 0.5% of gross domestic product.

Mass media and the Mexican Ministry of Health shared the responsibility to inform society and empower the population. They allowed people to gather information on the exceptional circumstances in Mexico and learn about influenza and preventive measures. Unfortunately, the frequency and intensity of influenza-related news also produced feelings of confusion and doubts about the magnitude and severity of the outbreak. The way the number of patients with A(H1N1)pdm09 was presented in the media created confusion and increased mistrust towards the government. The above could probably have been avoided if the difficulties and uncertainties encountered with a new and unknown virus had been better communicated.

21.3 Lessons and Ongoing Planning

A number of important lessons were identified during the response to the 2009 pandemic. The importance of preparedness plans considering hospital surge capacity (especially the number and availability of intensive care beds), a strategic stockpile of drugs for critically ill patients and a programme for patient referral to hospitals prepared to manage patients with influenza pneumonia and ventilatory support were all key factors, as patients with pneumonia and ILI require more care and enhanced infection control precautions. Intensive-care transfers between neighbouring hospitals provided aid in receiving a small number of patients, but this procedure was questioned by patients' relatives and was difficult to implement. The technology for accurate and fast diagnosis of influenza was limited to a few academic centres. Infrastructure and molecular diagnostic techniques (RT-PCR) for influenza and other respiratory viruses have since been increased and surveillance systems for influenza and other infections have also been reinforced. Preparedness and Response Plans for infectious and non-infectious emergency conditions are being revised incorporating these and other lessons identified from the A(H1N1)pdm09 epidemic.

In the face of an emergency, knowledge, intelligence and leadership all come under strain. Mexico's response at the beginning of a new influenza pandemic, when little was known on the biology and epidemiology of the new virus, was made with the aim to save human lives. For some critics, the Government response was exaggerated, but it slowed the spread of the virus and allowed the country to prepare for the second much bigger wave of the pandemic. The health system showed its strengths and weakness. It was clear that diagnostic capacity, epidemiological surveillance, intensive care infrastructure and communication resources at all levels, needed to be reinforced.

Further Reading

Córdoba-Villalobos, J.A., Sarti, E., Arzoz-Padrés, J., Manuell-Lee, G., Romero Méndez, J. and Kuri-Morales, P. (2009) The influenza A (H1N1) epidemic in Mexico. Lessons learned. *Health Research Policy and Systems* 7, 21.

Perez-Padilla, R., de la Rosa-Zamboni, D., Ponce de Leon, S., Hernandez, M., Quiñones-Falconi, F., Bautista, E., Ramirez-Venegas, A., Rojas-Serrano, J., Ormsby, C.E., Corrales, A., Higuera, A., Mondragon, E. and Cordova-Villalobos, J.A.; INER Working Group on Influenza (2009) Pneumonia and respiratory failure from swine-origin influenza A (H1N1) in Mexico. *New England Journal of Medicine* 361(7), 680–689.

Stern, A.M. and Markel, H. (2009) What Mexico taught the world about pandemic influenza preparedness and community mitigation. *Journal of the American Medical Association* 302(11), 1221–1222.

D. Vilar-Compte and P. Volkow

Case Study 2: Chile

JEANNETTE DABANCH

Universidad de los Andes Hospital Militar, Santiago, Chile

22.1 Introduction

Chile is a long (4329 km) and narrow country with 16.6 million people, located at the southern end of South America. Most of the country has a temperate climate and seasonal influenza activity typically occurs between April and September (autumn–winter).

22.2 Pandemic Preparedness

When the first wave of influenza A(H1N1)pdm09 started, the country was well advanced in its preparation plans for the influenza pandemic. Following World Health Organization (WHO) recommendations, in 2002 the Chilean Ministry of Health began developing a plan to cope with the potential emergence of a new influenza virus, with the aim of reducing both morbidity and mortality, and the consequent social and economic impact. In 2005, the government approved the first pandemic influenza plan, which was updated in 2007. Planning considered strengthening existing areas by identifying and correcting flaws and developing new strategies to facilitate an appropriate and timely response, and defining operational responsibilities.

One of the key reinforced areas was sentinel viral respiratory surveillance in humans. This was done by increasing the number of national sentinel units; monitoring data on emergency room visits and hospitalization for acute respiratory infection (in primary healthcare centres and hospitals); early detection and notification of acute respiratory infection outbreaks; expansion of the annual influenza immunization programme to new high-risk groups (pregnant women, children between 6 and 24 months of age and poultry workers); optimizing the organization and responsiveness of the public and private healthcare network; reinforcing healthcare-associated infection control measures; and enhancing the existing influenza surveillance programme in animals.

The low clinical suspicion of viral influenza as the aetiologic agent of severe acute respiratory infection and pneumonia in adults was one of the most deficient areas, together with low laboratory diagnostic capacity for respiratory viruses and an insufficient number of critical care beds.

The new response strategies consisted of pharmaceutical and non-pharmaceutical measures. The former included the establishment of a national antiviral stockpile, development of clinical influenza guidelines, a pandemic vaccination strategic plan and a national pneumococcal immunization programme for people 65 years and older. Non-pharmaceutical measures included public health interventions, such as infection control practices (including hand hygiene, respiratory etiquette and voluntary social distancing, aimed at reducing person-to-person transmission); a communication plan for different target audiences (public sector and healthcare workers); creation of an inter-sectoral advisory committee to coordinate decision making at a national level; and implementation of the 2005 WHO International Health Regulations. The plan considered various potential scenarios, with different estimated attack rates, severity of morbidity and mortality and differential responses according to the different pandemic phases.

22.3 Pandemic Response

In April 2009, after the pandemic phase change issued by WHO, the national plan was activated. Viral respiratory surveillance was intensified, the mandatory reporting of all influenza-like illness (ILI) cases (especially travellers from affected areas) began and the distribution of antivirals to all public and private national health services started.

On 17 May, Chile reported its first three cases. They were Chilean tourists travelling back from the Dominican Republic. These cases were followed by clusters of the infection in schools within the metropolitan region. By the end of May, 11 of the 15 national administrative regions had reported cases.

According to the national respiratory virus surveillance network, the total duration of the outbreak was 12 weeks. The pandemic virus replaced the circulating seasonal influenza virus, which accounted for less than 1% of confirmed influenza cases.

The Chilean government response was fast and included clinical guidelines and other measures supported by a panel of epidemiology and infectious disease experts. The first implemented strategy was a containment one including active surveillance for cases of ILI, voluntary isolation at home or in healthcare settings (depending on severity of illness) and treatment of all confirmed cases with antiviral drugs and prophylaxis for contacts. This changed to a mitigation strategy two weeks after the first case report. This second strategy was focused on early detection, laboratory confirmation of influenza (at the Chilean Institute of Public Health), adequate treatment of severe cases, antiviral treatment of all outpatients with ILI and active contact tracing, and post-exposure antiviral prophylaxis for high-risk groups. A communication strategy was started through different media channels in order to teach the population about the importance of early consultation and self-care measures.

During 2009, ILI consultations were five to six times higher than in the previous season. By the end of the first pandemic wave, 368,129 ILI cases were notified, representing a 1.2% influenza pandemic population attack rate. The first wave showed the highest incidence rate in children between 5 and 14 years of age (4.5%) and the lowest in people aged 60 years and over (0.4%). The majority of patients presented with mild and uncomplicated disease.

During the same period, 1622 laboratory-confirmed cases of pandemic influenza were hospitalized. Pneumonia was the most common diagnosis at admission and the median age of patients was 32 years (range 11 days to 94 years). The overall rate of hospitalization was 9.4 per 100,000 population. The case hospitalization rate was 0.6%, with the highest rate in adults over 60 years (3.5%) and the lowest in children aged 5 to 14 years (0.2%), consistent with those reported for seasonal influenza. Four per cent of hospitalized patients required admission to an intensive care unit. All inpatients received antiviral treatment according to national guidelines.

Out of all hospitalized patients, 155 died with an overall population mortality of 0.93 per 100,000,

the median age was 47 years (range 4 months to 89 years). Fifty per cent of deaths were due to severe respiratory failure. While the overall case fatality rate was 0.04%, it was 0.4% in adults 60 years and older, indicating the substantially increased likelihood of death in patients older than 60 years infected with A(H1N1)pdm09. Eighty-seven per cent of patients who died had underlying co-morbidities. Delay in medical care was also a risk factor for death. It is noteworthy that no deaths were reported in pregnant women.

During the outbreak, all public and private hospitals operated as a network and the increased need for beds was solved by using those assigned to elective surgery, which was suspended. Pandemic vaccine was not available at the time of the first wave of the outbreak.

Community mitigation measures included education about protective measures to reduce transmission and promotion of early consultation. Avoiding closed crowded places was the only social distancing measure recommended.

During the first pandemic wave, other South American countries reported varying impacts. For example Argentina reported an overall rate of hospitalization of 34 per 100,000 population of which 11% required intensive care, with an overall mortality of 1.5 per 100,000. In Brazil overall mortality was 1.1 per 100,000 population although this was highest in southern Brazil (3.3 per 100,000).

22.4   Forward Planning

The plan implemented in Chile included raised awareness, rapid identification of cases, antiviral treatment of all ILI cases, creation of a health network that included public and private hospitals and an educational strategy, all of which may have influenced the relatively benign course of the outbreak. The availability of updated information for public and healthcare providers during the pandemic period was also important. Notwithstanding these results, lessons were learned and improvements are required. In spite of the fact that the outbreak was mild the healthcare system was overwhelmed. We need to improve responsiveness to severe outbreaks and increase and improve the coordinated response among decision makers and healthcare providers in order to appropriately adapt the guidelines and measures according to the evolution of any future pandemic.

Further Reading

Dabanch, J., Perret, C., Nájera, M., Gonzalez, C., Guerrero, A., Olea, A., Fasce, R., Morales, C.; Advisory Committee of the Chilean Ministry of Health (2011) Age as risk factor for death from pandemic (H1N1) 2009, Chile. *Emerging Infectious Diseases* 17(7), 1256–1258.

Torres, J.P., O'Ryan, M., Herve, B., Espinoza, R., Acuña, G., Mañalich, J. and Chomalí M. (2010) Impact of the novel influenza A(H1N1) during the 2009 autumn–winter season in a large hospital setting in Santiago, Chile. *Clinical Infectious Diseases* 50, 860–868.

Van Kerkhove, M.D., Mounts, A.W., Mall, S., Vandemaele, K.A., Chamberland, M., dos Santos, T., Fitzner, J., Widdowson, M.A., Michalove, J., Bresee, J.,

Olsen, S.J., Quick, L., Baumeister, E., Carlino, L.O., Savy, V., Uez, O., Owen, R., Ghani, F., Paterson, B., Forde, A., Fasce, R., Torres, G., Andrade, W., Bustos, P., Mora, J., Gonzalez, C., Olea, A., Sotomayor, V., Najera De Ferrari, M., Burgos, A., Hunt, D., Huang, Q.S., Jennings, L.C., Macfarlane, M., Lopez, L.D., McArthur, C., Cohen, C., Archer, B., Blumberg, L., Cengimbo, A., Makunga, C., McAnerney, J., Msimang, V., Naidoo, D., Puren, A., Schoub, B., Thomas, J., Venter, M.; WHO Southern Hemisphere Influenza Comparison Study Working Group (2011) Epidemiologic and virologic assessment of the 2009 influenza A(H1N1) pandemic on selected temperate countries in the Southern Hemisphere: Argentina, Australia, Chile, New Zealand and South Africa. *Influenza and Other Respiratory Viruses* 5(6), e487–e498.

23 Case Study 3: New Zealand

LANCE C. JENNINGS

Canterbury Health Laboratories and University of Otago, Christchurch, New Zealand

23.1 Introduction

New Zealand was the first country in the southern hemisphere to report the importation of influenza A(H1N1)pdm09, following the return of a group of high school students from Mexico on 25 April 2009. The detection of these cases triggered the activation of New Zealand's Influenza Pandemic Action Plan (NZIPAP), and the public health response to this threat was perhaps the largest the country has ever mounted.

23.2 State of Previous Planning and Preparedness Entering 2009

New Zealand's pandemic planning has followed a comprehensive emergency management approach involving the whole of government, incorporating all available expertise and resources into an action plan, under the umbrella of New Zealand's National Health Emergency Plan. This approach has been taken because considerable expertise exists in New Zealand for emergency management using the New Zealand Coordinated Incident Management System model, developed for natural hazards such as earthquakes, fire and floods. Further, hospitals and health professionals are used to dealing with emergencies every day and planning is required to manage surges due to infectious diseases for example; however these have all been scaled up for an event of national proportions.

New Zealand's pandemic planning has evolved since 1997, from an initial response framework to the current advanced operational Action Plan (NZIPAP, version 2010). The NZIPAP 2006 version compared favourably with 29 European pandemic plans, however scope for further improvement was identified. Initiatives such as Exercise Virex in 2002, involving 21 District Health Boards (DHBs) and 13 Public Health Units (PHUs) in the first national response exercise to test a pandemic plan conducted globally; the use of the NZIPAP as the framework for the Ministry of Health's response to the outbreak of severe acute respiratory syndrome in 2003; then Exercise Cruickshank, a whole-of-government exercise in 2007, have ensured the Action Plan remains a live document and reflects evolving understanding. In response to the avian influenza threat, targeted research and other simulation exercises to test and refine planning tools have also been conducted.

The goals of the NZIPAP (Fig. 23.1) are to:

- minimize the impact of the disease and to mitigate its effects on the people of New Zealand;
- enable society to continue to function as normally as possible during and after a pandemic;
- minimize and mitigate the economic consequences of a pandemic in New Zealand.

These are underpinned by a six-stage strategy with associated trigger points that in summary is as follows:

1. Planning and preparedness – 'Plan For It' – interpandemic period.
2. Border management – 'Keep It Out' – human-to-human transmission overseas, or very high suspicion of human-to-human transmission, or Australia and/or Singapore close borders.
3. Cluster control – 'Stamp It Out' – human pandemic strains found in New Zealand.
4. Pandemic management – 'Manage It' – clusters in separate locations or spread within New Zealand.
5. Post-peak management – 'Manage It: Post-Peak'.
6. Recovery – 'Recover From It' – population protected by vaccination or pandemic abated.

Pivotal to the action plan is a whole-of-government response system. Overall coordination and collaboration is achieved through a cross-ministry advisory group, with a cross-ministry steering group (EM-SG) providing leadership and strategic oversight through to the Minister of Health. A standing Pandemic Influenza Technical Advisory Group provides expert clinical, virological, epidemiological,

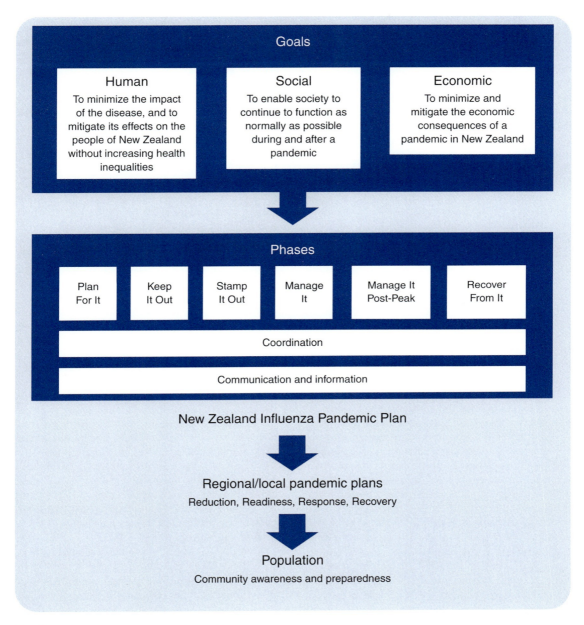

Fig. 23.1. New Zealand strategic approach to a pandemic.

infection control and ethical advice to inform the Ministry of Health's pandemic response planning, and advises on communicating key messages, public health interventions and other associated issues during a pandemic threat. The country's 21 DHBs are the lead agencies for planning and responding on a local and regional basis. The action plan explicitly recognizes that effective information flow between DHBs, ambulance services and the primary healthcare sector is required.

23.3 Reflection on What Happened in 2009

Between April and December 2009, New Zealand experienced the first wave of the influenza A(H1N1)-pdm09 pandemic. Influenza activity escalated during June, peaked during July and had waned by the end of August after about 8 weeks. The first imported cases were detected on 25 April, triggering the activation of the NZIPAP and implementation of the public health response. New Zealand declared influenza a notifiable and quarantinable disease on 30 April following the World Health Organization raising the global pandemic threat to Phase 5. A(H1N1)pdm09 vaccine was not available in New Zealand until 2010.

The initial response focused on 'containment' involving both border management 'Keep It Out' and cluster control 'Stamp It Out' strategies from 25 April until 22 June, when New Zealand formally switched to the 'Manage It' phase. Border management involved the public health service establishing a presence at international airports, with staff meeting each international flight and the establishment of manned information booths. Passenger locator forms were introduced on to incoming aircraft to provide information to passengers. They also provided additional passenger details and assisted with influenza case finding and contact tracing. Arriving passengers with an influenza-like illness (ILI) were assessed, treated with oseltamivir and placed in voluntary isolation, while their contacts were traced and given oseltamivir prophylaxis. Respiratory samples were also obtained for virological confirmation. Although most cases were reported from the community (with ILI cases contacting their doctor or the public health service), rather than at the borders, this overall strategy of 'containing' these cases or small clusters appeared to delay community transmission of A(H1N1)pdm09 by nearly 6 weeks through May into June.

Regardless of whether the long lead-in period was an epidemiological phenomenon or a result of a highly effective public health response, it bought valuable time for the EM-SG to assess the evolving global situation and to strengthen various elements of the response. These included surveillance, the public health service's front-line capacity, virus diagnostic capacity and other aspects of primary and secondary health care, and other government departments' responses. Above all, it allowed the EM-SG to develop simple public health messages about basic respiratory hygiene and social distancing, including staying away from work or school if sick (home isolation for mild cases) and seeking early medical advice. Public health messages were communicated by radio and television, regular media updates and other media such as posters and the use of websites. A national free-calling telephone health information or 'Healthline' was established with call triaging.

The community spread of A(H1N1)pdm09 became apparent in the three main population centres during the week of 16 June 2009, placing attempts at containment under severe pressure. No longer could all clusters be contained and both public health services and virus diagnostic services were stretched to full capacity. Although smaller population centres had not yet been affected, the national response was moved into the 'management' phase on 22 June. The management of cases with moderate to severe disease became a priority. Antiviral use was prioritized for the treatment of cases, particularly those at risk of severe outcomes, and routine prophylaxis of contacts ceased. Cluster control activities in the community ceased and 'Flu Centres' were established in some DHBs to manage ILI patients. The pharmacist prescribing of oseltamivir was also modified to allow remote telephone triaging.

Community mitigation measures included complete or partial school closures and public education on measures to protect individuals and reduce transmission. A number of schools (< 20) or early childcare centres formally closed, while others closed because of high absenteeism. However, the school holidays (4–19 July) coincided with the peak of the pandemic and may have lessened transmission during this period.

Surveillance, which was enhanced in accordance with the NZIPAP from April, was pivotal to managing the response. Two existing sentinel general practitioner systems capturing both epidemiological and virological data allowed estimation of the disease burden, circulating virus strains and real-time pandemic progression. The EM-SG also utilized a new HealthStat system (developed by the Ministry of Health) that captured ILI data electronically each week from >100 general practices. The notifiable disease surveillance system (EpiSurv) recorded individual laboratory-confirmed cases and cases from both primary and secondary care, which provided complementary information.

However, once the 'Manage It' phase was under way, routine virological testing was restricted to severe cases and this system was less useful, providing an underestimate of the true community disease burden. The capture of hospitalization and death data into EpiSurv was supplemented with daily monitoring of hospital and intensive care admissions and deaths.

Although New Zealand held a forward-purchasing agreement for pandemic vaccines with a regional manufacturer, another agreement was entered into for the supply of 300,000 doses of the non-adjuvanted cell culture-based monovalent A(H1N1)pdm09 vaccine (Celvapan® H1N1), to provide protection for people at higher risk of life-threatening complications and front-line healthcare workers, prior to a second 2010 pandemic wave. This vaccine was received late in 2009, but not made available until February 2010 in advance of the seasonal trivalent vaccine scheduled for April 2010. Front-line healthcare workers were offered it in the first instance and DHBs with well-organized immunization strategies achieved high coverage, while others opted to wait for the seasonal vaccine; overall the uptake was low. By May 2010, about 1 million of 4.4 million New Zealanders had received either one or both vaccines.

23.4 Forward Look

The pandemic lessons from countries in the southern hemisphere have been identified. Unique to these lessons was New Zealand's apparently successful containment, with a delay of approximately 6 weeks from the detection of the first imported cases to the establishment of community transmission. Public health activity at the borders is unlikely to have been effective on its own; however in combination with vigorous case cluster control may have contributed to delayed spread. Further evaluation of these interventions is required.

The communication of simple cost-effective mitigation measures during New Zealand's 'lag period' is likely to have had some benefit. A culture of staying home if sick developed and the public health messaging (including hand and respiratory hygiene) built on existing school-based 'SneezeSafe' hygiene initiatives.

The initiation of research as a pandemic evolves is required to help direct a national response. Late during the pandemic a serological survey was initiated to inform pandemic-specific vaccine usage in 2010 prior to a second wave. A pandemic influenza morbidity and mortality review committee was established to review all 2009 influenza-associated deaths, with a view to providing policy and clinical advice prior to the second wave. This review led to the eligibility criteria for subsidized 2010 seasonal vaccine being extended to include pregnant women, children under 5 years of age and obese individuals. The timely analysis of the first cases imported into New Zealand would have produced useful information to address the many uncertainties during initial stages of the evolving pandemic.

Many of the lessons identified have been incorporated into an updated NZIPAP. Previous New Zealand pandemic planning had been based on the severe 1918 scenario, essentially because of the national knowledge base on this pandemic and the importance of avian influenza A(H5N1) as a potential pandemic threat. However, the NZIPAP 2010 has been modified so the mix of actions at different phases can be customized to apply to a mild or moderate pandemic.

Further Reading

Bandaranayake, D., Jacobs, M., Baker, M., Hunt, D., Wood, T., Bissielo A., Macfarlane M., Lopez L., Mackereth G. and Huang Q. (2011) The second wave of 2009 pandemic influenza A(H1N1) in New Zealand, January–October 2010. *EuroSurveillance* 16(6), pii:19788. Available at: http://www.eurosurveillance.org/ViewArticle.aspx?Articleid=19788 (accessed 29 March 2012).

New Zealand Ministry of Health (2010) New Zealand Influenza Pandemic Plan: A Framework for Action. Available at: http://www.health.govt.nz/publication/new-zealand-influenza-pandemic-plan-framework-action (accessed 29 March 2012).

Williams, D., Begg, A., Burgess, K., Hider, M., Jennings, L., Martin-Smith, M., McCormack, P., Mitchell, J., Pithie, A., Schroeder, P. and Werno A. (2010) Influenza H1N1 2009 in Canterbury: a case study in pandemic response co-ordination. *Journal of Primary Health Care* 2(4), 323–329.

24 Case Study 4: Former Soviet Union

Irina Papieva

WHO Country Office, Yerevan, Armenia

24.1 Pandemic Preparedness

Experiences gained during the response to avian influenza outbreaks, and the capacities built afterwards, provided a platform from which the governments of Former Soviet Union (FSU) countries could promote and invest in pandemic preparedness planning. The opportunities to do so have been greatly increased by the enormous influx of funds and technical expertise coming from major international stakeholders, such as the World Health Organization (WHO), the United Nations Children's Fund (UNICEF), the World Bank (WB), the United States Agency for International Development (USAID) and the US Centers for Disease Control and Prevention (CDC). Moreover, major reforms in the health and economic sectors under way in countries after their independence from the Soviet Union have allowed governments to change agendas and re-prioritize many initiatives and interventions.

Many efforts were made to strengthen the capacities of the respective health systems, which are defined as 'comprising all the organizations, institutions, and resources that are devoted to producing actions principally aimed at improving, maintaining or restoring health'; however, the FSU countries still apply vertical management and address health needs mainly within the frames of specific programme areas and sectoral structures. There is still an absence of adequate horizontal linkages between sectors and management tiers. Cooperation and coordination mechanisms still require further development within the health sector as well as outside it, although major improvements are evident. On the other hand, there is clear understanding by governments that well-functioning health systems are essential to improving health and reaching specific goals. Thus, new approaches to addressing health needs from a health system perspective have been applied in many countries and within the frameworks of many programmes, including pandemic preparedness.

By early 2009, health systems were strengthened to enable FSU countries to respond to the pandemic. Most of the countries developed stand-alone pandemic preparedness plans, although a minority were still using revised avian influenza plans or amendments to more generic disaster preparedness plans. Although based on the WHO guidelines for pandemic preparedness planning and thus having an adequate structure, the completeness, flexibility and realism of some plans could have been questioned and still require more detailed work-up. Most of the plans did not address adequately a number of policy considerations, strategic approaches and operational arrangements associated with them. In addition to a somewhat limited number of national stakeholders (many plans were almost entirely focused solely on the Ministry of Health), the roles and responsibilities of different international stakeholders were also unclear. Political and economic developments across the region, ongoing institutional reforms in many sectors, inadequate state funding, as well as an absence of a coordinated approach to the funding provided by the international donor and development agencies also contributed to the incompleteness of many operational issues of the plans. In some of the FSU countries, the plans remained as secret government documents and were not publicly available.

However, many governments were beginning to accept the value of a multi-sectoral approach and were beginning to test plans through simulation exercises. For many, if not all, FSU countries the overall planning process with all its learning experiences was more important than the final plan.

24.2 Pandemic Response

Putting plans into action during the 2009 A(H1N1)-pdm09 pandemic proved to be extremely difficult across all countries of the region. Following the very first response actions outlined in the plans, it became apparent that many plans, as originally conceived, were not going to work. This was attributed to the fact of having the WHO phases of pandemic alert as a trigger for the response, without consideration of local developments, as well as the lack of flexibility and adaptability of the plans. However, the mechanisms and approaches presented in the plans did provide a framework capable of guiding governments throughout the response to the pandemic. The long and challenging planning process was a good foundation, which facilitated further communication and coordination between representatives of different institutions, organizations and professionals across many sectors and at different levels.

Selected parts of the plans, including the various standard operating procedures, access to treatment and laboratory diagnostics, triage, referral mechanisms, case management and infection control guidelines, were satisfactorily applied in the early stages of the pandemic. However, later on, as new evidence emerged almost continuously, it was impossible to adapt, communicate and apply new procedures with sufficient speed. The rigidity of national planning structures, in addition to overall system requirements (the need for issuing additional orders, performing additional training and communication campaigns, etc.), meant that the overall health services' response to the pandemic become disorganized and fragmented in places.

Most of the public health measures outlined in the plans were applied in the early stages of the pandemic. However, the approaches and the extent of their implementation were not coherent across the countries. The most notable differences related to the application of travel restrictions and border controls. Although the WHO guidance on these points served as a benchmark, national governments were compelled to apply public health measures based on political decision making and possible wider society impacts. Public health measures were not always widely understood outside the health sector, which at times caused additional problems and a lack of transparency. Furthermore, although countries had obligations under the International Health Regulations (IHR), the internal legal frameworks did not always support their smooth implementation.

Many governments had identified the maintenance of essential services as a high priority. However, how this would happen was not well described in planning documents, and consequently this did not work well during the pandemic. There were some problems with optimal use of healthcare facilities at all levels: primary, secondary and tertiary, particularly inefficient and insufficiently rehearsed referral mechanisms between tiers. The availability of resources, including health personnel, pharmaceutical products and essential medical equipment and their adequate distribution, was also an issue in some countries. Considering that the 2009 pandemic was generally mild, the extent to which FSU countries were able to address maintenance of other essential services, as identified in the plans, requires further work in case the next pandemic is more severe.

Many countries attempted to present plans for a range of interventions related to the use of antiviral drugs and vaccines. Most presented the importance of and approaches to the use of antiviral drugs. However, the operational issues, such as delivery modes from the central stockpile to the local level, prescription practices and follow-up issues, such as reporting back to the central level, and re-distribution and disposal of unused medications, were not tackled thoroughly. Another issue of concern related to whether physicians on the front line decided to adhere to the WHO's guidelines on antiviral drug use versus those of the manufacturer (for example, usage of oseltamivir in children under 1 year of age).

Many countries developed vaccination plans incorporating the most important components, such as priority groups, delivery modes at all levels and monitoring of the adverse events. However, insufficient financial considerations and the reliance on donor support hampered timely translation of the plans into action in some countries. Paradoxically, several countries that did not experience such problems still suffered relative failure of the vaccination campaigns due to public apathy or opposition. Inadequate communication strategies implemented prior to and during the pandemic played an important role in contributing to this unexpected outcome.

Communication was probably the poorest part of the response to the 2009 pandemic despite the fact that many countries developed separate communication plans. Misunderstanding about the pandemic threat, which stemmed from confusion with avian influenza, was still present in some population groups. Surprisingly, many healthcare workers played an important role in contributing to this situation in addition to the rumours, speculations and criticism widely articulated by media representatives during the pandemic. Moreover, those plans with precise templates for the use of nominated spokespersons, and the best in the region, still did not succeed in distinguishing communication strategies for different target groups. As a result, ongoing communication with different population groups added more confusion to the overall situation and drove the activation of other non-official and less scientifically reliable communication channels, such as social groups and informal networks. Limited involvement of the public, media representatives and healthcare workers in earlier pandemic preparedness planning was the main factor which led to communication failures during the actual response to the pandemic.

24.3   Ongoing Preparedness

The experiences gained during the response to the 2009 pandemic proved that plans themselves do not survive intact for very long after a real crisis begins. The plans simply provide a conceptual framework, which can serve as a starting point for governments to address different issues of concern in an ongoing, adaptive way. For initiatives to be effective and realistic, planning should be performed: within and across sectors; at national, sub-national and local levels; with involvement of a broader representation of national and international stakeholders, including international donor agencies, civil society organizations, private organizations and the media.

The appropriateness of generic planning was recognized by many governments and already had been applied in some countries. The response to the pandemic has helped many governments to identify much broader health system gaps that need to be addressed at a strategic level.

Given the very rapid rate of political and economic change in the FSU counties, it is of utmost importance to ensure that future pandemic preparedness plans are flexible and reviewed on a regular basis. Issues such as financial and human resources, monitoring and evaluation, human rights and ethical considerations should become an integral part of national plans. The existing capacities of health systems in different FSU countries vary, although they retain the same overall approaches and there is common commitment towards the strengthening of health systems in the region.

The physician and writer Orizon S. Marden stated that 'a good system shortens the road to the goal' and in the context of pandemic planning in the FSU countries it is worth reiterating the importance of investing in and building system capacities across all functions, including financing, resources, service delivery and stewardship, rather than focusing on specific issues in isolation. There is a commitment of the governments at all levels to address the issues and failures identified during the response to the 2009 pandemic. At the same time, there is clear understanding that any further efforts in strengthening the capacities of the health systems should be evidence-based and adequately balanced between the policy approach, operational capacities and available resources, which, for now, remain very different from those in countries in the Western world.

Further Reading

Hashim, A., Jean-Gilles, L., Hegermann-Lindencrone, M., Shaw, I., Brown, C. and Nguyen-Van-Tam, J.S. (2012) Did pandemic preparedness aid the response to pandemic (H1N1) 2009? A qualitative analysis in seven countries within the WHO European Region. *Journal of Infection and Public Health* 5(4), 286–296.

WHO Regional Office for Europe and University of Nottingham (2010) Recommendations for good practice in pandemic preparedness identified through evaluation of the response to pandemic (H1N1) 2009. Available at: http://www.euro.who.int/__data/assets/pdf_file/0017/128060/e94534.pdf (accessed 21 September 2012).

25 Case Study 5: Africa

ABDULSALAMI NASIDI

Nigeria Centre for Disease Control (NCDC), Abuja, Nigeria

25.1 Background

The African Region is already stretched with competing public health priorities and is still dominated by a very high burden of diseases and very high maternal and infant mortality. Currently, sub-Saharan Africa hosts 66% of the global burden of the HIV/AIDS pandemic, 31% of the global burden of tuberculosis and 86% of the global burden of malaria. Additionally, this region is prone to recurrent epidemics such as haemorrhagic fevers, meningitis and water-borne diseases such as cholera. The emergence of avian influenza A(H5N1) in 1997 and its recrudescence from late 2003, coupled with the recent A(H1N1)pdm09 influenza pandemic, has demonstrated an urgent need for countries in the region to have pandemic preparedness plans in place.

By mid-June 2007, Nigeria became the first country in the African Region to activate its pandemic response plan after an A(H5N1) avian influenza outbreak the previous year. The plan is a multisectoral integrated avian and pandemic influenza plan involving three major ministries, namely the Ministries of Health (human health), Agriculture (animal health) and Communication, and was prepared in conjunction with the development partners working in the country. Many other African countries followed Nigeria's example and have now developed pandemic preparedness and response plans of their own. However, by May 2009 only nine of the 46 African countries had influenza (pandemic) preparedness and response plans. The situation improved rapidly and, by August of the same year, 35 countries (76%) in the region had activated some form of national emergency preparedness and contingency response plan, and a crisis management team had been put in place by the WHO Regional Office for Africa in Brazzaville. By the end of 2009 all 46 countries had pandemic plans in place.

Nigeria was one of the first African countries to test its pandemic plan by holding national pandemic exercises in 2007, 2009 and 2011. The 2011 simulation was the largest ever government exercise in that country. It was carried out jointly with the military and US Department of Defense. This series of exercises helped the dissemination of positive information to healthcare professionals and the public.

25.2 Understanding the Burden of Influenza in Africa

The introduction of highly pathogenic avian influenza A(H5N1) into sub-Saharan Africa in 2006 heightened anxiety about the potential for the emergence of an A(H5N1) pandemic with the ability to transmit efficiently from person to person and cause severe morbidity and mortality. A number of factors that are unlikely to change in sub-Saharan Africa in the near future – poor nutritional status, high rates of co-morbid diseases such as HIV/AIDS, a young population, poverty, overcrowding and limited access to healthcare – could all contribute to unusually high mortality from a severe pandemic virus. However, influenza surveillance in Africa remains limited, especially in rural areas; thus, the epidemiology and seasonality of interpandemic influenza viruses are unclear for this region. The earlier perception that influenza does not cause substantial mortality in Africa may contribute to the underutilization of influenza vaccines, antivirals and other control measures. However a recent study has shown that overall rates of seasonal influenza-related excess mortality among adults aged ≥65 years in South Africa were substantially greater than those observed in the USA. Unusually severe outbreaks of influenza A(H3N2) occurred in Madagascar and the Democratic Republic of Congo in 2002, suggesting that populations in African countries may experience an increased risk of severe outcomes following influenza infection for the reasons outlined above. Several African countries are engaged in laboratory capacity building and influenza surveillance initiatives supported by the World Health Organization (WHO) and US Centers for Disease Control and Prevention (CDC). However due to the challenges the region is facing which are mainly as a result of limited financial and technical resources, these activities are limited even though greatly needed. For example, the WHO Regional Office for Africa stated in August 2009 that the region required US$31 million for the implementation of African pandemic preparedness and response plans, yet only US$700,000 was available.

25.3   Evolution of the Pandemic

The African Region reported its first confirmed case of A(H1N1)pdm09 on 18 June 2009 in South Africa some 6 weeks after recognition of the first cases in the USA and Mexico. Rapidly thereafter ten further cases of the new virus were detected in four additional countries: Cape Verde, Algeria, Ethiopia and Cote d'Ivoire. All the confirmed cases were imported with the exception of one case in Algeria where the patient was in close contact with an imported case that was confirmed locally. The regional WHO office immediately provided technical assistance and engaged countries to update their preparedness and response plans. In total during the pandemic, 26 African countries reported a total of 18,598 laboratory-confirmed cases, including 168 deaths. Thirty-four countries that had developed or started developing A(H5N1) response plans quickly adapted these to respond to A(H1N1)pdm09. Weak health infrastructures, limited disease surveillance capabilities, and a host of underlying health issues such as large populations of HIV-infected individuals, placed Africa in a situation that could have led to potentially devastating effects had the A(H1N1)-pdm09 virus been more virulent.

The continent, assisted by the WHO, made substantial progress and achieved the objective of developing a workable pandemic preparedness and response plan with government commitment in most countries. However, operating such a plan in countries with weak public structures and weak health system became a challenge. The need to embark on mass capacity building and health system strengthening in the post-pandemic era is an ongoing priority. Notwithstanding, the African Region initially reported a very low incidence of influenza A(H1N1)pdm09 and widespread activity took time to develop. By the end of July 2009, the

WHO Regional Office for Africa had reported only 157 cases, in comparison to the 87,000 cases reported by PAHO (WHO Regional Office for the Americas, the Pan American Health Organization). Confirmed cases peaked in September 2009 in East Africa but this was delayed until March 2010 in parts of West Africa. Overall, cases started to decline by June 2010, just before WHO declared that the pandemic was over on 10 August 2010. Although there may well have been under-ascertainment in Africa, these data indicate that the major A(H1N1)pdm09 pandemic wave in parts of Africa occurred as late as March 2010. These data are broadly consistent with the findings from a review of the 1968 A(H3N2) pandemic in Africa (see Further Reading).

25.4   Pharmaceutical and Public Health Interventions

WHO recommends that countries should consider stockpiling antiviral drugs in preparedness for a pandemic. African countries were limited in fulfilling this recommendation as only few could afford to procure limited supplies of antiviral drugs and vaccines. Although the WHO established a stockpile for a rapid containment response, this covered less than 5% of the regional population; as such poor-resource/low-income countries of Africa were left with little or no supplies of these vital drugs and vaccines to combat the A(H1N1)pdm09 pandemic. A review of the region's response plans towards the end of 2009 showed that although 45 of 46 countries anticipated the use of antiviral drugs, stockpiling was only mentioned by four. Some countries highlighted the need for further financial support to secure national stockpiles – but most provided few details. The logistical issues around storage and distribution of vaccines and drugs were scarcely addressed in most plans. Only one country (Central African Republic) explicitly stated that 1.5% of the population could be the potential target of antiviral treatment, and only two countries, Zambia and Tanzania, mentioned the use of existing delivery mechanisms for drug distribution.

African countries lack domestic self-reliance in vaccines and biologicals and to date, current global vaccine production is concentrated in industrialized countries. Within the African continent, Egypt and South Africa are the only countries currently planning to develop capacity for influenza vaccine production with the technical assistance of WHO.

Although aware that they would be unlikely to access pandemic vaccine due to limited availability and economic constraints, 25 countries expressed an intention to use pandemic vaccine in their plans. Most countries in the region that intended procuring the vaccine envisaged vaccination of not more than 10% of their population, with healthcare workers afforded highest priority. As a result of access issues, monovalent A(H1N1)pdm09 vaccines were not supplied to African countries (mainly on a donated basis) until the first quarter of 2010 despite the fact that the first cases in Africa were detected in June 2009. This triggered the speculation that the vaccines were being dumped on the continent due to short expiry dates. Some countries even deployed seasonal influenza vaccine in the hope that it would offer a degree of cross-protection. Lack of affordability and a reliance on donated stock from the United Nations meant that many African governments only began pandemic vaccination campaigns between late June 2010, and the end of August 2010, when the rest of the world was announcing the end of the pandemic.

With the paucity of drugs and vaccines in the region, several African countries recommended non-pharmaceutical personal measures to reduce transmission. These included personal hygiene/respiratory etiquette, avoidance of close contact with sick people, hand hygiene and social distancing. The global lack of availability of antivirals and pandemic influenza vaccines during 2009/10 led to an overall emphasis on non-pharmaceutical public health interventions by many African countries. To avoid similar occurrences in the future, African countries need to perfect their pandemic plans, improve on their capacity to respond to the pandemic and reduce their dependence on imported drugs and vaccines.

25.5 Summary

The African Region faced the 2009 pandemic against a backdrop of multiple unresolved health problems, competing health priorities for limited resources and generally under-developed healthcare systems and public health infrastructures. However, the impact in 2009/10 was still limited due to the low virulence of the 2009 pandemic virus but might not have been so if a more virulent virus had emerged, e.g. A(H5N1). Pandemic preparedness plans should be devised on the basis of local socio-economic conditions, and address issues such as limited capacity which are common to most developing countries' healthcare systems. Pandemic preparedness issues in the African Region are immense; however, most countries in the region have shown commitment to pandemic planning and, with the assistance and support of WHO and CDC, and financial support from other donors, the region has improved its state of preparedness. Influenza control strategies need to address a lack of surveillance and influenza awareness in the continent. In 2009 both antiviral drugs and vaccines were in short supply and the latter arrived almost too late in relation to disease activity. Partnerships and international solidarity are essential components of pandemic planning for the African Region, which especially requires improved access to antiviral drugs and influenza vaccines in the future.

Further Reading

Breiman, R.F., Nasidi, A., Katz, M.A., Kariuki Njenga, M. and Vertefeuille, J. (2007) Preparedness for highly pathogenic avian influenza pandemic in Africa. *Emerging Infectious Diseases* 13(10), 1453–1458.

Cohen, C., Simonsen, L., Kang, J.W., Miller, M., McAnerney, J., Blumberg, L., Schoub, B., Madhi, S.A. and Viboud, C. (2010) Elevated influenza-related excess mortality in South African elderly individuals, 1998–2005. *Clinical Infectious Diseases* 51(12), 1362–1369.

Ortiz, J.R., Lafond, K.E., Wong, T.A. and Uyeki, T.M. (2012) Pandemic influenza in Africa, lessons learned from 1968: a systematic review of the literature. *Influenza and Other Respiratory Viruses* 6(1), 11–24.

26 Case Study 6: Denmark

Kåre Mølbak

Statens Serum Institut, Copenhagen, Denmark

26.1 Introduction

Although there were many similarities in the course of the 2009 influenza pandemic among the countries of Europe, there were also notable differences. Most countries saw two pandemic waves in 2009. The first wave, in the early summer of 2009, gave rise to limited community transmission in most European countries, except in the UK and Spain where community transmission was clearly documented, particularly in school settings. In most of continental Europe, cases diagnosed over the summer were mainly imported cases of influenza A(H1N1)pdm09, e.g. from the USA, Mexico and countries of the southern hemisphere. However, as travel-associated cases were also found among young tourists travelling within Europe, it is likely that community transmission also occurred at crowded European travel resorts. The second wave in the autumn of 2009 was a result of sustained transmission within Europe and in most countries, the outbreak lasted from the second week of October to mid-December 2009. Again, the timing of this important outbreak differed between countries and regions in Europe.

Between the different European countries, there were various approaches in the initial attempts to manage and possibly contain the pandemic, diagnostic practices, case-management practices, communication to the public, and so forth. Perhaps the most striking difference was related to pandemic vaccination policy, reflected by differences in advance purchase agreements and vaccination programme implementation. In an assessment report prepared for the European Commission, it appeared that more than half of the responding member states had an advance purchase agreement with a vaccine manufacturer prior to the outbreak in 2009, and nearly two-thirds ordered pandemic vaccines when the World Health Organization (WHO) declared Pandemic Phase 6. A few countries including Poland and Lithuania chose not to vaccinate, while others such as Sweden and Finland immunized >50% of the population using monovalent, adjuvanted influenza A(H1N1)pdm09 vaccines.

26.2 Pandemic Preparedness and Response in Denmark

In 2006, the Danish National Board of Health issued a Pandemic Preparedness Plan that outlined strategies for the public health response according to the different WHO pandemic phases. The strategy in WHO Phases 3 to 5 included attempts to contain the pandemic by classic epidemic measures such as isolation and quarantine. In Phase 6, the strategy changed to focus on mitigation, e.g. case management of patients with severe illness, including treatment with antiviral drugs, and post-exposure antiviral treatment of patients with underlying illness. The plan provided guidance for use of antiviral drugs, antibiotics, immunization strategies, non-pharmaceutical measures and communication, as well as outlining roles and responsibilities of the different stakeholders. It was supported by detailed plans and action cards for the health sector and the Danish Emergency Management Agency (covering broader civil preparedness arrangements). Importantly, the Danish government had a flexible advance vaccine purchase agreement with a vaccine manufacturer, allowing the government to buy different numbers of vaccine doses depending on the initial risk assessment. As a consequence, the declaration of WHO Phase 6 did not automatically result in placing an order of vaccines for the entire population but only to cover an estimated number of people in specified at-risk groups.

Prior to the pandemic, several surveillance systems were established to monitor influenza, including the sentinel network of general practitioners, surveillance of influenza-like illness contacts at the Danish medical on-call service and monitoring of mortality. To obtain a more complete understanding of the course of the pandemic and to make a comprehensive assessment of the dimensions and severity of the disease, surveillance was enhanced with additional data collection schemes during the summer months of 2009.

To obtain population-based estimates of the clinical attack rate, data from the two different primary healthcare surveillance systems, national numbers of the proportion of positive influenza tests and data from a web-based interview on healthcare-seeking behaviour during the pandemic were combined. In total, it was estimated that 274,000 individuals (5%) in Denmark experienced clinical illness. The highest attack rate was found in children aged 5–14 years (15%). Data on hospital admissions (ICD-10 codes) for influenza-related conditions were obtained from the national hospital discharge registry. Admission to intensive care was monitored by a dedicated surveillance scheme. Compared with the expected number of hospital admissions, there was an unprecedented 80% increase in the number of influenza-related hospital admissions in children aged 5–14 years whereas the elderly were relatively spared. As the absolute number of admissions was few, the hospitals could cope with the pandemic. The number of patients admitted to intensive care approached 5% of the national capacity. Mortality was estimated among laboratory-confirmed cases but was also expressed as excess all-cause mortality attributed to influenza-like illness in a multivariable time-series analysis. Estimates of the number of deaths ranged from 30 to 312 (0.5–5.7 per 100,000 population) depending on the methodology. The wide range between these two estimates (the latter being based on all-cause mortality) underpins the challenge in putting exact numbers on influenza-related mortality.

Pandemic vaccines were available from the beginning of November 2009. As the initial numbers of deliveries were limited, the primary target group was individuals with underlying illness, with other target groups offered the vaccines later (in reality, this was when the outbreak was over). In total, 6% of the population was vaccinated with at least one dose of monovalent, adjuvanted, A(H1N1)pdm09 vaccine. Among individuals with chronic illness, the coverage was only around 20%. Vaccinations were registered in a national registry, and in a registry linkage study we determined vaccine effectiveness among the individuals with underlying illness. With the outcome confirmed influenza A(H1N1)pdm09 infection, effectiveness was 49% after one dose.

In conclusion, the pandemic was characterized by fairly high morbidity rates and unprecedented high numbers of admissions to hospitals for a range of influenza-related conditions affecting mainly school-children. None the less, the burden of illness and mortality was lower than assumed in planning scenarios, primarily because the elderly were more or less spared from the pandemic, unlike for seasonal influenza. Vaccines came late and the coverage was low. Vaccines protected against infection, even among those with chronic illness. However, it is unlikely that the vaccines had a large impact on the overall course of the pandemic, because of their late arrival.

To account for the fact that 20th century pandemics have had different severities, the Danish pandemic plan allowed for some flexibility in the response. It was clearly stated that public health measures had to be adopted based on specific risk assessments. Even so, the plan was prepared in the light of the spread of avian influenza A(H5N1) (causing very severe illness in the few individuals infected through contact with birds) and severe acute respiratory syndrome (a severe illness where traditional epidemic measures were effective in limiting the spread because infectivity was maximal well after symptom onset), as well as the historical and potential worst case scenario of the Spanish flu (A(H1N1) in 1918). Hence, independently of the risk assessment, the plan assumed that it was worthwhile to use resources on a 'containment phase'. The aim in this phase was not to stop the pandemic (as this is impossible), but to delay spread in order to limit damage for society and gain time for obtaining vaccines (Chapter 16). It remains an open question as to how effective this strategy was and if it was worth the effort; for example, in the UK the containment approach was very intensive and very protracted – from late April to early July 2009. It may be likely that in future planning, the 'containment phase' should be viewed as more optional, in case of a severe pandemic. In a milder scenario, the focus from the beginning may be on encouraging basic hygienic measures (hand hygiene, cough etiquette, absence from work in case of acute illness) and on the 'mitigation', i.e. on identifying groups at risk of severe illness, preventing infection where possible and treating to minimize complications.

26.3 Vaccination

Among countries in Europe, vaccination policies varied from no vaccination, through risk-group-based strategies, to mass vaccinations targeting the entire population. It is difficult to find evidence for these different choices, and a clear impact on public health of those different strategies remains to be demonstrated. In Denmark, only some 20% of the primary target group (people with chronic illnesses) were vaccinated, which is far from optimal. In contrast, in the Netherlands, coverage in the risk groups has been estimated to be 70%. The low coverage in Denmark may have resulted from the late arrival of vaccines. Limited stocks of vaccines were available in October 2009, and the ethical issues of an early delivery to selected groups need to be discussed in future planning. From a European perspective, vaccination campaigns were launched in the different countries between mid-October and late November, illustrating the variability in vaccine availability. The low vaccine uptake may also be related to the challenges for risk communication. As most infections were mild, there is at the individual level little difference between seasonal and pandemic influenza – the difference is only seen from a public health perspective. On the one hand, the aim of risk communication is to inform the population and avoid panic since it is 'only influenza'. On the other, it is important to strongly encourage individuals at risk of severe outcome to seek care and to get vaccinated when the vaccine has arrived. This message, which is scientifically sound, may be perceived by the media and the population as a 'mixed message' with opposing directions. Furthermore, risk communication was challenged by discussions and controversy about vaccine safety.

26.4 Morbidity and Mortality

The Danish pandemic plan outlined the need to monitor overall morbidity, hospital admissions and deaths due to influenza without providing many details on how this actually should be carried out or how such surveillance systems should be implemented and funded. Nevertheless it was possible to change priorities and redirect manpower to undertake most of these activities, which allowed for obtaining a fairly complete understanding of the course of the pandemic, including estimates of the clinical attack rate, burden of illness at the hospital level and vaccine effectiveness. Unfortunately however, no data on sero-conversion rates were available, which makes it difficult to validate the estimates of the clinical attack rate and to make a forward risk assessment regarding the coming years.

Only the UK possessed good data from serological surveys but even these were not available until September 2009.

26.5 Summary

In conclusion, Denmark and most of Europe was well prepared for the pandemic, but nevertheless a number of lessons were learned which may be valuable for the next pandemic. Most importantly, preparedness needs to be more flexible and adaptable based on evidence and risk assessments. Such an approach, where a risk assessment directly informs the management, requires more emphasis on timely national and international data collection, interpretation and analysis. As an example, a timely and comprehensive analysis of excess mortality and case fatality from Mexico would have been of importance for assessing the risk for public health. This aspect deserves more emphasis in future planning.

Finally, one of the most important outcomes was the revival of hygienic measures, including hand hygiene and cough etiquette. The 2009 pandemic brought these simple and acceptable measures into focus, and this may ultimately benefit the control and prevention of other infections as well.

Further Reading

Emborg, H.D., Krause, T.G., Hviid, A., Simonsen, J. and Mølbak, K. (2012) Effectiveness of vaccine against pandemic influenza A/H1N1 among people with underlying chronic diseases: cohort study, Denmark, 2009–2010. *British Medical Journal* 344, d7901. Available at: http://www.bmj.com/content/344/bmj.d7901?view=long&pmid=22277542 (accessed 29 March 2012).

European Centre for Disease Prevention and Control (2010) The 2009 A(H1N1) pandemic in Europe. Available at: http://ecdc.europa.eu/en/publications/Publications/101108_SPR_pandemic_experience.pdf (accessed 29 March 2012).

Health Protection Agency and CRISMART (2010) Assessment Report on EU-wide Pandemic Vaccine Strategies. Available at: http://ec.europa.eu/health/communicable_diseases/docs/assessment_vaccine_en.pdf (accessed 29 March 2012).

Mølbak, K., Widgren, K., Jensen, K.S., Ethelberg, S., Andersen, P.H., Christiansen, A.H., Emborg, H.D., Gubbels, S., Harder, K.M., Krause, T.G., Mazick, A., Nielsen, L.P., Nielsen, J., Valentiner-Branth, P. and Glismann, S. (2011) Burden of illness of the 2009 pandemic of influenza A (H1N1) in Denmark. *Vaccine* 29 (Suppl. 2) B63–B69.

27 Case Study 7: South-east Asia

VERNON LEE AND VINCENT J.X. PANG

National University of Singapore, Singapore

27.1 Introduction

The South-east Asia (SE Asia) region is a melting pot of more than half a billion people from different socio-cultural and ethnic groups. It includes the countries of Brunei, Cambodia, Indonesia, Laos, Malaysia, Myanmar, Philippines, Singapore, Thailand, Timor Leste and Vietnam. A substantial proportion of the population lives in urban areas, and socio-economic development in the region is vastly different among and within countries.

SE Asia has seen the emergence and re-emergence of many infectious diseases in recent years, including severe acute respiratory syndrome, Nipah virus, chikungunya, dengue and avian influenza A(H5N1), emphasizing the importance of disease management. At the same time, regional diversity poses challenges for public health planners.

27.2 Pandemic Preparedness

Assessments of the national influenza preparedness plans of SE Asia countries in 2006 and 2007 found that several plans had gaps similar to those in European countries, including the lack of operational details on implementation and management of limited resources. Later assessments in 2008 and 2009 showed improvement in areas such as surveillance, laboratory capacity, monitoring and evaluation, and public communication. However, concerns remained on preparedness beyond the early containment phase at the local level, particularly in lower-resourced countries. One challenge was the shortage of healthcare resources to meet demand during a pandemic, particularly in countries with existing healthcare infrastructure problems and inadequate healthcare financing.

Some countries have special coordination units to execute national response operations during a pandemic (e.g. Laos and Indonesia), while others rely on existing governance structures (e.g. Vietnam) or have a response structure within the national disaster response framework where decisions are made and managed centrally (e.g. Cambodia and Thailand). Most countries had held national operational readiness exercises, especially table top exercises, and some had progressed to live exercises – for example, Indonesia held a full-scale multi-sectoral containment exercise for an epicentre of novel human virus with pandemic potential in 2008, while Singapore had conducted several health-sector pandemic influenza exercises. Exercises in the region were mostly focused on preparedness for severe pandemic influenza, likely driven by A(H5N1) outbreaks in the region.

Most countries have surveillance and diagnostic capabilities that are integrated with the international community. There was also extensive public health education through various forms of media focusing on preventing avian influenza transmission. However, more emphasis was needed on advocating social responsibility such as respiratory hygiene and self-isolation, and instilling public confidence through assurance that healthcare resources and public health measures were adequate.

Pharmaceutical interventions pose a large financial burden to most countries considering stockpiles of vaccines and antiviral drugs due to limited supply and high cost. For example, antiviral stockpiles of Thailand and Indonesia covered about 1% of their population and Cambodia only 0.1%. In most countries, there was a policy to provide antiviral treatment to cases as well as prophylaxis for close contacts. However, few had a clear policy on rationing and prioritization for distribution of these drugs.

27.3 The 2009 Pandemic in South-east Asia

First detection of the 2009 pandemic virus in individual SE Asian countries was from May to June 2009, 1 to 2 months after its emergence in

Mexico and North America. Across all countries, the initial index cases were isolated and contact tracing performed. Close contacts were either quarantined or monitored for symptoms, and most countries made antiviral drugs available for treatment.

All countries created public awareness through the media – for example in Cambodia, the Ministry of Health informed the public of new updates including implementation of the national action plan. In Myanmar, there were increased efforts to educate the public as well as to engage other local partners to increase awareness on A(H1N1)pdm09 prevention methods. Countries also provided strong emphasis on personal hygiene, and advocated some form of self-isolation and self-restriction on travel when ill, and seeking medical treatment for influenza-like illness. In Singapore, a campaign was launched to educate the public on A(H1N1)pdm09 and the importance of personal hygiene and social responsibility such as temperature monitoring. In the Philippines, schools were provided with guidelines and recommendations to reduce spread.

All countries also instituted public health measures such as intensification of border control measures and increased hospital surveillance. Some countries advised the public to defer their travel plans to affected countries. Temperature and health screening was deployed at some borders even though the scientific effectiveness of these measures was uncertain. This was likely a visible public reassurance, and a possible deterrent to ill travellers. It is also possible that these containment measures may have delayed the onset of community transmission in SE Asian countries.

Although the actual timing of the surge in cases and their peak is not available in most countries, national responses to the local epidemics were generally similar in terms of transition to the mitigation phase that focused on reducing mortality and spread through outpatient treatment, health education and social distancing.

Most countries advised mild cases to be managed as outpatients without the need for antiviral drugs, and to self-isolate at home. Surge capacity in the primary healthcare setting was increased for this purpose, and antiviral treatment and hospitalization reserved for those at high-risk of complications or with severe illness. Contact tracing and quarantine were generally stopped.

The A(H1N1)pdm09 vaccine was broadly available in SE Asian countries as they received their first batch of vaccines between November 2009 and March 2010 – most developing countries received their vaccines through the World Health Organization or other donors. Initial administration of the vaccines was to high-risk groups and other priority groups such as healthcare workers. Reports have shown that vaccines were deployed to different regions within each country, and doses administered as a proportion of doses distributed ranged from 39 to 88% by the end of the campaigns.

Public health measures were also deployed. Within the community, most countries recommended social distancing measures such as reducing large gatherings or avoiding crowded places, and advocated the importance of social responsibility by adopting self-isolation and good personal hygiene habits. In some countries, individual schools that had potential outbreaks were closed to prevent further transmission; while in Hanoi, Vietnam, all schools were closed for 10 days after community transmission became established. In Singapore, front-line healthcare workers were provided with personal protective equipment, the number of visitors to healthcare facilities was regulated and temperature screening was deployed. These measures may have reduced the risk of healthcare workers being infected.

It was also important to ensure that the response was not out of proportion to the pandemic's severity and to enable life to continue. For example, the inaugural Asian Youth Games 2009 in Singapore and the 25th SE Asian Games 2009 in Vientiane, Laos, took place as planned without undermining mitigation strategies, due to detailed contingency planning and execution with effective communication.

Although there are no specific figures available for the economic impact of the 2009 pandemic, the Asian Development Bank had shown that a hypothetical moderate to severe pandemic could result in a reduction in gross domestic product from between 0.7 and 2.8% in Indonesia, to between 11 and 23% in Singapore, depending on the impact on supply and demand of goods and services in individual countries. Adequate preparedness and response is therefore essential to avert a health and economic disaster.

27.4 Ongoing Preparedness

The 2009 pandemic was relatively mild and served as a good rehearsal for future pandemics. Several countries are revisiting their preparedness plans to improve issues such as severity assessment and best use of resources. Moving forward, it is important for countries to consider the new evidence available on the effectiveness of different public health measures and to incorporate these into their plans.

For example, the poor accessibility and lack of clear distribution plans and communication on treatment guidelines for antiviral drugs were challenges in countries with limited stockpiles. However, such drugs are costly to stockpile, especially for less-resourced countries where their cost-effectiveness is less compelling. Similarly, pandemic vaccine is another critical issue that requires consideration if sufficient vaccines are to be available in a timely manner to less well-resourced countries.

It is also important for countries to plan not only for containment and initial epidemic spread, but for widespread epidemic and surge capacity. There is also a need for a coordinated multi-sectoral response beyond the health sector, to have clearly developed operational details and to test these through comprehensive exercises that engage local communities. The 2009 pandemic will hopefully result in stronger plans in the SE Asia region to mitigate a future pandemic.

Further Reading

Fisher, D., Hui, D.S., Gao, Z., Lee, C., Oh, M.D., Cao, B., Hien, T.T., Patlovich, K. and Farrar, J. (2011) Pandemic response lessons from influenza H1N1 2009 in Asia. *Respirology* 16(6), 876–882.

Hanvoravongchai, P., Adisasmito, W., Chau, P.N., Conseil, A., de Sa, J., Krumkamp, R., Mounier-Jack, S., Phommasack, B., Putthasri, W., Shih, C.S., Touch, S. and Coker, R.; AsiaFluCap Project (2010) Pandemic influenza preparedness and health systems challenges in Asia: results from rapid analyses in 6 Asian countries. *BMC Public Health* 10, 322.

Kamigaki, T. and Oshitani, H. (2010) Influenza pandemic preparedness and severity assessment of pandemic (H1N1) 2009 in South-east Asia. *Public Health* 124(1), 5–9.

28 Case Study 8: North America

DAN JERNIGAN

Centers for Disease Control and Prevention, Atlanta, Georgia, USA

28.1 Before the Pandemic in North America

Prior to the emergence of the 2009 pandemic influenza virus (A(H1N1)pdm09) in North America, a number of factors contributed to improving pandemic preparedness in Canada and the USA. In 2003, the outbreak of infection due to the Severe Acute Respiratory Syndrome coronavirus (SARS-CoV) in Toronto, Canada served as a stark example of how an unknown emerging respiratory virus could rapidly appear and cause significant illness and death, leading to considerable social and economic disruption thousands of miles away from where it had recently started. Following that, in 2004, cases of human infection from avian influenza A(H5N1) began increasing in South-east Asia; the case fatality rate was exceptionally high at around 60–70%. Following these experiences, public health officials began developing pandemic plans largely designed to respond to a severe global pandemic, similar to what was seen with the 1918 A(H1N1) pandemic with an estimated 500,000-600,000 deaths in the USA.

Pandemic planning efforts were based on several reasonable assumptions based on knowledge at the time: the pandemic would emerge from avian sources in South-east Asia and would cause high numbers of deaths. These plans and preparedness efforts accounted for several important components of the US response. For example, significant government resources were directed to:

- **Surveillance:** existing seasonal influenza surveillance systems were enhanced and expanded; federal funds led to development and deployment of new influenza diagnostic tests; 'novel influenza virus infection' was made a notifiable disease in support of the new World Health Organization (WHO) International Health Regulations (IHR); a 'pandemic severity index' (PSI) was established to communicate the likely fatality of the coming pandemic; financial and technical resources were provided to countries around the globe to improve capacity for laboratory testing, surveillance and pandemic response.
- **Pharmaceutical interventions:** stockpiles of antiviral drugs were established; federal funds were directed to develop new influenza vaccines and build additional vaccine manufacturing capacity.
- **Non-pharmaceutical interventions:** plans were made for efforts to slow the introduction and spread of pandemic influenza, including school closures, border closures and other formal efforts for social distancing in the workplace and community; hospitals developed surge treatment plans to account for possible rapid increases in patients needing care.
- **Communications:** messages to communicate risk and response recommendations were extensively tested and ready for use; mechanisms for use of broadcast, web and various social media were developed.
- **Coordination:** 'Emergency Operations Centers' were established at the federal, state and local levels to implement an 'incident command' approach for streamlining decision making and execution of action for control of the pandemic; multilateral agreements among Canada, the USA and Mexico were initiated to allow for rapid and unencumbered interaction among the partners; numerous exercises, sometimes lasting three full days with multiple state and federal agencies 'playing', led to considerable testing and revising of the pandemic plans.

What appeared in 2009, however, was emergence from swine sources in North America with illness burden predominantly in younger people with lower overall mortality. Despite these differences in assumptions, many preparedness efforts allowed for rapid and flexible reconfiguration for the response.

28.2 A Pandemic is Recognized

As part of pandemic preparedness efforts, the US Centers for Disease Control and Prevention (CDC) sponsored clinical trials to evaluate a new point-of-care influenza diagnostic device. On 30 March 2009, a 10-year-old boy with mild influenza-like illness was tested with the experimental device and was found to have an infection with an influenza A strain that could not be identified as either of the circulating influenza A subtypes (i.e. seasonal A(H1N1) or A(H3N2)). This 'unsubtypable' influenza A virus met the novel influenza case definition and was received at CDC on 15 April 2009 for further testing. One additional 'unsubtypable' case in southern California was identified and both were reported in the CDC's online *MMWR* publication on 21 April 2009. The report described the two infections caused by a novel influenza A virus with genes that originated from birds, swine and humans, and for which much of the population had limited immunity; both cases had mild illness and recovered without being hospitalized. Gene sequences from the viruses were immediately posted to public websites.

At about the same time, public health laboratory investigators in Canada, working with officials in Mexico on clusters of unexplained respiratory disease, determined that samples from Mexican cases had the same genetic sequences as those posted by CDC in public databases; however, the Mexican cases were associated with significant illness and death. Additional laboratory-confirmed cases in Mexico, Canada and the USA led to recognition of an emerging pandemic and prompted numerous response efforts.

28.3 Responding to the Pandemic

Public health officials in Canada, the USA and Mexico quickly established communication with each other, and with the Pan American Health Organization (PAHO) and WHO. In compliance with IHR requirements, each case was reported as a Public Health Emergency of International Concern (PHEIC). Emergency Operations Centers were started at federal, state/provincial and local levels. Given the differences between the reported case severity in the USA and Mexico, rapid investigations were needed to determine more about the characteristics of A(H1N1)pdm09 infection. Specific response efforts in the USA included:

- **Field investigations:** given the sporadic appearance of cases in different regions, federal, state and local public health officials deployed teams to evaluate the clinical illness of the cases and to determine household and community transmission in neighbourhoods and universities. These efforts were rapidly published and were instrumental in understanding the relatively low case fatality rate and sufficient human-to-human transmission of A(H1N1)pdm09. These and other data directed policy makers to greatly revise previous plans that had been developed for a 1918-like influenza pandemic.

- **Enhanced surveillance:** new surveillance systems and new molecular A(H1N1)pdm09 tests were developed and deployed at state and local health departments to aid in case detection and reveal the spread and severity of the pandemic. These efforts were critical in demonstrating three key features. First, the late spring wave of cases occurred sporadically across the USA. Second, a lower but persistent number of summer cases occurred. Third, as schools opened, a dramatic autumn wave occurred from August through November of 2009, approximately 3 months earlier than in a 'normal' winter season. By April 2010, an estimated 61 million cases, 274,000 hospitalizations and 12,470 deaths had occurred due to A(H1N1)pdm09 in the USA.

- **Communications:** the unfolding pandemic had many uncertainties, and communications were designed to convey this along with providing maximum transparency of response efforts and recommendations as they were refined according to emerging data.

- **Community mitigation:** early after recognition, the potential impact and severity of the emerging pandemic prompted consideration of planned non-pharmaceutical interventions. The PSI had been designed to assist officials in selecting mitigation efforts based on the case fatality rate of the emerging pandemic; however, A(H1N1)-pdm09 appeared to have a seasonal level of mortality, making the PSI difficult to use and requiring development of other means for evaluating the severity. For Canada, the USA and Mexico, A(H1N1)pdm09 cases were occurring in various regions, indicating that established transmission was under way. Given this, and contrary to prior plans, attempts at containment of A(H1N1)-pdm09 and border control were not warranted. Recommendations for school closure were also revised and in general were not implemented given the lower severity of A(H1N1)pdm09 compared to prior pandemics.

- **Antiviral treatment:** twenty-five per cent of the USA antiviral stockpile was distributed; however, commercial availability alleviated need for additional stockpile assets. Paediatric formulations were often in short supply and, in retrospect, needed to have been included in greater amount in the national stockpile.
- **Vaccines:** one of the first viruses detected in California was used by manufacturers globally to produce the A(H1N1)pdm09 monovalent vaccine. Because the pandemic started in the midst of northern hemisphere seasonal influenza vaccine production, vaccine manufacturers had to significantly increase production capacity to meet the requirement for A(H1N1)pdm09 vaccine, ultimately making 124 million doses; of which approximately 90 million were administered to people. Although vaccine was made in record time, it still did not arrive until the autumn wave was peaking in most parts of the USA, leading to less impact on prevention through immunization than desired. None the less, the tremendous coordination and logistic effort required for the A(H1N1)pdm09 vaccine campaign underscored the need for a well-resourced, strong public–private cooperation to achieve such a monumental endeavour.

In conclusion, pandemic preparedness efforts in North America prior to emergence of A(H1N1)-pdm09 clearly paid off through exercising coordination across multiple jurisdictions, improved epidemiologic and diagnostic infrastructure, and enhancements to existing federal, state and local public health systems. A focus on a severe, 1918-like pandemic was important for driving preparedness efforts; however, future pandemic planning should allow for a more flexible response that accounts for, and allows revision based on, an unfolding spectrum of severity and transmissibility.

Further Reading

Centers for Disease Control and Prevention (2010) The 2009 H1N1 Pandemic: Summary Highlights, April 2009–April 2010. Available at: http://www.cdc.gov/h1n1flu/cdcresponse.htm (accessed 29 March 2012).

Pan American Health Organization (2010) Response to Pandemic (H1N1) 2009 in the Americas: Lessons and Challenges. Available at: http://www.paho.org/ah1n1flu/ (accessed 29 March 2012).

Public Health Agency of Canada (2010) Lessons Learned Review: Public Health Agency of Canada and Health Canada Response to the 2009 H1N1 Pandemic. Available at: http://www.phac-aspc.gc.ca/about_apropos/evaluation/reports-rapports/2010–2011/h1n1/index-eng.php (accessed 29 March 2012).

D. Jernigan

Case Study 9: Saudi Arabia

ZIAD A. MEMISH[1,2] AND GWEN M. STEPHENS[1]

[1]Ministry of Health, Riyadh, Kingdom of Saudi Arabia;
[2]Alfaisal University, Riyadh, Kingdom of Saudi Arabia

29.1 Introduction

Saudi Arabia's pandemic influenza planning began, as it did for most Eastern Mediterranean member states, in the late 1990s. Within a few years, however, concern about the country's significant vulnerability to respiratory pandemics was underscored as the Saudi government interrupted its annual Hajj pilgrimage planning sessions to address an evolving respiratory outbreak that had appeared in southern China during the winter of 2002. By spring 2003 Saudi agencies responsible for the safety and well-being of 2 million Hajj visitors faced a dilemma. Fortunately severe acute respiratory syndrome, as this emerging infection came to be known, was to burn itself out in less than 1 year but it brought reality to modern influenza pandemic planning as no other infectious disease in recent memory. Attention turned to influenza, specifically avian influenza A(H5N1) with its high fatality rate and mounting case count in Egypt and Indonesia; both countries with large populations attending Hajj. Domestic influenza prevention and infection control policies were revisited. Efforts were made to expand seasonal influenza immunization of the local population and healthcare workers. During this time, Saudi Arabia continued to emphasize the absence of any structured international surveillance in the Eastern Mediterranean. When Mexico declared a national alert in April 2009, due to several cases of severe respiratory infections in young people caused by a novel influenza A virus, the Saudi Ministry of Health was already involved in international discussions about contingency plans for the 2009 upcoming Hajj.

29.2 Background

Over millennia, Muslim pilgrims had converged in Mecca in western Saudi Arabia in observance of the Hajj pilgrimage in what has become the largest mass gathering of its kind anywhere in the world.

Health hazards, particularly those associated with communicable disease, had escalated as attendance had grown from under 1 million in the late 1990s to more than 2 million by 2009. Pilgrims from more than 180 countries had typically attended Hajj; a gathering with enormous diversity in ethnicity, age and socio-economic status. A disproportionate number of pilgrims are middle-aged or older and co-morbidities are common. Some 200,000 pilgrims arrive from countries with minimal resources, many having foregone any pre-Hajj healthcare. Combine this with extremely crowded venues and the influx of livestock, butchers and abattoir workers, and the potential for communicable disease transmission (by human, animal or insect vectors) is readily appreciated. After 10 days, as the event nears its conclusion, these risks assume global significance as pilgrims begin their journey home.

29.3 Hajj Healthcare Infrastructure

The Hajj is conducted under the auspices of Saudi Arabia's government. As the Custodian of the Two Holy Mosques, Saudi Arabia's king has a unique responsibility for the safety and well-being of Hajj pilgrims each year. The Preventive Medicine Committee oversees all key public health and preventive matters during the Hajj and supervises staff working at all ports of entry. Public health teams are distributed throughout the Hajj site.

Most years, over 90% of Hajj pilgrims arrive in Jeddah by air while the rest travel by sea or travel overland to Hijaz often through Yemen. Saudi Arabia's aviation authority has created a separate pilgrim terminal at Jeddah International Airport, which includes health screening systems, customs and immigration security. The terminal also features large holding areas that permit verification of immunization and health status. Clinics are available to administer to the ill and to dispense prophylactic medications and vaccines as required.

Healthcare services are available free of charge to international pilgrims in the area in and around the Hajj. This includes over 2700 beds and over 10,000 doctors and nurses.

29.4 Public Health Security Planning in Advance of the November 2009 Hajj

Respiratory infections are well established as a primary cause of hospitalization at the Hajj; transmission of seasonal influenza is well documented. As the global pandemic unfolded in 2009, authorities were aware that the highest rates of illness were being reported in children and young adults. Early reports documented higher than expected rates of hospitalization and fully occupied intensive care beds. Seasonal influenza strains continued to circulate as well, and while vaccines against these would continue to be available, there was little evidence they provided protection against A(H1N1)pdm09.

In June 2009, the Saudi Arabia Ministry of Health called for international consultations with global health counterparts to review the country's preparedness plans and assist with implementation of World Health Organization (WHO) core guidance for mass gatherings. Goals were to mitigate disease transmission and safeguard the health of pilgrims. Global health partners met in Jeddah between 26 and 30 June and evaluated Hajj policies and procedures including command and control systems, communications, venue security and, more importantly for this particular Hajj (late November 2009), reviews of medical and public health priorities. These included pre-travel recommendations, visa and immunization requirements, and adequacy of Hajj-specific resources including surge capacity for pilgrim screening, epidemiology and surveillance, informatics, laboratory diagnostics, infection control, triage systems for hospital admissions and patient management.

Just 1 week prior to the WHO declaration of a pandemic in June 2009, Saudi Arabia diagnosed its first laboratory-confirmed case in a Filipino expatriate resident. As Saudi Arabia evaluated its first 100 laboratory-confirmed cases in the summer of 2009, patterns were emerging in the kingdom and the Eastern Mediterranean Region that were consistent with international trends. Children and young adults had higher rates of infection than older adults. Mild disease was common, gastrointestinal symptoms not usually associated with seasonal influenza were more prevalent in A(H1N1)pdm09 cases. Patients requiring hospitalization were more likely to have underlying conditions such as autoimmune disorders, asthma and diabetes. Pregnant women were considered at risk of severe disease.

29.5 Hajj Pilgrim Requirements

Recommendations following the kingdom's global preparedness conference were published in the WHO *Weekly Epidemiological Record*, November 2009. Perhaps the most important recommendation was an advisory for all Muslims at risk of influenza complications to defer Hajj. Pilgrims' countries of origin were to assure compliance as the kingdom would admit all arriving to perform Hajj regardless of age. Countries of origin would also be responsible for routine pre-travel immunizations. Where influenza vaccine was available, proof of immunization for seasonal and A(H1N1)-pdm09 was required before visas could be issued. Health authorities in pilgrims' countries of origin were also responsible for counselling pilgrims about basic hygiene and measures to prevent respiratory infections. Concerns about possible emergence of antiviral drug resistance dissuaded authorities from dispensing oseltamivir except in the management of suspected cases. Practical protocols were also developed to triage laboratory testing and hospital admissions.

29.6 Saudi Arabia Outcomes: Influenza Pandemic of 2009

Saudi Arabia experienced two waves of A(H1N1)-pdm09 influenza infections, the first during August and a second wave from October to December 2009. Although the first case was diagnosed in early June, hospitals did not experience significant increases in related admissions for several months. Admission rates were similar between summer and winter waves. As in other jurisdictions, disease incidence was higher in younger individuals. Case fatality rate was difficult to ascertain given uncertain denominators but likely between 0.1 and 0.5%. Some studies have suggested that pregnant women and individuals with chronic disease were more likely to be hospitalized; however these were not consistent findings across studies conducted in Saudi Arabia.

With regard to Hajj, influenza screening protocols were operational at major ports of entry.

Thermography was used at Jeddah International Airport to detect pilgrims with fever. Medical teams evaluated symptomatic individuals. Those with compatible symptoms were transported to an isolation hospital where they were managed with oseltamivir pending test results from dedicated laboratories. Patients with negative tests and those afebrile for 24 h and in recovery were released to participate in the Hajj. No cases of oseltamivir-resistant influenza were found in Saudi Arabia during or after 2009 Hajj. Although 1.5 million doses of A(H1N1)pdm09 vaccine had been secured by the Ministry of Health and made available at Hajj, uptake was low – estimated at 39%; with 50% immunized against seasonal strains.

Despite the potential for a much larger epidemic, Saudi Arabia experienced far fewer A(H1N1)-pdm09 cases than expected. Prior to the Hajj, 1 to 2 million pilgrims visited Mecca during August and September to observe a lesser Umrah pilgrimage during Ramadan. Only 26 cases of A(H1N1)-pdm09 were confirmed. A total of 73 cases were diagnosed during Hajj, and there were five fatalities. Studies comparing respiratory virus detection rates of inbound and outbound Hajj pilgrim populations showed insignificant differences. Some data suggest the 2009 Hajj experienced a modest decline in attendance, perhaps because fewer vulnerable pilgrims attended. The low number of pandemic cases is not readily explained. Again this might be seen as a 'near miss' event featuring global transmission of a highly infectious virus with limited virulence. Global health implications of the annual Hajj remain compelling. While Saudi Arabia authorities prepare for the future, they have renewed calls for structured surveillance systems based in the region. Health leaders in the kingdom have also called for a new medical discipline to address public health challenges associated with mass gatherings.

Further Reading

World Health Organization (2009) Health conditions for travellers to Saudi Arabia for the pilgrimage to Mecca (Hajj). *Weekly Epidemiological Record* 84(46), 477–480. Available at: http://www.who.int/wer/2009/wer8446.pdf (accessed 29 March 2012).

Index

antiviral drugs (*continued*)
    administration routes 123, 124, 129
    adverse effects 123, 126, 128
    in children 122, 129, 130, 222
    effectiveness 122, 124–125
    M2 channel blockers 22, 122–124
    manufacturing capacity 132, 177
    mode of action 23, 123
    modelling supply/usage 117, 121
    neuraminidase inhibitors 23, 64, 124–132,
        133, 136–137
        see also laninamivir; peramivir;
            oseltamivir; zanamivir
    prophylaxis 39, 126, 133
    public health effects 124, 125–126
    resistance 123–124, 126–129
    stockpiling and deployment strategies 126,
        129–133, 199, 212
        distribution to patients 82, 106–107,
            110, 133
Argentina 51, 202
AS03 adjuvant 143, 147
Asia
    as source of new viral strains 29, 32–33,
        36, 41
    South-east 217–219
Asian flu (1957 pandemic) 37, 42–44
asymptomatic illness 4, 10
    2009 pandemic 53–54
Australia 42, 50
autonomy 183
avian influenza
    1918 pandemic 28, 37, 42, 174, 177
    in birds 31–33, 38–39
    in humans 17, 36–37, 45–46
    as source of pandemic influenza 37–38
    viral subtypes 20
    see also A(H3N8); A(H5N1); A(H7N7);
        A(H9N2); A(H10N4)

B-cells 24
bacterial infections
    antibiotic use 134–136, 137, 177
    complications of influenza 3, 64,
        133–134
baculovirus expression vector system 145–146
basic reproduction number (R_0) 55
bats 35
bird flu *see* avian influenza
boarding schools 7
border controls/closures 164, 166–171
    on arrival 169, 170, 206, 223–224, 225
    pre-embarkation 168–169, 170, 224
Brazil 202
Burma (Myanmar) 218
business continuity planning (BCP) 93–95, 107

Cambodia 218
Canada 187, 220, 221
canine influenza 34–35
capacity planning 84
CAR *see* clinical attack rate
carnivorous mammals 34–35
case fatality rate (CFR) 55–56, 80
cell culture-based vaccine production 140
CFR *see* case fatality rate
chickens 31, 32, 38–39
children
    2009 pandemic 53, 54
    antiviral drug use 122, 129, 130, 222
    hand hygiene 73
    influenza type B 2
    seasonal influenza 2, 4
Chile 201–202
China 36, 41
    Severe Acute Respiratory Syndrome
        (SARS) 167, 192
ciprofloxacin 134–135
clarithromycin 134
cleaning
    environmental 71, 73
    hand hygiene 71, 73, 153, 155
clinical attack rate (CAR)
    2009 pandemic 55
    modelling 113
    seasonal influenza 3–4
clinical presentation 2–3, 10
    1918 pandemic 42
    1957 pandemic 43–44
    2009 pandemic 61, 64–65
co-amoxiclav 134
command and control in pandemic planning 83–84
command post exercises (CPX) 99–100, 101
common cold (influenza C) 2, 19
communication 108, 110, 189–197
    with healthcare workers 195, 196
    in preparedness planning 83, 91, 99–100,
        102, 189–191
    with the public 161, 191–195, 196–197,
        200, 209–210
    about vaccine production/use 144, 145, 149
    about vaccine safety 149, 150
complications
    2009 pandemic 61–62, 63–64
    effect of antiviral drug treatment 125, 130
    pneumonia 3, 63–64, 132–135
    seasonal influenza 3, 6
contact transmission 69–70
    control measures 71, 72, 74
containment 104–106, 120
    see also prophylaxis; social distancing
Cooperative Arrangement for the Prevention of Spread
    of Communicable Disease through Air Travel
    (CAPSCA) 167

viral structure 19–21
voluntary sector 107

washing of hands (hand washing) 71, 73,
    153, 155
waterbirds 32
websites in communication 190, 193, 194–195
white blood cells 23–24
WHO *see* World Health Organization
wild birds 31, 32, 38
workplace absenteeism 176
    due to school closure 117, 158, 160, 178
workplace closure 156, 162

World Health Organization (WHO)
    IHR (International Health Regulations (2005)) 77,
        165–167, 168
    Outbreak Communication guidelines 190–191
    preparedness planning 47, 78, 85, 86, 182
    on vaccines 140, 146, 148

years of life lost (YLL) 56–57

zanamivir (Relenza®) 20, 23, 64, 123, 124, 136
    see also neuraminidase inhibitors (NAIs)
zoonotic influenza 17, 20, 35–39